Nutritional Care of the Patient with Celiac Disease

Nutritional Care of the Patient with Celiac Disease

Editor: Hervey Weiss

AMERICAN
MEDICAL PUBLISHERS
www.americanmedicalpublishers.com

AMERICAN
MEDICAL PUBLISHERS
www.americanmedicalpublishers.com

Cataloging-in-Publication Data

Nutritional care of the patient with celiac disease / edited by Hervey Weiss.
p. cm.
Includes bibliographical references and index.
ISBN 978-1-63927-765-0
1. Celiac disease. 2. Celiac disease--Patients--Nutrition. 3. Celiac disease--Patients--Nutrition--Requirements.
4. Celiac disease--Nutritional aspects. 5. Gluten-free diet. I. Weiss, Hervey.
RC862.C44 N88 2023
616.399--dc23

American Medical Publishers,
41 Flatbush Avenue,
1st Floor, New York,
NY 11217, USA

ISBN 978-1-63927-765-0 (Hardback)

Contents

Preface

Celiac Disease is a type of autoimmune disease which is permanent in nature. It is majorly caused through gluten ingestion in genetically predisposed individuals. In celiac disease, villous atrophy and intestinal inflammation is caused in small intestines due to permanent gluten intolerance resulting in severe malabsorption. Nutrition has a vital role in managing celiac disease. Gluten free diet is essential for managing this disease. There does not exist any cure for this disease, only following a lifelong gluten free diet can be beneficial in the treatment. Gluten free diet should be followed with care to balance the nutrient requirements for preventing deficiencies and maintaining a person's health. This book explores the important role of nutrition in gastrointestinal tract disorders. It strives to provide a fair idea about celiac disease and to help develop a better understanding of the latest advances in its clinical management. A number of latest researches have been included to keep the readers up-to-date with the global concepts on this medical condition.

Significant researches are present in this book. Intensive efforts have been employed by authors to make this book an outstanding discourse. This book contains the enlightening chapters which have been written on the basis of significant researches done by the experts.

Finally, I would also like to thank all the members involved in this book for being a team and meeting all the deadlines for the submission of their respective works. I would also like to thank my friends and family for being supportive in my efforts.

Editor

1

Cereal-Based Gluten-Free Food: How to Reconcile Nutritional and Technological Properties of Wheat Proteins with Safety for Celiac Disease Patients

Carmela Lamacchia [1], Alessandra Camarca [2], Stefania Picascia [2], Aldo Di Luccia [1] and Carmen Gianfrani [2,3,*]

[1] Department of Food Science, University of Foggia, Via Napoli 25, 71100 - Foggia, Italy. E-Mails: c.lamacchia@unifg.it (C.L.); a.diluccia@unifg.it (A.D.L.)

[2] Institute of Food Sciences-CNR, Carmen Gianfrani, ISA-CNR, Via Roma 64, 83100 - Avellino, Italy; E-Mails: acamarca@isa.cnr.it (A.C.); s.picascia@isa.cnr.it (S.P.)

[3] Institute of Protein Biochemistry-CNR, Via P. Castellino, 111, 80131 – Naples, Italy.

* Author to whom correspondence should be addressed; E-Mail: cgianfrani@isa.cnr.it;

Abstract: The gluten-free diet is, to date, the only efficacious treatment for patients with Celiac Disease. In recent years, the impressive rise of Celiac Disease incidence, dramatically prompted changes in the dietary habit of an increasingly large population, with a rise in demand of gluten-free products. The formulation of gluten-free bakery products presents a formidable challenge to cereal technologists. As wheat gluten contributes to the formation of a strong protein network, that confers visco-elasticity to the dough and allows the wheat flour to be processed into a wide range of products, the preparation of cereal-based gluten-free products is a somehow difficult process. This review focuses on nutritional and technological quality of products made with gluten-free cereals available on the market. The possibility of using flour from naturally low toxic ancient wheat species or detoxified wheat for the diet of celiacs is also discussed.

Keywords: Celiac Disease; cereals; wheat gluten; dough; immune toxicity

---

1. Introduction

In the past 100 years, the human being has experienced a biological transformation with a speed greater than the trend of the last millennia. Over the past seventy years, the diet of Western man has been totally revolutionized: farm food, once characterized for being fresh and free of toxin residues, additives and preservatives, has been almost completely replaced by food products of an industrial chain that is, in the great majority of cases, oriented towards profit and the creation of induced needs. All this has radically changed, and still continues to change, the biological systems in humans leading to metabolic syndrome, allergies and intolerances, among both children and adults, in developed and developing countries.

In this context, in the last two decades, a series of epidemiologic studies have shown a particular increase in Celiac Disease (CD), a life-long intolerance to gluten proteins (the seed storage proteins) present in most cereals [1], both in the United States and Europe, and in developing countries [2,3]. In these subjects, the consumption of cereals containing gluten causes a chronic inflammatory process leading to lesions in the small intestine and a dysfunction in nutrient absorption [1]. The CD treatment, therefore, is based on a strict gluten-free diet throughout the patient's lifetime. Though this dietary regimen guarantees the full recovery of small intestine architecture and functions, for many patients it is strongly restrictive, especially for social events and during travelling. In addition, it is a great task for the food industry to provide safe food that partly resembles in taste and appearance pasta, bread and other baked goods. Furthermore, the nutritional importance of wheat proteins should not be underestimated, particularly in less developed countries where bread, noodles and other products (e.g., bulgur, couscous) may represent substantial diet components.

2. Celiac Disease

Celiac disease is the most common food induced enteropathy in humans. CD is strongly associated with particular HLA genotypes, as only individuals carrying the DQA1*0501 and DQB1*0201 (DQ2), or DQA1*0301 and DQB1*0302 (DQ8) alleles develop the disease. Gluten intolerance presents a large variety of symptoms including gastrointestinal and extra-intestinal manifestations, though in some patients, particularly of pediatric age, the disease is completely symptomless [4,5]. Typical clinical manifestations of CD include chronic diarrhea, weight loss and anemia, mainly caused by malabsorption, as a direct consequence of intestinal villous atrophy. However, a significant proportion of patients have "atypical" form, characterized by extra-digestive symptoms, including skin lesions, isolated hypertransaminasemia, bone pains and fractures, and infertility [6]. Several serological screening detecting the CD-associated anti-tissue transglutaminase (or anti-endomysium) IgA antibodies, and followed by endoscopy, have shown that approximately 1% of the general population have celiac disease [7,8]. However, Maki and co-workers found that the total prevalence of CD is even higher, reaching 1.99% in the Finnish population [9]. The wide spectrum of clinical manifestations, together with the absence of clear symptoms in some cases, could explain why the prevalence of CD is so underestimated. Regarding the pathogenic mechanisms, it is widely accepted that CD is an immune mediated disorder, in which intestinal CD4+ T cells, highly reactive to dietary gluten, have a pivotal role in disease pathogenesis [10]. In addition, recent studies have indicated the prominent role of both innate immune cells and adaptive CD8+ T cells in damaging the mucosal tissue [10,11]. To date, the only treatment for celiac disease patients is the lifelong complete exclusion of the gluten from the diet. With such a dietary restriction, clinical symptoms, serological markers, and duodenal mucosa histology normalize [12], however gluten reactive T cells remain in the small intestine of patients on gluten-free diet, and re-exposure to the gluten results in immune activation and in mucosal damage. As a consequence, gluten avoidance is strongly recommended; nevertheless, dietary compliance is imperfect in a large number of patients for several reasons, including the need of flavor and palatability of gluten-free cereal-based food [13].

3. Gluten, the Dough "Treasure"

Gluten is one of the earliest protein fractions described by chemists, (a first description by Beccari was in 1728), and it is defined as the "cohesive, visco-elastic proteinaceous material" that remains when wheat dough is washed to remove starch granules and water soluble constituents [14,15]. Gluten is formed by storage proteins necessary for plant germination [16]. In these respects, the wheat storage proteins may not differ much from those of other cereals [14,17], however, the distinctive feature that makes wheat unique is, precisely, the visco-elasticity of gluten. When the grain is milled and mixed with water, storage proteins form a dough, capable of retaining gas bubbles. These properties make wheat suitable for the preparation of a great diversity of food products, including breads, noodles, pasta, and cookies, and it has been the subject of extensive attention by the food industry. Of note, in order to meet the consumer needs, food industries have made in the last fifty years an indiscriminate use of wheat gluten even in food that is naturally devoid, as sauces, chips, cold cuts.

Gluten contains hundreds of proteins, which are present either as monomers or as oligo- and polymers, linked by inter-chain disulphide bonds [15,17], and characterized by high contents of glutamine and proline (namely prolamins), and by low contents of charged amino acids. The new system of classification, based on the availability of complete amino acid sequences, divided the gluten proteins in three broad groups: sulphur-rich (S-rich), sulphur-poor (S-poor), and high molecular weight (HMW) prolamins ([18], Figure 1). Traditionally, gluten proteins have been divided according to their solubility in alcohol-water solutions (e.g., 60% ethanol), as the soluble gliadins and the insoluble glutenins [19]. These properties are largely determined by the inter-chain disulphide bonds, with the glutenins consisting of disulphide-stabilized polymers. Reduction of these inter-chain bonds allows the separation of the glutenin subunits into low molecular weight (LMW) and high molecular weight (HMW) groups (Figure 2). In contrast, the alcohol-soluble gliadin fraction consists mainly of monomeric proteins, which either lack cysteine (ω-gliadins), or have only intra-chain disulphide bonds (α-type and γ-type gliadins) (Figure 2). However, small amounts of polymers related to the glutenins are also present in the gliadin fraction. These appear to differ from the alcohol-insoluble glutenins, as they have lower M_rs and higher contents of LMW subunits [20–22].

Figure 1. Schematic representation of types and peculiarities of wheat gluten proteins (gliadins and glutenins-GS; modified from [17]).

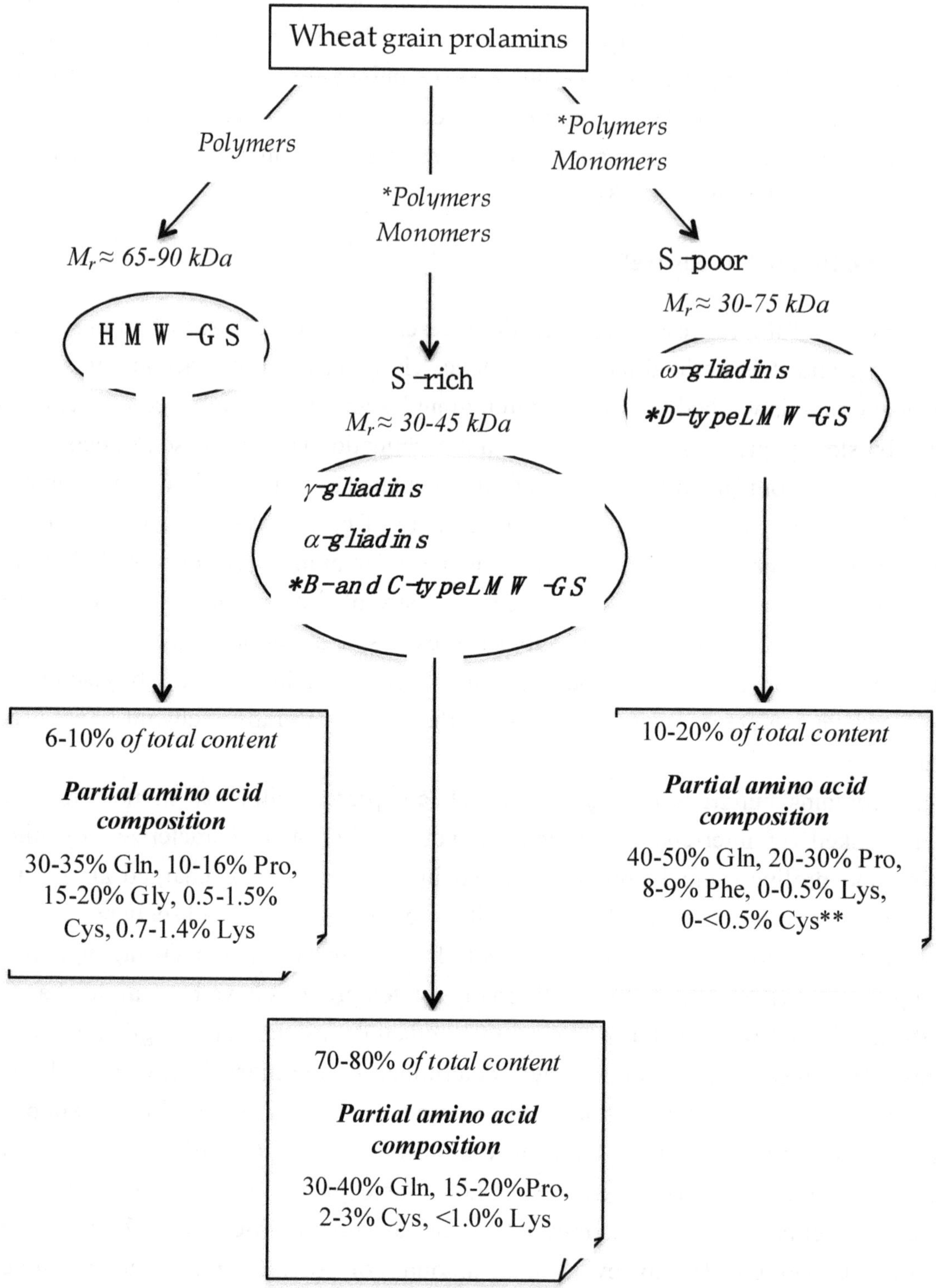

*C-type LMW subunits are essentially polymeric forms of α- and γ-gliadins and D-type LMW subunits polymeric ω-gliadins. The B-type LMW subunits constitute a discrete group of S-rich prolamins.
**Cys is present in D-type LMW subunits, but not ω-gliadins.

Figure 2. Gluten proteins: fractions and technological properties [23].

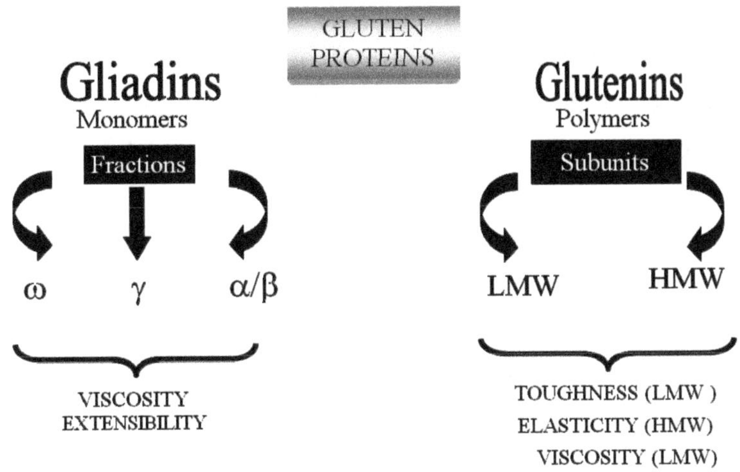

Both fractions are important contributors to the rheological properties of dough (Figure 2), though their functions are divergent. Hydrated gliadins have little elasticity and are less cohesive than glutenins, and contribute mainly to the viscosity and extensibility of the dough. In contrast, hydrated glutenins are both cohesive and elastic and are responsible for dough strength and elasticity [24,25]. A proper mixture of both fractions is essential for the quality of the end product. However, of particular importance are the glutenin polymers, and it is well established that strong (*i.e.*, highly visco-elastic) doughs contain high proportions of HMW glutenin polymers [24]. Numerous studies are consistent with the hypothesis that the HMW subunits form an elastomeric polymer network which provides a "backbone" for interactions with other glutenin subunits and with gliadins (Figure 3) [26,27]. There is no doubt that this network is mainly stabilized by inter-chain disulphide bonds [28,29]. Additional covalent bonds formed during dough making are tyrosine-tyrosine and thiyl-tyrosine crosslinks between gluten proteins [30–32]. However, the covalent structure of the gluten network is superimposed by non-covalent bonds (hydrogen bonds, ionic bonds, hydrophobic bonds) [33].

Figure 3. A structural model for wheat gluten in which the HMW subunits provide a disulphide-bonded backbone that interacts with other gluten proteins by disulphide bonds (LMW subunits) and non-covalent interactions (gliadins) (modified from [26]).

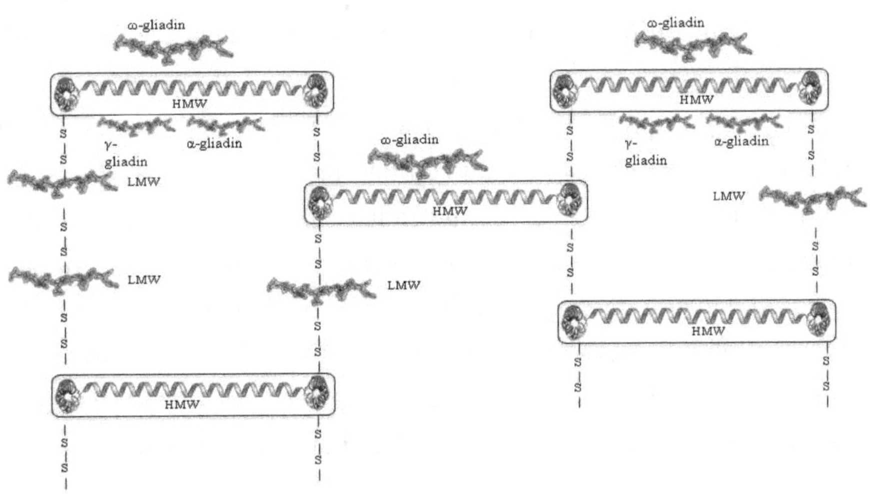

4. Formulation and Nutritional Value of Gluten-free Products

The food not allowed in the gluten free diet include: (a) all types of bread and food prepared with wheat flour, including kamut and spelt, rye, barley, triticale, or with ingredients from these flours; (b) food that contains wheat, or derivatives of gluten used as thickeners, such as hot dogs, salad dressing, sauces, canned, some types of cheese and cold cuts; (c) medicinal products that use gluten as binder in the pills or tablets.

Though from a nutritional point of view, gluten exclusion does not entail particular problems, being a mixture of proteins with low nutritional and biological value, the gluten-free diet creates enormous limitations, above all in the social activities related to food. In addition, this dietary therapy has, often low content of vitamins and ions, such as vitamins B and D, calcium, iron, zinc, and magnesium, as well as fiber [34–36]. Furthermore, one of the major risks is the risk to develop obesity and diseases related to metabolic syndrome [37]. However, the high technological value renders gluten almost indispensable in baked products, and its replacement, as structure-building protein, presents a major technological challenge for the food industry. Although many advances have been made in the preparation processes of gluten-free products, using starches, hydrocolloids, gums and novel ingredients [38], many gluten-free industrial products available on the market exhibit a low nutritional quality, poor mouth feel or flavor [39] and, no less important, are particularly expensive. As a consequence, the research interest to develop gluten-free products has significantly increased in recent years. The pilot study by Rotsch [40] showed that bread could be prepared from starch and gel-forming substances, since starch, combined with water, at a temperature included between 60 and 80 °C, increases in volume, in a sort of swelling (a process called gelatinization) [41–43]. This process increases the product consistency by mimicking the gluten viscoelastic properties. Thickeners and gums/hydrocolloids, derived from various seeds, fruits, or plant extracts, could be also added in these formulations to improve water retention, texture and appearance properties [44–47]. Among different types of flours, present on the market and rich in starch, rice and corn flour are the best suited to the gelatinization process. These starches, are polysaccharides composed of amylose and amylopectin, present in the original product in the percentages equal to 20%–30% and 70%–80%, respectively.

The amylose is a linear polymer of glucose in which the glucose units are held together by α (1→4) bonds, whilst the amylopectin is a branched polymer of glucose, similar to amylose, structured with side chains that are grafted every 24–30 glucose units through α (1→6) bonds. Amylopectin is the most responsible for the gelatinization of starch granules in the presence of water and heat. During this process a fraction of both amylopectin and amylose goes into solution, however, the starch gelatinization is inversely proportional to the amylose content [48,49]. From a nutritional perspective, the more starch is gelatinized (because of its reduced amount of amylose), the more it is hydrolysable by alpha-amylase, with an increase of the glycemic index [50,51]. In contrast, with a greater amylose content, the gelatinization process is reduced, as well as the glycemic index. Gluten-free food prepared with corn and rice starch have a high glycemic index [52,53] and increase the risk to develop metabolic syndromes in celiac patients [54,55]. In fact, it is well known from epidemiological studies that the daily consumption of high glycemic index food is correlated with the risk to develop cardiovascular disease, obesity and diabetes [56–60]. Furthermore, the use of palm oil, cream powder, microencapsulated high-fat powder, and low-fat dairy powders [39,40], aimed to improve the palatability of cereal-based gluten-free products, renders these products highly caloric.

5. Recent Advances in Formulation of Cereal-Based Gluten-Free Food

In addition to the high glycemic index and caloric density of cereal-based gluten-free food, these products generally are not enriched/fortified, so that, they may not contain the same levels of nutrients, as the natural wheat grains. Therefore, uncertainty still exists whether celiac patients compliant with gluten-free therapy have a nutritionally balanced diet. Grehn *et al.* screened the intake of nutrients and foods of 49 adults diagnosed with coeliac disease and following a strict gluten-free diet [61]. They had a lower intake of fibre when compared to a control group on a normal diet. In their studies with coeliac adolescents, Mariani *et al.* [62] concluded that adherence to a gluten-free diet worsens the nutritionally unbalanced diet in adolescents, as it has been thereafter confirmed by Thompson *et al.* [63]. For these reasons several studies investigated the preparation of a new generation of cereal-based gluten-free food. The enrichment of baked products with dietary fibres and devoid of gluten has been the goal of various technologist teams. Gallagher *et al.* incorporated inulin (8% inclusion level) into a wheat starch-based gluten-free formulation [64]. Inulin is a non-digestible polysaccharide that is classified as a dietary fibre. It also acts as a prebiotic by stimulating the growth of "healthy" bacteria in the colon [65]. When added to wheat bread, inulin improves loaf volume, increases dough stability and produces a uniform, and finely grained, crumb texture [66].

Gambus *et al.* replaced corn starch with amaranth flour to enhance the protein and fibre contents of gluten-free breads [67]. At a 10% replacement level, protein and fibre levels increased by 32% and 152% respectively, whilst sensory quality was unaffected. Taylor and Parker discussed the use of quinoa in the production of enriched gluten-free bakery goods [68]. Both quinoa and amaranth are *dicotyledonous* species that are not related to the actual cereals (*monocotyledons*), such as wheat, barley and rice. They are also called pseudocereals, since these species produce small seeds that resemble those of cereals. The grain of pseudocereals does not contain gluten proteins but it is rich in proteins with high biological value (albumins and globulins) and contains carbohydrates that can be considered nutraceuticals, as they have cholesterol- [69,70] and glycemic-lowering effects, and induce a reduction of free fatty acids [52]. Importantly, the total absence of immune toxicity of amaranth storage protein for celiacs patients has been demonstrated [71], and several studies were carried out in order to improve the structural properties of quinoa and amaranth as ingredients for bread, pasta and crackers [72–74].

6. Nutritional Quality of Wheat Flour: Advantages in Introducing a Cereal-Based Gluten-Free Food in Diet of Celiacs

The therapy with gluten-free products, besides the risk of nutrient deficiency and metabolic syndrome, as described above, entails the difficulty of maintaining the cure over time. Reduced palatability and taste of gluten-free food create enormous limitations in the diet of patients. To solve these issues, numerous studies are currently devoted to the use of *in vitro* detoxified flour or flour from ancient wheat cultivars, in the formulation of pasta and baked goods.

6.1. Nutritional and Health Properties of Hexaploid and Tetraploid Wheat

Worldwide, the number of people who eat wheat for a substantial part of their diet reaches several billions. Because of the high content of starch, (about 60%–70% of the whole grain and 65%–75% of white flour) wheat is often considered no more than a source of calories. Despite its relatively low protein content (usually 8%–15%), wheat still provides as much protein for human and livestock nutrition as the total soybean crop (as calculated in reference [75]. However, the lysine content of wheat is low and varies significantly from grain to flour [15]. Grain of high protein content has very low content of lysine approximately 30 mg g^{-1} protein [76]. Wheat is a source of minerals such as Zn (20–30 mg Kg^{-1}) and Fe (30–36 mg Kg^{-1}), contributing to 44% of the daily intake of iron (15% in bread), and 25% of the daily intake of zinc (11% in bread) in the UK [77] Wheat is also a source of selenium which varies widely from about 10 μg Kg^{-1} to over 2000 μg Kg^{-1} (FAO/WHO, 2001; [78]). The concentration of selenium in wheat is largely determined by the availability of this element in the soil. Wheat produced in Western Europe may contain only one-tenth of the selenium that is present in wheat grown in North America. Wheat also contains a range of components with established health benefits that are concentrated, or solely located, in the bran. In addition, the following components are either present in low amounts, or completely absent, and with a large variation in their concentrations:

- **lignans**, a group of polyphenols with phytoestrogen-like activity, present at levels up to 10 μg g^{-1} in wholemeal wheat and almost 20 μg g^{-1} in the bran [79];
- **phenolic acids** that in wholemeal range up to almost 1200 μg g^{-1} [80]. They represent, quantitatively, the major group of phytochemicals in the wheat grain and are derivatives of either hydroxibenzoic acid or hydroxycinnamic acid. Epidemiological studies indicate that phenolic acids have a number of health benefits which may relate to their antioxidant activity; furthermore, a high correlation between the total antioxidant activities of grain and their phenolic acid contents has been reported [81,82];
- **folates** that in wholemeal varied from 364 to 774 ng g^{-1} dry weight in winter wheats and from 323 to 741 ng g^{-1} dry weight in spring wheats, and positively correlated with the bran yield [83];
- **dietary fibre** derives from polymers of wheat endosperm cell wall: they are constituted mainly by arabinoxylans (approximately 70%) and (1-3) (1-4)β-D-glucans (approximately 20%). The arabinoxylans are present in both soluble and insoluble forms, being the former considered to have health benefits [84,85]. However, insoluble fibre may also favour the delivering phenolic antioxidants into the colon, with a reduction of colon-rectal cancer risk [86]. Gebruers *et al.* showed wide variation in the contents of total and water-extractable arabinoxylans in both white flour and bran fractions [87]. Similarly Ordaz-Ortiz *et al.* showed variation from 0.26% to 0.75% dry weight in the content of water-extractable arabinoxylan in 20 French wheat cultivars and from 1.66% to 2.87% dry weight in total arabinoxylans [88].

6.2. Ancient Wheats

Triticum monococcum, was the first wheat to be cultivated by man and is a diploid species characterized by the presence of the AA genome. Due to the simplicity of its genome, *Triticum monococcum* has attracted the interest of the scientific community on nutritional and health aspects in relation to celiac disease. If we consider, in fact, that for each genome (AA, BB and DD) there are dozens of genes coding for prolamins in wheat caryopses, it is evident that in *Triticum monococcum* the mere presence of the AA genome encodes for a reduced variety of gluten proteins (and of potential immune toxic peptides). Recent evidence shows that prolamins of some *Triticum monococcum* cause a reduced inflammatory effect in celiac patients [89–92], particularly for the inability to activate the innate branch of immune cells [89], or to induce apoptosis of enterocytes [93]. The reduced, or absent, toxicity of *Triticum monococcum* prolamins can then be interpreted in two ways, namely via (*i*) a low presence of toxic peptides; (*ii*) an abundant presence of protective sequences. However, other *in vitro* and *in vivo* studies have warned about the safety of some monococcum cultivars for celiac patients [94,95], thus suggesting that the immune toxicity for celiacs might strictly depend on the specific *Triticum monococcum* varieties.

The search of naturally detoxified, or less toxic, ancient grains is of great interest for their potential use in the general diet to prevent disease in those individuals at high risk to develop gluten intolerance.

Regarding the technological properties, though some studies have considered *Triticum monococcum* not suitable for bread and pasta production [96,97], it has been demonstrated that the aptitude to bread-making is extremely different and depends on the specific varieties analyzed [98,99]. Studies carried out at an industrial level have shown that pasta made with 100% of *Triticum monococcum* flour has very low loss of starch during cooking comparable to that made from durum wheat semolina [23]. These findings on the bread- and pasta-making aptitude of *Triticum monococcum* flours are encouraging, and indicate a real chance to select for ancient varieties with superior technological characteristics and reduced toxicity for celiacs.

6.3. Detoxification of Wheat Gluten

Numerous studies are currently devoted to prepare pasta and baked goods made from wheat flours modified in order to eliminate, or reduce, the immune toxicity of gluten proteins (detoxification process).

A first method, using endopeptidase of bacterial origin during the preparation of wheat flour dough, results in the complete degradation of gluten peptides including those that are strongly immune toxic for celiacs [100]. Such an approach, carrying out a total destruction of the gluten network, reduces the technological properties (viscoelasticity) of dough and, consequently, of pasta or baked goods, unless the flour is integrated with structuring agents, as pre-gelatinized starch, emulsifiers or hydrocolloids.

Another method to detoxify gluten proteins uses the specific transdamidation of toxic epitopes done by the tissue-transglutaminase of microbial origin (*Streptomyces mobaraensis)* in the presence of lysine methyl ester [101]. This method has the great advantage of blocking the immunogenicity of T cell epitopes (as demonstrated in an *in vitro* assays using intestinal T cell from celiacs), and more importantly, it keeps intact the gluten network and preserves the technological properties of the flour. Furthermore, this procedure uses an enzyme largely employed in the food industry for improving the texture of foods. A preliminary 90-days trial made with CD subjects in remission consuming bread slices with transamidated gluten indicated that only a subgroup of celiacs exhibited clinical symptoms compared to subjects consuming the toxic gluten [102]. The researchers have now implemented the transamidation reaction in order to reach protection in the great majority of CD volunteers that eat detoxified wheat flour.

7. Conclusions

The gluten proteins contained in wheat flour are crucial during the bread and pasta making process, since they confers to the dough its viscosity and elasticity. In addition, wheat flour provides to foodstuffs important nutritional components, including dietary fibre, vitamins, and minerals. These properties account for wheat being cultivated by man in such enormous quantities throughout the world. However, gluten proteins are also responsible for a very common, and in most cases very severe, intolerance in a large number of individuals. To date the only safe and efficacious therapy for people with celiac disease is the long-life avoidance of gluten from the diet.

The replacement of the unique technological properties of wheat gluten represents the major task of industry for providing high quality gluten-free foods, such as pasta, bread and baked products, in terms of structure, loss of starch during cooking, and optimal cooking time.

Nutritional studies on people with CD on a gluten-free diet revealed several nutrient deficiencies, particularly of vitamins and minerals, as well as an increased of obesity risk, this latter due to the high glycemic index of the gluten-free diet. However, despite the numerous studies, it has not yet been possible to offer celiac patients an alternative diet therapy, based on high nutritional and tasty cereals that are naturally gluten-free. Foodstuffs made with technologically detoxified wheat flour, or with wheat varieties with naturally low content of toxic gluten sequences, or more suitable to gastrointestinal enzymatic degradation, would be a much-desired dietary therapeutic alternative. An extensive production of foodstuffs made with detoxified wheat flour that could be commonly consumed not only by those people suffering gluten intolerance, but also by the rest of the population could be envisaged; the large diffusion of such products could have the goal, in a totally innovative way, of reducing the immune sensitization to gluten and, likely, decreasing the incidence of celiac disease.

Acknowledgments

This work has been partly supported by a grant from the Italian Ministry of Research PRIN 2009—"Interaction between innate and adaptive immunity in the pathogenesis of CD"—CUP: E61J11000300001, and by "ProAliFun" project P.O.N Ricerca e Competitività 2007–2013.

References

1. Shuppan, D.; Tennis, M.D.; Kelly, C.P. Celiac disease: Epidemiology, pathogenesis, diagnosis, and nutritional management. *Nutr. Clin. Care* **2005**, *8*, 54–69.
2. Hill, I.; Fasano, A.; Schwartz, R.; Counts, D.; Glock, M.; Horvath, K. Prevalence of celiac disease in at risk groups of children in United States. *Pediatr. Res.* **2000**, *136*, 86–90.

3. Barada, K.; Abu Daya, H.; Rostami, K.; Catassi, C. Celiac disease in the developing world. Gastrointest. *Endosc. Clin. N. Am.* **2012**, *22*, 773–796.
4. Paparo, F.; Petrone, E.; Tosco, A.; Maglio, M.; Borrelli, M.; Salvati, V.M.; Miele, E.; Greco, L.; Auricchio, S.; Troncone, R. Clinical, HLA, and small bowel immunohistochemical features of children with positive serum antiendomysium antibodies and architecturally normal small intestinal mucosa. *Am. J. Gastroenterol.* **2005**, *100*, 2294–2298.
5. Biagi, F.; Trotta, L.; Alfano, C.; Balduzzi, D.; Staffieri, V.; Bianchi, P.I.; Marchese, A.; Vattiato, C.; Zilli, A.; Luinetti, O.; *et al.* Prevalence and natural history of potential celiac disease in adult patients. *Scand. J. Gastroenterol.* **2013**, *48*, 537–542.
6. Di Sabatino, A.; Corazza, G.R. Coeliac disease. *Lancet* **2009**, *373*, 1480–1493.
7. White, L.E.; Merrick, V.M.; Bannerman, E.; Russell, R.K.; Basude, D.; Henderson, P.; Wilson, D.C.; Gillett, P.M. The rising incidence of celiac disease in scotland. *Pediatrics* **2013**, *132*, 924–931.
8. Kang, J.Y.; Kang, A.H.; Green, A.; Gwee, K.A.; Ho, K.Y. Systematic review: Worldwide variation in the frequency of coeliac disease and changes over time. *Aliment. Pharmacol. Ther.* **2013**, *38*, 226–459.
9. Lohi, S.; Mustalahti, K.; Kaukinen, K.;, Laurila, K.; Collin, P.; Rissanen, H.; Lohi, O.; Bravi, E.; Gasparin, M.; Reunanen, A.; *et al.* Increasing prevalence of coeliac disease over time. *Aliment. Pharmacol. Ther.* **2007**, *26*, 1217–1225.
10. Meresse, B.; Malamut, G.; Cerf-Bensussan, N. Celiac disease: An immunological jigsaw. *Immunity* **2012**, *36*, 907–919.
11. Mazzarella, G.; Stefanile, R.; Camarca, A.; Giliberti, P.; Casentini, E.; Marano, C.; Iaquinto, G.; Giardullo, N.; Auricchio, S.; Sette, A.; *et al.* Gliadin activates HLA Class-I restricted CD8+ T cells in celiac disease intestinal mucosa and induces the enterocyte apoptosis. *Gastroenterology* **2008**, *134*, 1017–1027.
12. Biagi, F.; Bianchi, P.I.; Marchese, A.; Trotta, L.; Vattiato C.; Balduzzi, D.; Brusco, G.; Andrealli, A.; Cisarò, F.; Astegiano, M.; *et al.* A score that verifies adherence to a gluten-free diet: A cross-sectional, multicentre validation in real clinical life. *Br. J. Nutr.* **2012**, *108*, 1884–1888.
13. Mazzeo, T.; Brambillasca, F.; Pellegrini, N.; Valmarana, R.; Corti, F.; Colombo, C.; Agostoni, C. Evaluation of visual and taste preferences of some gluten-free commercial products in a group of celiac children. *Int. J. Food Sci. Nutr.* **2014**, *65*, 112–116.
14. Shewry, P.R. Wheat. *J. Exp. Bot.* **2009**, *60*, 1537–1553.
15. Wieser, H. Chemistry of gluten proteins. *Food Microb.* **2007**, *24*, 115–119.
16. Shewry, P.R. The synthesis, processing, and deposition of gluten proteins in developing grain. *Cereal Food World* **1999**, *44*, 587–589.
17. Shewry, P.R.; Halford, N.G. Cereal seed storage proteins: Structures, properties and role in grain utilization. *J. Exp. Bot.* **2002**, *53*, 947–958.
18. Shewry, P.R.; Tatham, A.S. The prolamin storage proteins of cereal seeds: Structure and evolution. *Biochem. J.* **1990**, *267*, 1–12.
19. Osborne T.B. The vegetable proteins. *J. Soc. Chem. Ind.* **1924**, *43*, 440.
20. Bietz, J.A.; Wall, J.S. Isolation and characterization of gliadin-like subunits from glutenin. *Cereal Chem.* **1973**, *50*, 537–547.

21. Bietz, J.A.; Wall, J.S. Identity of high molecula weight gliadin and ethanol-soluble glutenin subunits of wheat: Relation to gluten structure. *Cereal Chem.* **1980**, *57*, 415–421.
22. Kanazawa, H.; Yonezawa, D. Studies on polypeptide composition of low molecular weight glutenin. *J. Agr. Chem. Soc. Jpn.* **1973**, *47*, 17–22.
23. Lamacchia, C.; La Gatta, B.; Schiavulli, A.; Pati, S.; Petrella, G.; di Luccia, A. *Triticum monococcum* species, a chance for pasta business. *Prof. Pasta* **2013**, *April-June,* 12–27.
24. Field, J.M; Shewry, P.R.; Miflin, B.J. Solubilization and characterization of wheat gluten proteins; correlations between the amount of aggregated proteins and baking quality. *J. Sci. Food Agric.* **1983**, *34*, 370–377.
25. Payne, P.I. Genetics of wheat storage and the effect of allelic variation on breadmaking quality. *Annu. Rev. Plant Phys.* **1987**, *38*, 141–153.
26. Shewry, P.R.; Popineau, Y.; Lafiandra, D.; Belton, P. Wheat glutenin subunits and dough elasticity: Findings of the EUROWHEAT project. *Trends Food Sci. Technol.* **2001**, *11*, 433–441.
27. Lindsay, M.P.; Skerritt, J.H. The glutenin macropolymer of wheat flour doughs: Structure-function perspective. *Trends Food Sci. Tech.* **1999**, *10*, 247–253.
28. Shewry, P.R.; Tatham, A.S. Disulphide bonds in wheat gluten proteins. *J. Cereal Sci.* **1997**, *25*, 207–227.
29. Wieser, H. The Use of Redox Agents. In *Bread Making-Improving Quality*; Cauvain, S.P., Ed.; Woodhead Publishing Ltd.: Cambridge, UK, **2003**; pp. 424–446.
30. Tilley, K.A.; Benjamin, R.E.; Bagorogoza, K.E.; Okot-Kotber, B.M.; Prakash, O.; Kwen, H. Tyrosine cross-links: Molecular basis of gluten structure and function. *J. Agric. Food Chem.* **2001**, *49*, 2627–2632.
31. Lamacchia, C.; di Luccia, A.; Baiano, A.; Gambacorta, G.; La Gatta, B.; Pati, S.; La Notte, E. Changes in pasta proteins induced by drying cycles and their relationship to coking behavior. *J. Cereal Sci.* **2007**, *46*, 58–63.
32. Lamacchia, C.; Baiano, A.; Lamparelli, S.; Terracone, C.; Trani, A.; Di Luccia, A. Formation of polymeri proteins during pasta-making in barley and semolina mixture and predictions of its effects on cooking behavior and acceptability. *Food Chem.* **2011**, *129*, 319–328.
33. Wieser H.; Bushuk W.; Mac Ritchie F. The Polymeric Glutenins. In *Gliadin and Glutenin: The Unique Balance of Wheat Quality. St. Paul American Association of Cereal Chemistry*; Wrigley, C., Bekes, F., Bushuk, W., Eds.; American. Association of Cereal Chemists: St. Paul MN, USA, 2006; pp. 213–240.
34. Shepherd, S.J.; Gibson, P.R. Nutritional inadequacies of the gluten-free diet in both recently-diagnosed and long-term patients with celiac disease. *J. Hum. Nutr. Diet.* **2013**, *26*, 349–358.
35. Hallert, C.; Grant, C.; Grehn, S.; Grännö, C.; Hultén, S.; Midhagen, G.; Ström, M.; Svensson, H.; Valdimarsson, T. Evidence of poor vitamin status in coeliac patients on a gluten-free diet for 10 years. *Aliment. Pharmacol. Ther.* **2002**, *16*, 1333–1339.
36. Wierdsma, N.J.; van Bokhorst-de van der Schueren, M.A.; Berkenpas, M.; Mulder, C.J.; van Bodegraven, A.A. Vitamin and mineral deficiencies are highly prevalent in newly diagnosed celiac disease patients. *Nutrients* **2013**, *5*, 3975–3992.

37. Kabbani, T.A.; Gldberg, A.; Kelly, C.P.; Pallav, K.; Tariq, S.; Peer, A.; Hansen, J.; Dennis, M.; Leffler, D.A. Body mass index and risk of obesity in celiac disease treated with the gluten-free diet. *Aliment. Pharmacol. Ther.* **2012**, *35*, 723–729.
38. Zannini, E.; Jones, J.M.; Renzetti, S.; Arendt, E.K. Functional replacements for gluten. *Annu. Rev. Food Sci. Technol.* **2012**, *3*, 227–245.
39. Arendt, E.K.; O'Brien, C.M.; Schober, T.; Gormley, T.R.; Gallagher, E. Development of gluten-free cereal products. *Farm Food* **2002**, *12*, 21–27.
40. Rotsch, A. Chemische und technische Untersuchungen an künstlichen Teigen. *Brot. Gebaeck.* **1954**, *8*, 129.
41. Anon. Hydrocolloids improve shelf-life and moisture retention of shelf-stable bagels. *Food Technol.* **2002**, *56*, 50.
42. Laureys, C. A natural choice for texture: Rice derivatives. *Food Technol. Eur.* **1996**, *3*, 68–71.
43. Ward, F.M.; Andon, S.A. Hydrocolloids as film formers, adhesives and gelling agents for bakery and cereal products. *Cereal Food World.* **2002**, *47*, 52–55.
44. Chillo, S.; Suriano, N.; Lamacchia, C.; Del Nobile, M.A. Effects of additives on the rheological and mechanical properties of non-conventional fresh handmade tagliatelle. *J. Cereal Sci.* **2009**, *49*, 163–170.
45. Gan, J.; Rafael, L.G.B.; Cato, L.; Small, D.M. Evaluation of the Potential of Different Rice Flours in Bakery Formulations. In Proceedings of the 51st Australian Cereal Chemistry Conference, Cooge, New South Wales, 9-13 September 2001; pp. 309–312.
46. Norton, I.T.; Foster, T.J. Hydrocolloids in Real Food Systems. In *Gums and Stabilisers in the Food Industry II*; Royal Society of Chemistry: Cambridge, UK, 2002; pp. 187–200.
47. Ranhorta, G.S.; Loewe, R.J.; Puyat, L.V. Preparation and fortification of soy-fortified gluten-free bread. *J. Food Sci.* **1975**, *40*, 62–64.
48. Frederickson, H.; Silverio, J.; Andersson, R.; Eliasson, A.C.; Aman, P. The influence of amylose and amylopectin characteristics on gelatinisation and retrogradation properties of different starches. *Carbohydr. Polym.* **1998**, *35*, 119–134.
49. Sasaki, T.; Yasui, T.; Matsuki, J. Effect of amylose content on gelatinisation, retrogradation, and pasting properties from waxy and nonwaxy wheat and their F1 seeds. *Cereal Chem.* **2000**, *77*, 58–63.
50. Holm, J.; Lundquist, I.; Bjorck, I.; Eliasson, A.C..; Asp, N.G. Degree of starch gelatinization, digestion rate of starch *in vitro*, and metabolic response in rats. *Am. J. Clin. Nutr.* **1988**, *47*, 1010–1016.
51. Bird, A.R.; Lopez-Rubio, A.; Shrestha, A.K.; Gidley, M.J. Resistant Starch *in vitro* and *in vivo*: Factors Determining Yield, Structure and Physiological Relevance. In *Modern Biopolymer Science*; Academic Press, Elsevier Inc: London, UK, 2009; pp. 449–510.
52. Berti, C.; Riso, P.; Monti, L.D.; Porrini, M. *In vitro* starch digestibility and *in vivo* glucose response of gluten free foods and their counterparts. *Eur. J. Nutr.* **2004**, *43*, 198–204.
53. Eliasson, A.; Larsson, K. *Cereals in Breadmaking*; Marcel Dekker: NY, USA, **1993**.
54. Scaramuzza, A.E.; Mantegazza, C.; Bosetti, A.; Zuccotti, G.V. Type 1 diabetes and celiac disease: The effects of gluten free diet on metabolic control. *World J. Diabetes* **2013**, *4*, 130–134.

55. Norsa, L.; Shamir, R.; Zevit, N.; Verduci, E.; Hartman, C.; Ghisleni, D.; Riva E.; Giovannini, M. Cardiovascular disease risk factor profiles in children with celiac disease on gluten free diets. *World J. Gastroenterol.* **2013**, *19*, 5658–5664.
56. Livesey, G.; Taylor, R.; Livesey, H.; Liu, S. Is there a dose-response relation of dietary glycemic load to risk of type 2 diabetes? Meta-analysis of prospective cohort studies. *Am. J. Clin. Nutr.* **2013**, *97*, 584–596.
57. Liu, S.; Willett, W.C., Stampfer, M.J.; Hu, F.B.; Franz, M.; Sampson, L.; Hennekens, C.H.; Manson, J.E.A. prospective study of dietary glycemic load, carbohydrate intake, and risk of coronary heart disease in US women. *Am. J. Clin. Nutr.* **2000**, *71*, 1455–1461.
58. Brand-Miller, J.C.; Holt, S.H.; Pawlak, D.B.; McMillan, J. Glycemic index and obesity. *Am. J. Clin. Nutr.* **2013**, *76*, 281S–285S.
59. Tosi, E.A.; Ciappini, M.C.; Masciarelli, R. Utilisation of whole amaranthus (*Amaranthus cruentus*) flour in the manufacture of biscuits for coeliacs. *Alimentaria* **1996**, *34*, 49–51.
60. Ferrara, P.; Cicala, M.; Tiberi, E.; Spadaccio, C.; Marcella, L.; Gatto, A.; Calzolari, P.; Castellucci, G. High fat consumption in children with celiac disease. *Acta Gastroenterol. Belg.* **2009**, *72*, 296–300.
61. Grehn, S.; Fridell, K.; Lilliecreutz, M.; Hallert, C. Dietary habits of Swedish adult coeliac patients treated by a gluten-free diet for 10 years. *Scand. J. Food Nutr.* **2001**, *45*, 178–182.
62. Mariani, P.; Viti, M.G.; Montuori, M.; La Vecchia, A.; Cipolletta, E.; Calvani, L.; Bonamico, M. The gluten-free diet: A nutritional risk factor for adolescents with celiac disease? *J. Pediatr. Gastroenterol. Nutr.* **1998**, *27*, 519–523.
63. Thompson, T. Thiamin, riboflavin, and niacin contents of the gluten-free diet: Is there cause for concern? *J. Am. Diet. Assoc.* **1999**, *99*, 858–862.
64. Gallagher, E.; Polenghi, O.; Gormley, T.R. Novel Rice Starches in Gluten-Free Bread. In Proceedings of the International Association of Cereal Chemists Conference, Budapest, Hungary, May 26-29, **2002**; pp. 24–26.
65. Gibson, G.R.; Roberfroid, M.B. Dietary modulation of the human colonic microbiota: Introducing the concept of prebiotics. *J. Nutr.* **1995**, *125*, 1401–1412.
66. Anon, E. Inulin: Added value. *Eur. Bak.***1999**, *32*, 40–44.
67. Gambus, H.; Gambus, F.; Sabat, R. The research on quality improvement of gluten-free bread by amaranthus flour addition. *Zywnosc* **2002**, *9*, 99–112.
68. Taylor, J.R.N.; Parker, M.L. Quinoa. In *Pseudocereals and Less Common Cereals, Grain Properties and Utilization Potential*; Springer: Verlag, Berlin, **2002**; pp. 93–122.
69. Danz, R.A.; Lupton, J.R. Physiological effects of dietary amaranth (*Amarantus cruentus*) on rats. *Cereal Food World* **1992**, *37*, 489–494.
70. Qureshi, A.A.; Lehamn, J.W.; Peterson, D.M. Amaranth and its oil inhibit cholesterol biosynthesis in 6-week-old female chickens. *J. Nutr.* **1996**, *126*, 1972–1978.
71. Bergamo, P.; Maurano, F.; Mazzarella, G.; Iaquinto, G.; Vocca, I.; Rivelli, A.R.; de Falco, E.; Gianfrani, C.; Rossi, M. Immunological evaluation of the alcohol-soluble protein fraction from gluten-free grains in relation to celiac disease. *Mol. Nutr. Food Res.* **2011**, *55*, 1266–1270.
72. Alvarez-Jubete, L.; Arendt, E.K.; Gallagher, E. Nutritive value of pseudocereals and their increassing use as functional glutenfree ingredients. *Trends Food Sci. Tech.* **2010**, *21*, 106–113.

73. Lamacchia, C.; Chillo, S.; Lamparelli, S.; Suriano, N.; Del Nobile, M.A. Amaranth, quinoa and oat doughs: Mechanical and rheological behaviour, polymeric size distribution and extractability. *J. Food Eng.* **2010**, *96*, 97–106.
74. Caperuto, L.; Amaya-Farfan, J.; Camargo, C. Performance of quinoa (*Chenopodium quinoa* Willd.) flour in the manufacture of gluten free spaghetti. *J. Sci. Food Agric.* **2000**, *81*, 95–101.
75. Shewry, P.R. Seed Proteins. In *Seed Technology and Its Biological Basis*; Black, M., Bewley, J.D., Eds.; Sheffield Academic Press: Sheffield, UK, **2000**; pp. 42–84.
76. Mossè, J.; Huet, J.C. Aminoacid composition and nutritional score for ten cereals and six legumes or oilseeds: Causes and ranges of variation according to species and to seed nitrogen content. *Sci. Aliment.* **1990**, *10*, 151–173.
77. Andersson, H.; Nävert, B.; Bingham, S.A.; Englyst H.N.; Cummings, J.H. The effects of breads containing similar amounts of phytate but different amounts of wheat bran on calcium, zinc and iron balance in man. *Br. J. Nutr.* **1983**, *50*, 503–510.
78. Combs, G.F. Selenium in global food systems. *Br. J. Nutr.* **2001**, *85*, 517–547.
79. Nagy-Scholz, E.; Ercsey, K. Lignan Analysis of Cereal Samples by GC/MS Method. In *The HEALTHGRAIN Methods Book*; Shewry, P.R., Ward, J., Eds.; St. Paul, MN USA, **2009**.
80. Li, L.; Shewry, P.R.; Ward, J.L. Phenolic acids in wheat varieties in the HEALTHGRAIN diversity screen. *J. Agric. Food Chem.* **2008**, *56*, 9732–9739.
81. Drankham, K.; Carter, J.; Madl, R.; Klopfenstein, C.; Padula, F.; Lu, Y.; Warren, T.; Schmitz, N.; Takemoto, D.J. Antitumor activity of wheats with high orthophenolic content. *Nutr. Cancer* **2003**, *47*, 188–194.
82. Wende, L.; Fang, S.; Shancheng, S.; Corke, H.; Beta, T. Free radical scavenging properties and phenolic content of Chinese black-grained wheat. *J. Agric. Food Chem.* **2005**, *53*, 8533–8536.
83. Piironen, V.; Edelmann, M.; Kariluoto, S.; Bedo, Z. Folate in wheat genotypes in the HEALTHGRAIN diversity screen. *J. Agric. Food Chem.* **2008**, *56*, 9726–9731.
84. Moore, M.A.; Beom Park, C.; Tsuda, H. Soluble and insoluble fiber influences on cancer development. *Crit. Rev. Oncol. Hematol.* **1998**, *27*, 229–242.
85. Lewis, S.J.; Heaton, K.W. The metabolic consequences of slow colonic transit. *Am. J. Gastr.* **1999**, *94*, 2010–2016.
86. Vitaglione, P.; Napolitano, A.; Fogliano, V. Cereal dietary fibre: A natural functional ingredient to deliver phenolic compounds into the gut. *Trends Food Sci. Tech.* **2008**, *19*, 451–463.
87. Gebruers, K.; Domez, E.; Boros, D.; Fras, A.; Dynkowska, W.; Bedo, Z.; Rakszegi, M.; Delcour, J.A.; Courtin, C.M. Variation in the content of dietary fiber and components thereof in wheats in the HEALTHGRAIN diversity screen. *J. Agric. Food Chem.* **2008**, *56*, 9740–9749.
88. Ordaz-Ortiz, J.J.; Devaux, M.F.; Saulnier, L. Classification of wheat varieties based on structural features of arabinoxylans as revealed by endoxylanase treatment of flour and grain. *J. Agric. Food Chem.* **2005**, *53*, 8349–8356.
89. Gianfrani, C.; Maglio, M.; Rotondi Aufiero, V.; Camarca, A.; Vocca, I.; Iaquinto, G.; Giardullo, N.; Pogna, N.; Troncone, R.; Auricchio, S.; *et al.* Immunogenicity of *monococcum* wheat in celiac disease patients. *Am. J. Clin. Nutr.* **2012**, *96*, 1339–1345.

90. De Vincenzi, M.; Luchetti, R.; Giovannini, C.; Pogna, N.E.; Saponaro, C.; Galterio, G.; Gasbarrini, G. *In vitro* toxicity testing of alcohol-soluble proteins from diploid wheat *Triticum monococcum* in celiac disease. *J. Biochem. Toxicol.* **1996**, *11*, 313–318.
91. Lundin, K.E.; Sollid, M.N. Mapping of gluten T-cell epitopes in the bread wheat ancestors: Implication for celiac diseases. *Gastroenterology* **2005**, *128*, 393–401.
92. Pizzuti, D.; Buda, A.; D'Odorico, A.; D'Inca, R.; Chiarelli, S.; Curioni, A.; Martines, D. Lack of intestinal mucosal toxicity of Triticum monococcum in celiac disease patients. *Scand. J. Gastroenterol.* **2006**, *41*, 1305–1311.
93. Vincentini, O.; Maialetti, F.; Gazza, L.; Silano, M.; Dessì, M.; De Vincenzi, M.; Pogna, N.E. The environmental factors of celiac disease: Cytotoxicity of hulled species *Triticum monococcum, Triticumturgidum* ssp dicoccum and *T. aestivum* ssp spelta. *J. Gastroenterol. Hepatol.* **2007**, *22*, 1861–1822.
94. Vaccino, P.; Becker, H.A.; Brandolini, A.; Salamini, F.; Kilian, B. A catalogue of *Triticum monococcum* genes encoding toxic and immunogenic peptides for celiac disease patients. *Mol. Genet. Genomics*. **2009**, *281*, 289–300.
95. Suligoj, T.; Gregorini, A.; Colomba, M.; Ellis, H.J.; Ciclitira, P.J. Evaluation of the safety of ancient strains of wheat in coeliac disease reveals heterogeneous small intestinal T cell responses suggestive of coeliac toxicity. *Clin. Nutr.* **2013**, *32*, 1043–1049.
96. Brandolini, A.; Marturini, M.; Plizzari, L.; Hidalgo, J.C.; Pompei, C.; Hidalgo, A. Chimical and technological properties of *Triticum monococcum, Triticum turgidum* and *Triticum aestivum. Tec. Molit. Int.* **2008**, *59*, 85–93.
97. D'Egidio, M.G.; Nardi, S.; Vallega, V. Grain, flour and dough characteristics of selected strains of diploid wheats *Triticum monococcum* L. *Cereal Chem.* **1993**, *70*, 298–303.
98. Corbellini, M.; Empilli, S.; Vaccino, P.; Brandolini, A.; Borghi, B.; Heun, M.; Salamini, F. Einkorn characterizationfor bread and cookie production in relation to protein subunit composition. *Cereal Chem.* **1999**, *76*, 727–733.
99. Borghi, B.; Castagna, R.; Corbellini, M.; Heun, M.; Salamini, F. Breadmaking quality of einkorn wheat (*Triticum monococcum* ssp. *monococcum*). *Cereal Chem.* **1996**, *73*, 208–214.
100. Rizzello, C.G.; de Angelis, M.; di Cagno, R.; Camarca, A.; Silano, M.; Losito, I.; de Vincenzi, D.; de Bari, M.D.; Palmisano, F.; Maurano, F.; *et al.* Highly efficient gluten degradation by lactobacilli and fungal proteases during food processing: New perspectives for Celiac Disease. *Appl. Environ. Microbiol.* **2007**, *73*, 4499–4507.
101. Gianfrani, C.; Siciliano, R.A.; Facchiano, A.M.; Camarca, A.; Mazzeo, M.F.; Costantini, S.; Salvati, V.M.; Maurano, F.; Mazzarella, G.; Iaquinto, G.; *et al.* Transamidation inhibits the intestinal immune response to gliadin *in vitro*. *Gastroenterology* **2007**, *133*, 780–789.
102. Mazzarella, G.; Salvati, V.M.; Iaquinto, G.; Stefanile, R.; Capobianco, F.; Luongo, D.; Bergamo, P.; Maurano, F.; Giardullo, N.; Malamisura, B.; *et al.* Reintroduction of gluten following flour transdamidation in adult celiac patients: A randomized, controlled clinical study. *Clin. Dev. Immunol.* **2012**, *2012*, 329150.

2

Celiac Disease and Overweight in Children

Antonella Diamanti [1,*], Teresa Capriati [1,2], Maria Sole Basso [1], Fabio Panetta [1], Vincenzo Maria Di Ciommo Laurora [3], Francesca Bellucci [1], Fernanda Cristofori [2] and Ruggiero Francavilla [2]

[1] Gastroenterology-Hepatology and Nutrition Unit, "Bambino Gesù" Children's Hospital, Piazza Sant'Onofrio 4, Rome 00165, Italy; E-Mails: teresa.capriati@gmail.com (T.C.); msole.basso@opbg.net (M.S.B.); fabio.panetta@opbg.net (F.P.); francesca.bellucci@opbg.net (F.B.)

[2] Gastroenterology Unit, Pediatric Clinic of University, Piazza Giulio Cesare 11, Bari 70124, Italy; E-Mails: fernandacristofori@gmail.com (F.C.); rfrancavilla@gmail.com (R.F.)

[3] Epidemiology and Biostatistics Unit, "Bambino Gesù" Children's Hospital, Piazza Sant'Onofrio 4, Rome 00165, Italy; E-Mail: vmaria.diciommo@opbg.net

* Author to whom correspondence should be addressed; E-Mail: antonella.diamanti@opbg.net;

Abstract: The clinical presentation of celiac disease in children is very variable and differs with age. The prevalence of atypical presentations of celiac disease has increased over the past 2 decades. Several studies in adults and children with celiac disease indicate that obesity/overweight at disease onset is not unusual. In addition, there is a trend towards the development of overweight/obesity in celiac patients who strictly comply with a gluten-free diet. However, the pathogenesis and clinical implications of the coexistence of classic malabsorption (e.g., celiac disease) and overweight/obesity remain unclear. This review investigated the causes and main clinical factors associated with overweight/obesity at the diagnosis of celiac disease and clarified whether gluten withdrawal affects the current trends of the nutritional status of celiac disease patients.

Keywords: celiac disease; overweight; obesity; gluten free diet

---

1. Introduction

Celiac disease (CD) is a life-long condition that affects the small intestine in genetically susceptible individuals [1]. The global prevalence ranges from 1% to 2% [2,3]. In children, the symptoms upon CD presentation are highly variable and are influenced by age. Very young children often present with "classic" symptoms including diarrhea, abdominal distension, and growth retardation [4–6]. Diarrhea and malabsorption represent the typical presentation of CD in young children [7], while abdominal pain, vomiting, and constipation are atypical gastrointestinal symptoms more common in older children and teenagers. Furthermore, in children, CD can be diagnosed on the basis of the occurrence of extra-intestinal conditions such as arthritis, neurological diseases, and anemia [8,9] or on the basis of screening procedures in the absence of gastrointestinal symptoms (typical or atypical) and in child or adolescent with CD- associated conditions [10].

The presentation of CD has changed over time. In the last 2 decades, diarrhea and malabsorption have progressively decreased as the mode of CD onset among both adults and children, whereas atypical manifestations have increased. Interestingly, many reports indicate that CD can be associated with overweight or normal weight; hence, malnutrition is not always present at CD presentation [4,6,11,12]. Therefore, CD and obesity can coexist during both childhood and adolescence. After the first 2 cases reported by Semeraro [13] and Conti-Nibali [14] in 1986 and 1987, respectively, there have been several reports of the coexistence of CD and obesity/overweight in children and adolescents in the last 2 decades [15–19].

At present, in pediatric [20–27] and adult [28–33] case series of CD, the body mass index (BMI) at diagnosis is within the normal range in many patients. Nevertheless, the pathogenesis and clinical implications of the coexistence of CD and overweight/obesity remain unclear. The clinical relevance of this association is highlighted by the observation that CD patients with normal weight or overweight at diagnosis have a higher risk of developing obesity after starting a gluten-free diet (GFD), which definitely improves intestinal absorption in these patients. Moreover, the GFD regimen appears to be associated with high lipid and protein intake, particularly in adolescents [20,29].

The key studies concerning the pathogenesis and clinical evidence of the association between CD and overweight/obesity in subjects aged <18 years are discussed below. This review investigated the causes and main clinical factors associated with overweight/obesity at CD diagnosis. In addition, this review aims to clarify if gluten withdrawal affects the trend of the nutritional status of CD patients.

2. Clinical Evidence of CD and Overweight/Obesity

2.1. Summary of the Main Case Reports

The first pediatric case report [13] by Semeraro *et al.*, in 1986 describes an obese 14-year-old girl who had been diagnosed with CD at the age of 1 year on the basis of a clinical condition characterized by malabsorption, diarrhea, and stunted growth (*i.e.*, weight in the 7th percentile). The girl was started on a GFD, and had a normal weight at 2 years of age; however, she was overweight at 5 years of age and obese at 10. She had a negative family history for endocrine diseases and CD but a positive family history for obesity.

There are other reports of the development of obesity in children on a GFD who initially had malabsorption. For example Czaja-Bulsa *et al.* [15] describe the case of an 18-year-old boy with growth failure (*i.e.*, <3rd percentile) and chronic diarrhea following gluten introduction and before CD diagnosis. However, after gluten withdrawal, his weight increased to the 97th percentile at 5 years of age despite persistent mucosal atrophy. More recently, Balamtekin *et al.* [19] reported a similar case of a 21-month-old child with the classic condition of malabsorption (*i.e.*, chronic diarrhea, failure to thrive, and abdominal distension) at CD onset. After 11 years on a GFD, the child became obese (weight, >97th percentile).

Meanwhile, there are other reports of children with overweight/obesity at the time of CD diagnosis. The first published report describes a 5-year-old girl with obesity, short stature, and recurrent abdominal pain. The diagnosis of CD was suspected on the basis of family history, *i.e.*, a sister with CD. A GFD attenuated the symptoms and improved height and weight growth [14]. Furthermore, in 2001, Franzese *et al.* [16] reported the case of a patient with steatohepatitis associated with obesity resistant to a low-calorie diet, in which CD was diagnosed on the basis of moderate persistent hypertransaminasemia. In 2006, Oso and Fraser [17] diagnosed CD in an obese teenager who had recurrent episodes of diarrhea, especially after eating spaghetti. At diagnosis, blood tests revealed low iron, GFD feeding normalized iron level, and the symptoms disappeared. However, the patient continued to gain weight (10 kg over 6 months) during follow-up. In 2009, Arslan *et al.* [18] reported the case of a 7-year-old obese patient with CD (weight, >95th percentile; weight/height ratio, 167%) suspected of having Hashimoto's thyroiditis and affected by hypochromic anemia unresponsive to iron therapy. Moreover, Balamtekin *et al.* [19] describe the case of a 17-year-old obese girl with weight >97th percentile and a BMI of 32.9 with epigastric pain and vomiting. CD was diagnosed on the basis of the gastrointestinal symptoms, and the symptoms disappeared after a GFD was started. Nevertheless, her weight continued to increase.

2.2. Summary of Case Series

At present, few case series have been published on this topic. Valletta *et al.* [24] report the prevalence of overweight (BMI z-score > +1) and obesity (BMI z-score > +2) to be 11% and 3%, respectively, in 149 children newly diagnosed with CD between 1991 and 2007. The authors found that after initiating a GFD, the BMI z-score increased significantly and the percentage of overweight subjects almost doubled. In a retrospective study, Venkatasubramani *et al.* [22] report 5% of patients had a BMI > 95th percentile among 143 patients with CD diagnosed between 1986 and 2003. Among the obese patients, the most common symptoms at onset were abdominal pain, diabetes, and diarrhea.

Brambilla *et al.* [25] compared 150 children with CD on a GFD with 288 healthy sex- and age-matched children. They also retrospectively evaluated changes in BMI from CD diagnosis to the last clinical evaluation. The median BMI of CD patients was significantly lower than that of the healthy controls. In particular, children with CD were less frequently overweight or obese (12% *vs.* 23.3%) and more frequently underweight (16% *vs.* 4.5%) than the controls. However, after GFD feeding, the number of underweight subjects decreased significantly, while the number of overweight subjects increased slightly.

Reilly *et al.* [26] studied 142 children with newly diagnosed CD from 2000 to 2008. Nearly 19% of patients had a high BMI at diagnosis (12.6% overweight and 6% obese), while 74.5% had a normal BMI. Meanwhile, the BMI of 75% of the patients with high BMI at diagnosis decreased on a GFD. Among patients with a normal BMI at diagnosis, weight *z*-scores increased significantly after diet treatment and 13% became overweight. Interestingly, in that survey, the initial symptom in 28% of overweight CD patients was abdominal pain and the diagnosis was made on the basis of the screening test in a asymptomatic portion of the population by 28%. Venkatasubramani *et al.* [22] also found abdominal pain is one of the most common features of CD presentation in overweight patients. Another important aspect of their survey results is that the CD diagnosis was made on the basis of the screening test in at least 25% of overweight patients. Brambilla *et al.* [25] suggest that identifying CD patients on the basis of screening tests, and not symptoms, may increase the probability of finding overweight or obese subjects at CD diagnosis.

In a cross-sectional multicenter study, Norsa *et al.* [27] enrolled 114 children with CD in serologic remission, who were on a GFD for at least 1 year. The anthropometric measurements at diagnosis revealed that 9.6%, 76.3%, 8.8%, and 5.3% were underweight (BMI < 5th percentile), had normal weight (BMI = 5–85th percentile), were overweight (BMI = 85–95th percentile), and were obese (BMI > 95th percentile), respectively. After gluten withdrawal, the prevalence of overweight and obesity increased to 11.4% and 8%, respectively.

In a prospective case–control study, Barera *et al.* [34] found reduced fat mass, decreased bone mineral content, and lower lean body mass in the limbs of 29 children newly diagnosed with CD compared to healthy controls; all patients were normalized (*i.e.*, approaching corresponding parameters in the control population) on a GFD. Table 1 summarizes the main results of the abovementioned reports.

Table 1. Prevalence of overweight/obesity in CD.

Author (Year)	Country (Sample Size)	Overweight/Obesity at Presentation (%)	Overweight/Obesity after Initiating a GFD (%)	Reference
Aurangzeb (2010)	Australia & New Zealand ($n = 25$)	20.8/0	ND/ND	[21]
Venkatasubramani (2010)	Milwaukee, WI, USA ($n = 143$)	ND/5	ND/3	[22]
Balamtekin (2010)	Ankara, Turkey ($n = 220$)	ND/0.5	ND/ND	[23]
Valletta *et al.* (2010)	Italy ($n = 149$)	11/3	21/4	[24]
Reilly *et al.* (2010)	NY, USA ($n = 142$)	12.6/6	20/4	[26]
Norsa *et al.* (2011)	Italy & Israel ($n = 114$)	8.8/5.3	11.5/8.8	[27]
Brambilla *et al.* (2011)	Italy ($n = 150$)	11.3/0.7	9.4/0	[25]

GFD: gluten-free diet; ND: not done.

A clarification regarding the methodology of these studies should be made: in adults and children, the main criterion for defining overweight/obesity is BMI (or Quetelet index), which is calculated by dividing weight (in kg) by height (in m) squared. BMI is an expression of the weight "adjusted" to stature and is an index of adiposity; it is most strongly correlated with body fat and less correlated with stature. Despite its limitations, BMI is easy to calculate and widely used, especially in large-scale studies, to assess the risks of diseases. The internationally accepted age- and sex-standardized threshold values of BMI for nutritional status in adults are those proposed by the World Health Organization [35]. However, the curves of children's weight and height vary with growth, following development during puberty (with its consequences on body composition), and sex. Therefore, references for different age groups (*i.e.*, the distribution of percentiles with cut-off points) are necessary. There are many different percentile tables based on data from reference populations that also have very different anthropometric characteristics. Ideally, the study population should be compared with tables based on national curves. Alternatively, the International Obesity Task Force (IOTF), which is the main organization of childhood obesity scholars, have validated tables with mean percentiles derived from cross-sectional studies of different populations (e.g., the USA, Brazil, Hong Kong, Singapore, Holland, and Great Britain) to enable international comparisons [36].

In this regard, the abovementioned studies have a discrete methodological heterogeneity. Although all are based on the calculation of BMI, they used different categorizations in various case series, such as the BMI percentile, BMI *z*-score, and IOTF cut-off point. In addition, different studies were conducted on geographically diverse populations, and only a few studies compared the case population with a control population [21,25].

3. Pathogenetic Link between CD and Overweight/Obesity

3.1. Overweight and Obesity in Newly Diagnosed CD Patients: The "Compensatory" Hypothesis

Semeraro first hypothesized that the atrophy of the duodenum—jejunum in CD patients could be compensated by enhanced absorption in the distal intestinal segments [13]. The fat absorption coefficient could in fact be preserved in a patient with a partially atrophic bowel [13]. This process could be similar to that occurring in the residual bowel after surgical resection, which involves structural changes that lead to an increased absorptive attitude of the intestine. The intestinal adaptation consists of morphological changes of the mucosa, including increased villus height, crypt depth, and epithelial cell number. In CD patients, atrophy determines the loss of normal intestinal function. This can hypothetically induce increased absorption of the functionally preserved intestinal tract. If this process overcompensates, it could lead to the extraction of energy exceeding the child's needs, thus increasing the risk of overweight/obesity [13].

This compensatory hypothesis appears to be supported by some of the first published cases of adolescents affected by CD who continued to present with overweight or obesity despite persistent villous atrophy on jejunal biopsies [14,15]. The compensatory surface area of the small intestine appears to increase with patient age. Therefore, the intestine may develop the ability to absorb an adequate amount of compensatory energy [13]. This notion is corroborated by the particular distribution of symptoms upon CD diagnosis, which appears to be related to age [5–7]. Children aged less than 2 years often exhibit the classic CD presentation, which includes malabsorption. In contrast, older children, adolescents, and adults often present with atypical symptoms. This appears to be concordant with the compensatory hypothesis. In fact, the classic symptoms may be due to a lack of intestinal adaptation, which is less developed in young children as mentioned above. The absence of intestinal adaptation induces the occurrence of severe and classic symptoms including malabsorption and celiac crisis, which can be found in very young children newly diagnosed with CD. As intestinal adaptation is a time-dependent phenomenon, the probability that an individual's mucosa is modified increases with age. Therefore, CD symptoms could be attenuated in older children and adolescents.

Concordant with this hypothesis, there is no correlation between the presentation of CD and the degree of villous atrophy [37] or the extent of the intestine involved as visualized through video-capsule endoscopic procedures [38]. The morphological appearance of the mucosa may be unrelated to its functional expression responsible for the severity of the presenting symptoms.

In addition, the nutritional status of the underlying population is clearly very important for the correct interpretation of BMI in children with CD at diagnosis. CD may indeed develop in patients with overweight/obesity, reflecting an individual's predisposition (*i.e.*, genetic, nutritional, and environmental factors). The worldwide prevalence of overweight/obesity in children has increased over the last 2 decades; an estimated 60 million children will be overweight or obese by 2020 [39]. In this scenario, the symptoms of malabsorption that could manifest in overweight patients at CD onset may reduce the prevalence of overweight/obesity in CD patients compared to the reference population but increase it in comparison to what is usually expected in CD patients.

3.2. The Effect of Gluten Withdrawal on Overweight/Obese CD Patients

Overweight or obesity may develop in CD patients after gluten withdrawal. The main surveys on children discussed above report the normalization of BMI in underweight and overweight patients on a GFD, although they also report the development of overweight and obesity independent of baseline nutritional status [21–27,34]. In consideration of the abovementioned "compensatory" hypothesis, it can be supposed the mucosal healing following gluten withdrawal is responsible for the normalization of BMI in both underweight and overweight patients as a result of the recovery of energy balance. Therefore, the restoration of the absorptive functions of the whole bowel could constitute a physiological redistribution of the absorptive attitude in whole bowel mucosa. This could result in an increased energetic yield in patients with symptoms of malabsorption. However, in patients with a mucosa adapted to supply a higher energetic yield, the improved absorptive function of the whole bowel could induce the normalization of caloric balance. Nevertheless, it remains to be determined if a GFD itself is a cause of the development of overweight/obesity in CD patients.

The unpalatability of some gluten-free foods may induce a preference toward hyperproteic and hyperlipidemic foods [20,29,40]. This may consequently lead to increased energy intake followed by excessive weight gain [41]. Mariani *et al.* [20] examined the eating habits and diet composition of 47 adolescents with CD and compared them to those of 47 healthy age-matched control subjects. They divided the CD patients into 2 subgroups according to compliance with a GFD: group 1A patients rigorously adhered to a GFD, while group 1B patients did not comply with a GFD. Compared to Recommended Dietary Allowances, total energy, lipid, and protein intake were higher and carbohydrate intake was lower in CD patients and controls. Total caloric intake and lipid and protein consumption were higher in group 1A than in group 1B. As a consequence, overweight/obesity was more frequent in group 1A (72%) than in group 1B (51%) and the controls (47%).

Several studies confirm long-term GFDs may not be nutritionally balanced. Indeed, there is clinical evidence indicating high simple sugar, protein, and saturated fat intake as well as low complex carbohydrate and fiber intake in such diets [20,42,43]. Concordant with this pediatric evidence, higher total caloric [44], carbohydrate, and fat [45] intake is reported among adults with CD than among healthy control subjects. In contrast, a few studies in adults [46,47] and children [48] report reduced caloric intake in CD patients on a GFD.

Besides increased total caloric intake, the macronutrient composition of the diet may be involved in the pathogenesis of overweight and obesity in patients with CD. Carbohydrates are the major energy source in the diet of children in developed countries and are the dietary components that most strongly affect blood glycemia. Both the quantity and type of carbohydrates are the determinants of postprandial glycemia [49]. The glycemic index (GI) is a parameter used to classify foods according to their postprandial glycemic response [50].

Many gluten-free foods are characterized by a GI higher than that of equivalent gluten-containing foods [50,51], although this is refuted by some authors [52]. Gluten-free foods have a higher GI, because gluten protein does not allow the easy access of amylase to hydrolyze starch granules in the lumen of the small intestine [50]. However, many foods with a high GI have been shown to only slightly increase blood glucose and vice versa [51,53]. Thus, the GI provides a measurement of the quality but not the quantity of the carbohydrates consumed. Meanwhile, blood glycemia is influenced by the synergistic interaction between the quantity and quality of carbohydrates. Therefore, epidemiological studies are utilizing a new concept to assess outcomes as a result of glucose metabolism: the glycemic load (GL). The GL may be calculated with the product of GI (as a percentage) of available carbohydrates, representing both the quality and quantity of carbohydrates consumed. The GL may be interpreted as a measure of insulin requested in free-living conditions, because the amount of carbohydrates consumed at each meal usually varies in such conditions [51,54,55]. Nevertheless, if the blood glucose response to food is a determinant of body weight remains controversial [56].

Several studies conducted in overweight or obese children show discordant results regarding the associations of GI and GL with obesity. One cross-sectional study reports no association of body fat with GI or GL [57]. Others studies show positive associations of GI and GL with waist circumference, BMI, and the sum of 4 skinfolds [58,59]. However, other cohort studies report inconclusive results [60–62]. A meta-analysis [63] that identified six eligible randomized clinic trials including a total of 202 participants concludes that low-GI or low-GL diets confer marked benefits on weight, BMI, total fat mass, and lipid profile. Regardless, further research on long-term improvements is required. A more recent systematic review provides evidence that long-term interventions with a low-GI/GL diet confer beneficial effects on fasting insulin and pro-inflammatory markers such as C-reactive protein; such interventions might prove to be helpful in the primary prevention of obesity-associated diseases [64]. These aspects could help explain the occurrence of overweight/obesity in celiac patients on a GFD.

On the other hand, several studies evaluating the effects of a GFD on metabolic control, growth, and nutritional status in celiac patients with type I diabetes provide a natural model of the interactions between diet, glycemic response, and nutritional status, demonstrating how this interrelationship can be much more complex. However, these studies have completely discordant results. Some studies [65] indicate improvements in BMI and glycosylated hemoglobin (HbA1c) levels in patients with CD and type I diabetes on a GFD. Meanwhile, Novòa Medina *et al.* [66] report no effect on the metabolic control, height, or weight of such patients. Other studies evaluated the influence of GFDs on metabolic parameters including insulin dose, HbA1c, glucose excretion, and hypoglycemic episodes. Saadah *et al.* [67] report that a GFD resulted in a significant improvement of growth and influenced diabetic control, particularly higher insulin levels in patients with CD than the levels at baseline. Other authors [68,69] found no significant difference in the insulin dose, HbA1c, 24-h urinary glucose excretion, or the number of hypoglycemic episodes. Abid *et al.* [70] found that a GFD reduced gastrointestinal symptoms in the short term and particularly episodes of severe hypoglycemia in children with type I diabetes with CD; however, there were no changes in the standard deviation scores for height, weight, BMI, or the average HbA1c before and after GFD consumption. Furthermore, epidemiological studies show energy intake is predictor of weight gain [71]. Thus, the GI and GL of the previous meal can theoretically influence energy intake in the next meal. A recent meta-analysis on this topic suggests that the GI, but not the GL might influence the energy intake of the next meal [72]. This may be because low-GI foods result in sustained blood glucose levels and hunger is delayed as compared with that after a high-GI meal [73]. Furthermore, recent evidence suggests energy intake is associated with changes in the resting metabolic rate [74]. The mechanism involved in this phenomenon may be the specific effect of blood glucose level on satiety (*i.e.*, the glucostatic theory) or of other stimuli (e.g., peptides) involved in the control of appetite. Insulin and glucose stimulate the release of the leptin hormone that produces satiety and suppress the release of the ghrelin hormone that stimulates the appetite. Regardless, this does not precisely characterize relationships among GI, satiogenic leptin, and appetitic ghrelin. Furthermore, several gastrointestinal hormones called incretins are involved in the physiological control of hunger and satiety; they are involved in glucose metabolism and can act on pancreatic beta cells to stimulate insulin secretion. Among these hormones there is glucagon-like peptide-1 (GLP-1), which acts directly on the central nervous system and indirectly by slowing gastric emptying, inhibiting appetite and food intake, and inducing body weight reduction. The stimulation of insulin secretion by incretins is typically glucose dependent and manifests when glycemic levels are high but not when normal or low. Therefore, incretins have the potential to reduce hyperglycemia without causing hypoglycemia. A recent study revealed children with CD have a secretion pattern of gut-brain axis hormones that differs from that of controls. Alterations in this axis were more pronounced in children with both CD and type I diabetes mellitus; nevertheless, the roles of these gut-brain axis hormones in food intake and glycemic control in patients with CD and type I diabetes mellitus must be clarified [75].

Overall existing clinical evidence explains the variability of the anthropometric trends in CD patients after gluten withdrawal. However, it does not clarify why some CD patients develop overweight/obesity after beginning a GFD. Furthermore, as is the case in newly diagnosed CD patients, the global trend toward increased overweight/obesity could explain why CD patients on a GFD may become overweight. The changes in nutritional habits that induce the development of obesity are probably shared by CD patients and the general population. Table 2 summarizes the main pathogenetic links between CD and overweight/obesity.

Table 2. Suggested pathogenetic links between CD and overweight/obesity.

Time of Overweight/Obesity Diagnosis in Celiac Patients	Pathogenetic Link	Reference
Overweight/Obesity at CD Presentation	"Compensatory hypothesis": high energetic yield due to the slow adaptation of the atrophic mucosa	[13]
	Global trend toward overweight/obesity in children	[39]
	Diagnosis not based on clinical symptoms but on screening test	[25,26]
Overweight/Obesity on a GFD	"Compensatory hypothesis": normalization of caloric balance due to the restoration of mucosal functions	[13]
	Worldwide trend toward overweight/obesity in children	[39]
	Unpalatability of gluten-free foods, prompting the consumption of foods with high caloric content (*i.e.*, fat and protein).	[20,29,40]
	High GI/GL of GFD?	[49–74]
	Altered secretion of gut–brain axis hormones?	[75]

CD: celiac disease; GFD: gluten-free diet; GI: glycemic index; GL: glycemic load.

4. Conclusions

Overweight/obesity is more common in children with CD than previously recognized. The prevalence of overweight in CD patients at diagnosis ranges from 8.8% to 20.8% [21,24–27], whereas that in CD patients on a GFD ranges from 9.4% to 21% [23–26]. Meanwhile, the prevalence of obesity in CD patients at diagnosis ranges from 0% to 6% [21–27], whereas that in CD patients on a GFD ranges from 0% to 8.8% [22,24–27]. Overweight/obesity is more frequent in newly diagnosed CD patients diagnosed on the basis of abdominal pain [22,26] and on the basis of screening procedures [25,26]. During follow-up, it is possible the unpalatability of gluten-free foods leads a preference for foods with high caloric fat and protein contents. However, the occurrence of overweight may be explained by the global trend toward overweight/obesity in children [39] including CD patients. An unconfirmed but nonetheless interesting hypothesis is that the development of overnutrition status is due to the compensatory high energetic yield secondary to the slow functional adaptation of the atrophic mucosa [13]. Therefore, mounting evidence suggests CD should be considered even in overweight/obese children in appropriate clinical settings.

References

1. Green, P.H.; Cellier, C. Celiac disease. *N. Engl. J. Med.* **2007**, *357*, 1731–1743.
2. Hill, I.D.; Dirks, M.H.; Liptak, G.S.; Colletti, R.B.; Fasano, A.; Guandalini, S.; Hoffenberg, E.J.; Horvath, K.; Murray, J.A.; Pivor, M.; *et al.* Guideline for the diagnosis and treatment of celiac disease in children: Recommendations of the North American Society for Pediatric Gastroenterology, Hepatology and Nutrition. *J. Pediatr. Gastroenterol. Nutr.* **2005**, *40*, 1–19.

3. Mearin, M.L.; Ivarsson, A.; Dickey, W. Coeliac disease: Is it time for mass screening? *Best Pract. Res. Clin. Gastroenterol.* **2005**, *19*, 441–452.
4. Rampertab, S.D.; Pooran, N.; Brar, P.; Singh, P.; Green, P.H. Trends in the presentation of celiac disease. *Am. J. Med.* **2006**, *119*, e9–e14.
5. Vivas, S.; Ruiz de Morales, J.M.; Fernandez, M.; Hernando, M.; Herrero, B.; Casqueiro, J.; Gutierrez, S. Age-related clinical, serological, and histopathological features of celiac disease. *Am. J. Gastroenterol*. **2008**, *103*, 2360–2365.
6. Telega, G.; Bennet, T.R.; Werlin, S. Emerging new clinical patterns in the presentation of celiac disease. *Arch. Pediatr. Adolesc. Med.* **2008**, *162*, 164–168.
7. Llorente-Alonso, M.; Fernandez-Acenero, M.J.; Sebastian, M. Gluten intolerance: Gender and age-related features. *Can. J. Gastroenterol.* **2006**, *20*, 719–722.
8. Branski, D.; Troncone, R. Celiac disease: A reappraisal. *J. Pediatr.* **1998**, *133*, 181–187.
9. Ludvigsson, J.F.; Ansved, P.; Falth-Magnusson, K.; Hammersjö, J.A.; Johansson, C.; Edvardsson, S.; Ljungkrantz, M.; Stenhammar, L.; Ludvigsson, J. Symptoms and signs haven changed in Swedish children with coeliac disease. *J. Pediatr. Gastroenterol. Nutr.* **2004**, *38*, 181–186.
10. Husby, S.; Koletzko, S.; Korponay-Szabó, I.R.; Mearin, M.L.; Phillips, A.; Shamir, R.; Troncone, R.; Giersiepen, K.; Branski, D.; Catassi, C.; *et al.* European Society for Pediatric Gastroenterology, Hepatology, and Nutrition Guidelines for the diagnosis of coeliac disease. *J. Pediatr. Gastroenterol. Nutr.* **2012**, *54*, 136–160.
11. McGowan, K.E.; Castiglione, D.A.; Butzner, J.D. The changing face of childhood celiac disease in North America: Impact of serological testing. *Pediatrics* **2009**, *124*, 1572–1578.
12. Lo, W.; Sano, K.; Lebwohl, B.; Diamond, B.; Green, P.H. Changing presentation of adult celiac disease. *Dig. Dis. Sci.* **2003**, *48*, 395–398.
13. Semeraro, L.A.; Barwick, K.W.; Griboski, J.D. Obesity in celiac disease. *J. Clin. Gastroenterol.* **1986**, *8*, 177–180.
14. Conti Nibali, S.; Magazzù, G.; De Luca, F. Obesity in a child with untreated coeliac disease. *Helv. Paediatr. Acta* **1987**, *42*, 45–48.
15. Czaja-Bulsa, G.; Garanty-Bogacka, B.; Syrenicz, M.; Gebala, A. Obesity in an 18-year-old boy with untreated celiac disease. *J. Pediatr. Gastroenterol. Nutr.* **2001**, *32*, 226.
16. Franzese, A.; Iannucci, M.P.; Valerio, G.; Ciccimarra, E.; Spaziano, M.; Mandato, C.; Vajro, P. Atypical celiac disease presenting as obesity-related liver dysfunction. *J. Pediatr. Gastroenterol. Nutr.* **2001**, *33*, 329–332.
17. Oso, O.; Fraser, N.C. A boy with coeliac disease and obesity. *Acta Paediatr.* **2006**, *95*, 618–619.
18. Arslan, N.; Esen, I.; Demircioglu, F.; Yilmaz, S.; Unuvar, T.; Bober, E. The changing face of celiac disease: A girl with obesity and celiac disease. *J. Paediatr. Child Health* **2009**, *45*, 317–318.
19. Balamtekin, N.; Demir, H.; Baysoy, G.; Uslu, N.; Yuce, A. Obesity in adolescents with celiac disease: Two adolescents and two different presentations. *Turk. J. Pediatr.* **2011**, *53*, 314–316.
20. Mariani, P.; Viti, M.G.; Montouri, M.; La Vecchia, A.; Cipolletta, E.; Calvani, L.; Bonamico, M. The gluten free diet: A nutritional risk factor for adolescents with celiac disease? *J. Pediatr. Gastroenterol. Nutr.* **1998**, *27*, 519–523.

21. Aurangzeb, B.; Leach, S.T.; Lemberg, D.A.; Day, A.S. Nutritional status of children with coeliac disease. *Acta Padiatr.* **2010**, *99*, 1020–1025.
22. Venkatasubramani, N.; Telega, G.; Werlin, S.L. Obesity in pediatric celiac disease. *J. Pediatr. Gastroenterol. Nutr.* **2010**, *51*, 295–297.
23. Balamtekin, N.; Uslu, N.; Baysoy, G.; Usta, Y.; Demir, H.; Saltik-Temizel, I.N.; Ozen, H.; Gürakan, F.; Yüce, A. The presentation of celiac disease in 220 Turkish children. *Turk. J. Pediatr.* **2010**, *52*, 239–244.
24. Valletta, E.; Fornaro, M.; Cipolli, M.; Conte, S.; Bissolo, F.; Danchielli, C. Celiac disease and obesity: Need for nutritional follow-up after diagnosis. *Eur. J. Clin. Nutr.* **2010**, *64*, 1371–1372.
25. Brambilla, P.; Picca, M.; Dilillo, D.; Meneghin, F.; Cravidi, C.; Tischer, M.C.; Vivaldo, T.; Bedogni, G.; Zuccotti, G.V. Changes of body mass index in celiac children on a gluten-free diet. *Nutr. Metab. Cardiovasc. Dis.* **2013**, *23*, 177–182.
26. Reilly, N.R.; Aguilar, K.; Hassid, B.G.; Cheng, J.; Defelice, A.R.; Kazlow, P.; Bhagat, G.; Green, P.H. Celiac disease in normal-weight and overweight children: Clinical features and growth outcomes following a gluten-free diet. *J. Pediatr. Gastroenterol. Nutr.* **2011**, *53*, 528–531.
27. Norsa, L.; Shamir, R.; Zevit, N.; Verduci, E.; Hartman, C.; Ghisleni, D.; Riva, E.; Giovannini, M. Cardiovascular disease risk factor profiles in children with celiac disease on gluten-free diets. *World J. Gastroenterol.* **2013**, *19*, 5658–5664.
28. West, J.; Logan R.F.; Card, T.R.; Smith, C.; Hubbard, R. Risk of vascular disease in adults with diagnosed coeliac disease: A population-based study. *Aliment. Pharmacol. Ther.* **2004**, *20*, 73–79.
29. Dickey, W.; Kearney, N. Overweight in celiac disease: Prevalence, clinical characteristics, and effect of a gluten-free diet. *Am. J. Gastroenterol.* **2006**, *101*, 2356–2359.
30. Olén, O.; Montgomery, S.M.; Marcus, C.; Ekbom, A.; Ludvigsson, J.F. Coeliac disease and body mass index: A study of two Swedish general population-based registers. *Scand. J. Gastroenterol.* **2009**, *44*, 1198–1206.
31. Cheng, J.; Brar, P.S.; Lee, A.R.; Green, P.H. Body mass index in celiac disease: Beneficial effect of a gluten-free diet. *J. Clin. Gastroenterol.* **2010**, *44*, 267–271.
32. Kabbani, T.A.; Goldberg, A.; Kelly, C.P.; Pallav, K.; Tariq, S.; Peer, A.; Hansen, J.; Dennis, M.; Leffler, D.A. Body mass index and the risk of obesity in coeliac disease treated with the gluten-free diet. *Aliment. Pharmacol. Ther.* **2012**, *35*, 723–729.
33. Tucker, E.; Rostami, K.; Prabhakaran, S.; Al Dulaimi, D. Patients with celiac disease are increasingly overweight or obese on presentation. *J. Gastrointest. Liver Dis.* **2012**, *21*, 11–15.
34. Barera, G.; Mora, S.; Brambilla, P.; Ricotti, A.; Menni, L.; Beccio, S.; Bianchi, C. Body composition in children with celiac disease and the effects of a gluten-free diet: A prospective case-control study. *Am. J. Clin. Nutr.* **2000**, *72*, 71–75.
35. Bailey, K.V.; Ferro-Luzzi, A. Use of body mass index of adults in assessing individual and community nutritional status. *Bull. World Health Org.* **1995**, *73*, 673–680.
36. Cole, T.J.; Bellizzi, M.C.; Flegal, K.M.; Dietz, W.H. Establishing a standard definition for child overweight and obesity worldwide: International survey. *BMJ* **2000**, *6*, 1240–1243.
37. Brar, P.; Kwon, G.Y.; Egbuna, I.I.; Holleran, S.; Ramakrishnan, R.; Bhagat, G.; Green, P.H. Lack of correlation of degree of villous atrophy with severity of clinical presentation of coeliac disease. *Dig. Liver Dis.* **2007**, *39*, 26–29.

38. Murray, J.A.; Rubio-Tapia, A.; van Dyke, C.T.; Brogan, D.L.; Knipschield, M.A.; Lahr, B.; Rumalla, A.; Zinsmeister, A.R.; Gostout, C.J. Mucosal atrophy in celiac disease: Extent of involvement, correlation with clinical presentation, and response to treatment. *Clin. Gastroenterol. Hepatol.* **2008**, *6*, 186–193.
39. De Onis, M.; Blössner, M.; Borghi, E. Global prevalence and trends of overweight and obesity among preschool children. *Am. J. Clin. Nutr.* **2010**, *92*, 1257–1264.
40. Ferrara, P.; Cicala, M.; Tiberi, E.; Spadaccio, C.; Marcella, L.; Gatto, A.; Calzolari, P.; Castellucci, G. High fat consumption in children with celiac disease. *Acta Gastroenterol. Belg.* **2009**, *72*, 296–300.
41. Kupper, C. Dietary guidelines and implementation for celiac disease. *Gastroenterology* **2005**, *128*, S121–S127.
42. Ohlund, K.; Olsson, C.; Hernell, O.; Ohlund, I. Dietary shortcomings in children on a gluten-free diet. *J. Hum. Nutr. Diet.* **2010**, *23*, 294–300.
43. Hopman, E.G.; Le Cessie, S.; von Blomberg, B.M.; Mearin, M.L. Nutritional management of the gluten-free diet in young people with celiac disease in The Netherlands. *J. Pediatr. Gastroenterol. Nutr.* **2006**, *43*, 102–108.
44. Kemppainen, T.; Uusitupa, M.; Janatuinen, E.; Järvinen, R.; Julkunen, R.; Pikkarainen, P. Intakes of nutrients and nutritional status in coeliac patients. *Scand. J. Gastroenterol.* **1995**, *30*, 575–579.
45. Capristo, E.; Addolorato, G.; Mingrone, G.; de Gaetano, A.; Greco, A.V.; Tataranni, P.A.; Gasbarrini, G. Changes in body composition, substrate oxidation, and resting metabolic rate in adult celiac disease patients after a 1-year gluten-free diet treatment. *Am. J. Clin. Nutr.* **2000**, *72*, 76–81.
46. Björkman, A.C.; Mobacken, H.; Kastrup, W.; Andersson, H. Changes in food consumption and its nutritional quality when on a gluten-free diet for dermatitis herpetiformis. *Hum. Nutr. Appl. Nutr.* **1985**, *39*, 124–129.
47. Bardella, M.T.; Fredella, C.; Prampolini, L.; Molteni, N.; Giunta, A.M.; Bianchi, P.A. Body composition and dietary intakes in adult celiac disease patients consuming a strict gluten-free diet. *Am. J. Clin. Nutr.* **2000**, *72*, 937–939.
48. Dell'Olio, D.; Palma, L.; Malorgio, E.; Ansaldi Balocco, N. What do celiac children eat? Dietary analysis of a group of children with celiac disease on a diet. *Minerva Gastroenterol. Dietol.* **1995**, *41*, 269–273.
49. American Diabetes Association. Nutrition recommendations and interventions for diabetes. A position statement of the American Diabetes Association. *Diabetes Care* **2008**, *31*, S61–S74.
50. Jenkins, D.J.A.; Thorne, M.J.; Wolever, T.M.S.; Jenkins, A.L.; Venketschwer, R.; Thompson, L.U. The effect of starch-protein interaction in wheat on the glycemic response and rate of *in vitro* digestion. *Am. J. Clin. Nutr.* **1987**, *45*, 946–951.
51. Foster-Powell, K.; Holt, S.H.A.; Brand-Miller, J.C. International table of glycemic index and glycemic load values. *Am. J. Clin. Nutr.* **2002**, *76*, 5–56.
52. Packer, S.C.; Dornhorst, A.; Frost, G.S. The glycaemic index of a range of gluten-free foods. *Diabetes* **2000**, *17*, 657–660.

53. Monro, J.A. Glycaemic glucose equivalent: Combining carbohydrate content, quantity and glycaemic index of foods for precision in glycaemia management. *Asia Pac. J. Clin. Nutr.* **2002**, *11*, 217–225.
54. Salmerón, J.; Ascherio, A.; Rimm, E.B.; Colditz, G.A.; Spiegelman, D.; Jenkins, D.J.; Stampfer, M.J.; Wing, A.L.; Willett, W.C. Dietary fiber, glycemic load, and risk of NIDDM in men. *Diabetes Care* **1997**, *20*, 545–550.
55. Salmerón, J.; Manson, J.E.; Stampfer, M.J.; Colditz, G.A.; Wing, A.L.; Willett, W.C. Dietary fiber, glycemic load, and risk of non-insulin-dependent diabetes mellitus in women. *JAMA* **1997**, *277*, 472–477.
56. Livesey, G. Low-glycaemic diets and health: implications for obesity Satellite Symposium on "The role of low-glycaemic diets in obesity and health". *Proc. Nutr. Soc.* **2005**, *64*, 105–113.
57. Das, S.K.; Gilhooly, C.H.; Golden, J.K.; Pittas, A.G.; Fuss, P.J.; Dallal, G.E.; McCrory, M.A.; Saltzman, E.; Roberts, S.B. Long term effects of energy-restricted diets differing in glycemic load on metabolic adaptation and body composition. *Open Nutr. J.* **2007**, *85*, 1023–1030.
58. Barba, G.; Sieri, S.; Russo, M.D.; Donatiello, E.; Formisano, A.; Lauria, F.; Sparano, S.; Nappo, A.; Russo, P.; Brighenti, F.; *et al.* Glycaemic index and body fat distribution in children: The results of the ARCA project. *Nutr. Metab. Cardiovasc. Dis.* **2012**, *22*, 28–34.
59. Nielsen, B.M.; Bjørnsbo, K.S.; Tetens, I.; Heitmann, B.L. Dietary glycaemic index and glycaemic load in Danish children in relation to body fatness. *Br. J. Nutr.* **2005**, *94*, 992–997.
60. Buyken, A.E.; Trauner, K.; Günther, A.L.; Kroke, A.; Remer, T. Breakfast glycemic index affects subsequent daily energy intake in free-living healthy children. *Am. J. Clin. Nutr.* **2007**, *86*, 980–987.
61. Buyken, A.E.; Cheng, G.; Günther, A.L.; Liese, A.D.; Remer, T.; Karaolis-Danckert, N. Relation of dietary glycemic index, glycemic load, added sugar intake, or fiber intake to the development of body composition between ages 2 and 7 year. *Am. J. Clin. Nutr.* **2008**, *88*, 755–762.
62. Boye, K.R.; Dimitriou, T.; Manz, F.; Schoenau, E.; Neu, C.; Wudy, S.; Remer, T. Anthropometric assessment of muscularity during growth: Estimating fat-free mass with 2 skinfold-thickness measurements is superior to measuring mid-upper arm muscle area in healthy prepubertal children. *Am. J. Clin. Nutr.* **2002**, *76*, 628–632.
63. Thomas, D.E.; Elliott, E.J.; Baur, L. Low glycaemic index or low glycaemic load diets for overweight and obesity. *Cochrane Database Syst. Rev.* **2007**, *18*, CD005105.
64. Schwingshackl, L.; Hoffmann, G. Long-term effects of low glycemic index/load *vs.* high glycemic index/load diets on parameters of obesity and obesity-associated risks: A systematic review and meta-analysis. *Nutr. Metab. Cardiovasc. Dis.* **2013**, *23*, 699–706.
65. Acerini, C.L.; Ahmed, M.L.; Ross, K.M.; Sullivan, P.B.; Bird, G.; Dunger, D.B. Coeliac disease in children and adolescents with IDDM: Clinical characteristics and response to gluten-free diet. *Diabet. Med.* **1998**, *15*, 38–44.
66. Nóvoa Medina, Y.; López-Capapé, M.; Lara Orejas, E.; Alonso Blanco, M.; Camarero Salces, C.; Barrio Castellanos, R. Impact of diagnosis of celiac disease on metabolic control of type 1 diabetes. *Ann. Pediatr.* **2008**, *68*, 13–17.

67. Saadah, O.I.; Zacharin, M.; O'Callaghan, A.; Oliver, M.R.; Catto-Smith, A.G. Effect of gluten-free diet and adherence on growth and diabetic control in diabetics with coeliac disease. *Arch. Dis. Child* **2004**, *89*, 871–876.
68. Marchese, A.; Lovati, E.; Biagi, F.; Corazza, G.R. Coeliac disease and type 1 diabetes mellitus: Epidemiology, clinical implications and effects of gluten-free diet. *Endocrine* **2013**, *43*, 1–2.
69. Savilahti, E.; Simell, O.; Koskimies, S.; Rilva, A.; Akerblom, H.K. Celiac disease in insulin-dependent diabetes mellitus. *J. Pediatr.* **1986**, *108*, 690–693.
70. Abid, N.; McGlone, O.; Cardwell, C.; McCallion, W.; Carson, D. Clinical and metabolic effects of gluten free diet in children with type 1 diabetes and coeliac disease. *Pediatr. Diabetes* **2011**, *12*, 322–325.
71. Stubbs, C.O.; Lee, A.J. The obesity epidemic: both energy intake and physical activity contribute. *Med. J. Aust.* **2004**, *181*, 489–491.
72. Rouhani, M.H.; Salehi-Abargouei, A.; Azadbakht, L. Effect of glycemic index and glycemic load on energy intake in children. *Nutrition* **2013**, *29*, 1100–1105.
73. Anderson, G.H.; Woodend, D. Effect of glycemic carbohydrates on short-term satiety and food intake. *Nutr. Rev.* **2003**, *61*, S17–S26.
74. Caudwell, P.; Finlayson, G.; Gibbons, C.; Hopkins, M.; King, N.; Näslund, E.; Blundell, J.E. Resting metabolic rate is associated with hunger, self-determined meal size, and daily energy intake and may represent a marker for appetite. *Am. J. Clin. Nutr.* **2013**, *97*, 7–14.
75. Papastamataki, M.; Papassotiriou, I.; Bartzeliotou, A.; Vazeou, A.; Roma, E.; Chrousos, G.P.; Kanaka-Gantenbein, C. Incretins, amylin and other gut-brain axis hormones in children with coeliac disease. *Eur. J. Clin. Investig.* **2013**, *44*, 74–82.

3

Problems and Challenges to Adaptation of Gluten Free Diet by Indian Patients with Celiac Disease

Preeti Rajpoot and Govind K. Makharia *

Departments of Gastroenterology and Human Nutrition, All India Institute of Medical Sciences, New Delhi 110029, India; E-Mail: prajpoot15@gmail.com

* Author to whom correspondence should be addressed;
E-Mail: govindmakharia@gmail.com or govindmakharia@aiims.ac.in;

Abstract: Celiac disease is emerging in India and has become a public health problem. Almost 6–8 million Indians are estimated to have celiac disease. While there is a large pool of patients with celiac disease in India, until now, only a fraction of them have been diagnosed. With increasing awareness about celiac disease amongst health care providers and the general population, a massive increase in the number of patients with celiac disease is expected now and in the subsequent decade in India. While the number of patients with celiac disease is increasing, the country's preparedness towards the emerging epidemic of this disease is minimal. There are a number of issues, which requires urgent attention. Some of the key issues include increased awareness amongst health care professionals and the general public about the disease and its management, team-based management of patients with celiac disease, proper counseling and supervision of patients, training of dietitians in the management of patients with celiac disease, industrial production of reliable and affordable gluten-free food, and food labeling for gluten contents.

Keywords: nutrition; India; wheat; barriers; compliance, counseling

---

1. Introduction

Celiac disease (CeD) is an immune-mediated enteropathy caused by exposure to gluten in genetically susceptible individuals [1,2]. Once thought to be a rare disease and believed to occur only in Western Europe, CeD is now a global disease and affects almost 0.6%–1% of the world's population [3,4]. After Europe, America (both North and South), and the Middle East, it is now emerging in the East, including many Asian countries [5–13]. Also, once thought to be a disease of children and therefore to be managed mainly by pediatricians; CeD is now known to affect all the age groups including the elderly [14]. While CeD is emerging, the level of the awareness it too low amongst health care professionals, even amongst those most closely involved such as general physicians, family physicians, internists, gastroenterologist and pathologists [7,9].

2. Emergence of CeD in India

An increase in number of patients with CeD has been observed from many centers in India including ours [15,16]. Furthermore, two community based prevalence studies have been reported, both from the Northern part of India. In the first report from Ludhiana (Punjab), a questionnaire based survey of 4347 school children (3–17 years), Sood *et al.* [17] reported prevalence of CeD to be 1 in 310. In another community-based study including 10,488 subjects, both children and adults, we reported the prevalence of CeD in the Northern part of India to be 1.04% (1 in 96) and the prevalence of seropositivity (anti-tTG ab) to be 1.44% (1 in 69) [18]. Based on these two general population based studies, 5–8 millions of Indians are expected to have CeD. Of such a large pool of patients, only a fraction has been diagnosed to have CeD. The results of these studies suggest that CeD is a much greater problem in India than has been previously thought [18].

At present, only those with the most typical manifestations of CeD come to clinical attention and are ultimately diagnosed to have CeD. Now screening programs within populations indicate that celiac disease is under-diagnosed and what we detect clinically represents only the tip of the iceberg. With an appreciation of the existence of an iceberg of CeD in any society, and with increased awareness of CeD, patients with even milder symptoms are likely to be diagnosed in the coming years [19,20]. Currently, most celiac specific serology ELISA kits in India are imported from Europe. Their diagnostic cut-off values of antibody concentrations are based on Caucasian population data. With the difference and diversity in gluten ingestion, the cut-off values for a positive test in India may not be similar to those reported in the Caucasians.

3. Evolution of Dietary Management of CeD

Dietary management was a mainstay of treatment of CeD even in the early part of the 20th century [21]. During 1930s, clinical improvement was observed with several differing diets including an oyster diet suggested by Gee and the banana diet popularized by Haas [22]. Stools of such patients were quite greasy and worsening of their diarrhea after a carbohydrate diet led to another dietary approaches such as reduction or almost complete elimination of dietary fat or carbohydrates. A remarkable observation by a Dutch pediatrician, Willem Dicke [23], gave the birth to an idea from listening to one of his child patients' mothers. The mother of the patient told Willem Dicke that her child used to become better if he did not eat porridge. From a clinical observation of one child and through years of clinical questioning and dietary therapy, he concluded that wheat was the toxic agent leading to CeD [23,24]. Toward the end of World War II, the so-called "winter of starvation" when even bread was not available in Holland; children with CeD paradoxically improved even though they were consuming a starvation diet (almost devoid of wheat products). When bread was airdropped in Holland, deterioration was noticed in these children [23]. Such an observation further strengthened the idea that some of the ingredients of wheat were the toxic agents for CeD.

4. What Is Gluten?

The protein content of wheat varies between 8% and 17%, depending on the genetic make-up and external factors associated with the crop. When wheat flour is washed with water, the insoluble protein fraction forms a viscoelastic protein mass, called gluten. Gluten, which comprises roughly 78% to 85% of the total wheat protein, is a very large complex mainly composed of polymeric (multiple polypeptide chains linked by disulphide bonds and monomeric (single-chain polypeptides) proteins. Gluten plays a key role in determining the unique-baking quality of wheat by conferring water absorption capacity, cohesively, viscosity and elasticity on dough [25–27].

Gluten is classified into two main fractions according to their solubility in aqueous alcohols: the fraction which is soluble in aqueous alcohol is gliadin and those insoluble are called glutenins. Both the fractions consist of numerous, closely related polypeptides that are rich in glutamine and proline amino acids. Gliadins are mainly monomeric proteins with molecular weights around 28,000–55,000 and they are further subclassified as α/β-, γ- and ω-type according to differences in their primary structures. Glutenins consist of glutenin subunits of high (M_W 67,000–88,000) or low molecular weight (M_W 32,000–35,000) that are connected by intermolecular disulphide bonds. Non-covalent bonds such as hydrogen bonds, ionic bonds and hydrophobic bonds bind gliadins and glutenins, which provide structure and physical properties of the gluten. Glutenins confer elasticity, while gliadins mainly confer viscosity and extensibility to the gluten complex [25–27].

Gliadins and glutenins contain domains with numerous repetitive sequences rich in these amino acids [28]. The gliadins have high proline and glutamine content and humans inherently lack endopeptidases to cleave bonds between proline and glutamines. The incomplete digestion of gliadin by digestive tract enzymes leads to the generation of many polypeptides, which are immunogenic to patients genetically susceptible to CeD.

5. What Is a Gluten Free Diet (GFD)?

The absence of gluten in natural and processed foods represents a key aspect of the GFD (gluten free diet). The current Codex Standard for gluten free foods was adopted by the Codex Alimentarius Commission of the World Health Organization (Geneva, Switzerland) and by the Food and Agricultural Organization (Rome, Italy) in 1976 and amended in 1983. In 2000, the Codex Alimentarius Commission of the World Health Organization and the Food and Agriculture Organization described gluten free foods with a gluten level not exceeding 20 ppm and consisting of, or made only from ingredients which do not contain any prolamines from wheat or any Triticum species, such as spelt, kamut or durum wheat, rye, barley, oats, or their crossbred varieties [29,30].

Gluten intake varies from population to population and depends upon dietary practices. In a double blind, placebo controlled prospective study; Catassi *et al.* [31] demonstrated that an intake of as little as 50 mg of gluten per day for 3 months was sufficient to cause a significant decrease in the intestinal mucosal mucosal villous height/crypt depth ratio. Furthermore, a daily intake of gluten of lower than

10 mg is unlikely to produce significant histological abnormalities [32]. The GFD with the threshold at less than 20 ppm of gluten ensures an intake of less than 50 mg/day and provides a sufficient safety margin [33].

6. Indian Dietary Habits and Gluten in the Indian Diet

India is a country of diversity in terms of culture, language, living standards and dietary practices. Until a few decades ago, Indians used to prefer natural foods to refined foods. In general, Indian families cook most of their meals at home on a daily basis and eat freshly cooked warm food. Most Indians do not prefer frozen or packaged food and tend to prepare their food from fresh ingredients. Indians are also less likely to visit restaurants. The family and social bond is very strong and they like to have food together with family members. Most of the meals contain a combination of cereals, pulses, spices and vegetables. Those who can afford, also uses dairy products, fruits and non-vegetarian food.

The "Green Revolution" in 1970s and onwards, promoted record grain promoted and ensured self-sufficiency in cereal grains [34,35]. During the past two decades, a shift from traditional to modern technologies, globalization, industrialization, constant travels across the world, and a fast growing economy led to the use of processed and fast foods at least in the urbanized part of India. While on one hand, there is poverty and hunger causing under-nutrition and its related disorders; a substantial increase in the intake of fast food is on the other hand leading to over-nutrition related disorders such as obesity and diabetes [36–38]. Therefore, the effects of malabsorption secondary to CeD could be severe in those who already have poor nutritional status due tounderlying poverty and ignorance.

Gluten intake varies from population to population and depends upon dietary practices. Wheat is the staple cereal in the northern part of India and flat bread made from wheat flour is the one of the most important constituents of almost every meal. In the southern and northeastern part of India, rice is a staple cereal. A typical North Indian diet, where flat bread is the usual meal, contains about 25–30 g of gluten per day; whereas average gluten intake in the West varies from 10 to 20 g/day [39].

7. Barriers in Maintaining a Strict GFD in India

There are many barriers to maintenance of a GFD; some of them are universal and some of them are unique to Indian patients with CeD. Patients with CeD are challenged with barriers in maintenance of a strict GFD because of factors such as inadequate information and education about the disease, food contamination, and inadequate/no food labeling on the packaged food items [40,41].

Because of viscoelastic properties, as discussed earlier, gluten is used extensively in the food industry. In fact, efforts have been made to increase the gluten content of the wheat and globally the gluten industry is very big. It may be surprising to know that gluten is present in daily use items such as lipsticks, postage stamps, beer, ice-creams, sweets, confectionary foods spreads and seasonings, soups and sauces, malted beverages and many more [42]. Due to the lack of gluten labeling on food items in India, it is difficult for anyone to know if a particular food product is gluten free or not [43,44].

Contamination of food with gluten is another concern. The contamination of food with gluten can occur: during milling if the same mill is used without proper cleaning for grinding gluten-containing and gluten-free grains; at the grocery store, if the same spatula is used to pick gluten containing and gluten free grains/flours; at factories producing commercial food products if same production line and equipment are used for both gluten-containing and GF (gluten free) food products; during preparation of commercial food products where gluten is added as fillers, stabilizing agents or processing aids such as thickener in soups, canned vegetables and other processed foods; at home, if the same utensils are used for storing, cooking and handling (rolling pin, surface griddle, dusters and oil for frying) gluten-containing and GF cereal flours and products; and while eating out, if addition of thickeners fillers/binders had been used which may unintentionally contain gluten.

Successful management of CeD requires a team approach, including patient, family, physicians, and dietitian. After a diagnosis is made, all the patients should be referred to a dietician for nutritional assessment, diet education, meal planning, and assistance with the social and emotional adaptation to the GF lifestyle. A delay in referral, or no referral at all, increases the likelihood of the patient obtaining inaccurate information from the Internet, health food stores, alternative health practitioners, family, friends, and other sources, which may be outdated, inaccurate, and/or conflicting. This results in confusion, frustration, and insufficient knowledge regarding CeD and the GFD. The poorly informed patients might unnecessarily restrict certain foods, thus limiting the variety and nutritional quality of their diet [45].

Adherence to GFD is the most critical factor for remission of CeD. Adherence to GFD is complex and is influenced by knowledge, country or region of residence, availability of GF food, determination, and social support [46–49]. Furthermore, attitude and behaviors of significant others such as family, teachers and friends also affect the decision to comply with GFD. Compliance to GFD is best maintained when residing at home; and eating out with friends or at school are the most difficult places to comply with GFD [40]. Lack of background awareness about the CeD and its strict dietary restriction in the community creates a problem for the patient and the family of patients with CeD [1,40]. Furthermore, it has been observed that girls face compliance issues after marriage. The compliance to GFD is better if CeD is diagnosed in their early part of life compared to those in whom the diagnosis is made later in life. Patients having minimal symptoms or those diagnosed on screening comply less well than those who have overt symptoms [50,51]. As the patient grows from childhood to adulthood and become asymptomatic, the compliance to GFD gets worse. Non-appearance of acute symptoms after inadvertent or deliberate ingestion of gluten might make the patient more confident and induce them to try gluten at other occasions also. Many patients in remission might try gluten to see what happens to them with gluten intake [46–50].

Non-Availability of GF (Gluten Free) Food Products

Because of the perception that CeD is uncommon in India and a low absolute number of patients with CeD in India, the need for making a GFD available has not been perceived. The diagnosis of CeD presently is limited to only at the secondary and tertiary care centers and often more so in the northern part of India. There is some small-scale production of GFD (mainly flour and biscuits) food in certain sectors in the northern part of India, which relies upon mixing of non-wheat and non-barley cereals. There is a possibility of contamination at various levels such as during harvesting, storage and packaging of grain bags by the farmers. In fact all of these should be taken into consideration before the grains are used for making gluten free flour. Whichever gluten free flour/products are available do not undergo rigorous quality check for their gluten contents. The production of GFD in India till now has been small-scale industry based only, and the varieties and choices of GFD are also extremely limited.

Availability of GF foods is a factor, which determines compliance to GFD. Furthermore, difficulty in obtaining GF food also interrupts compliance to GFD. Even in countries where CeD is common, 10%–15% patients report difficulty in getting a continuous supply of GF food [52]. Non-availability of GFD outside their home environment restricts their travel, occupation and profession.

GF food items are considerably more expensive than regular gluten-containing food [53]. A nutritionally-balanced GF market basket, based on foods typically consumed by the Scottish population, costs more than a standard market basket [54]. Therefore, patients with CeD have additional financial requirement for purchasing of GFD for their living.

8. Measures to Break the Barriers to GFD

8.1. Patient Education and Awareness

The management of CeD is unique and different from the treatment of other medical or surgical diseases. At present, life-long and complete avoidance of gluten from the diet is the most effective treatment of CeD. While prescribing GFD is easy; the key to the success is the dietary counseling by a dietician and maintenance of compliance by the patient [44,46–48]. Like any other chronic disease management, education of the patients and their families about the disease and dietary restrictions is of immense importance. It is generally not possible to explain everything about the dietary restrictions in one visit from the nutrition specialist. The understanding and maintenance of GFD requires consistent supervision and guidance, which is best provided to the patients and families on multiple visits. At every visit to the hospital/clinic, the level of compliance to gluten avoidance should be checked and appropriate guidance should be provided.

8.2. Training of Nutritionist in CeD Management and Counseling of Patients

The dietary councilor should have sufficient knowledge about the GF food and food products. It is not only about prescribing GFD but it is essential to provide for the patient a specific well-balanced diet. The dietitian is the most qualified health care professional to provide nutrition therapy. Dietitians have extensive academic and practical experience including in-depth knowledge of nutrition, nutritional needs, nutrition composition and food preparation information and educational factors that affect food and nutrition behavior of people. They are also skilled to translate scientific information into laymen's terms and assist individuals in gaining knowledge, self-understanding, improved decision making, and behavioral changes. Although other health care professionals can disseminate nutrition advice, they do not have the training in nutrition sciences and food composition to be able to translate complex medical nutrition concepts and issues into attainable dietary changes [42,44,46–48].

8.3. Celiac Disease Support Groups

Celiac disease support groups provides a platform for patients to discuss their problems amongst themselves and learn from each other, provides information about GF products and their availability, but also can act as an advocacy for gluten labeling and other issues to the Government and regulatory bodies [55–57]. Furthermore, it has been observed that the adherence to a GFD increases when individuals are members of a patient support group [55–59].

8.4. Development of Reliable GFD at a Large Scale

While the number of patients with CeD is small at present in India, the absolute number of patients is rising day after day. As awareness about the disease increase, there is a likelihood of an exponential increase in the number of patients with CeD and hence the demand of GFD is likely to increase in the near future. Therefore, there is need for large-scale industrial level production of reliable and affordable GF food, including choices of food products ranging from snacks, flour, sweets, ice-creams and ready-to-eat packets.

All GF food products should be tested for their quality before releasing for patient's use. In fact, there should be certified gluten check laboratories where food items may be checked for their gluten contents. This is an important step to ensure quality of food for its gluten content until the gluten labeling legislation is enforced.

These foods, which are available at present in India, are not labeled for their gluten content. As mentioned above, gluten is used extensively in the food industry. Furthermore, even a small amount of gluten can maintain the disease activity [31–33]. It is therefore essential that food products, which are available, should be labeled for gluten content.

9. Combining Diabetes and Gluten Free Dietary Management Guidelines

Eight to fifteen percent of patients with CeD have type I diabetes [58,59]. Planning of a dietary management for such patients is a challenge for endocrinologists and dietitians. Disclosure of dietary restrictions with a diagnosis of CeD in a patient with type I diabetes may be received as a shock to the patient and the family. The objectives of diet planning for such patients are to provide a balanced nutritive diet with restrictions posed by diabetes and CeD. A healthy eating plan for diabetes should always be individualized based on the patient's need and metabolic outcome goals (HbA1C, weight/height, lipid profile, blood pressure, *etc.*) [60]. It is therefore essential that rather than making two dietary plans for control of CeD and diabetes, the dietitian should make one unified dietary plan for both the co-existing conditions.

10. Conclusions

CeD is a public health problem and 6–8 million Indians are estimated to have CeD. While there is a large pool of patients with CeD in India, only a fraction of them are currently diagnosed. With increasing awareness about CeD amongst health care providers and the general population, a massive increase in the number of patients with CeD is expected in the present and subsequent decade in India. While the number of patients with CeD is increasing, the country's preparedness towards this disease management is extremely minimal. There are a number of issues, which require urgent attention. Some of the key issues include team-based management of patients with CeD, proper counseling and supervision of patients, training of dietitians in the management of patients with CeD, industrial production of reliable and affordable GF food, food labeling for gluten contents and increase in awareness amongst health care professionals and the general public about the disease and its management.

References

1. Fasano, A.; Catassi, C. Clinical practice. Celiac disease. *N. Engl. J. Med.* **2012**, *367*, 2419–2426.
2. Schuppan, D.; Junker, Y.; Barisani, D. Celiac disease: From pathogenesis to novel therapies. *Gastroenterology* **2009**, *137*, 1912–1933.
3. Rewers, M. Epidemiology of celiac disease: What are the prevalence, incidence, and progression of celiac disease? *Gastroenterology* **2005**, *128*, S47–S51.
4. Fasano, A.; Berti, I.; Gerarduzzi, T.; Not, T.; Colletti, R.B.; Drago, S.; Elitsur, Y.; Green, P.H.; Guandalini, S.; Hill, I.D.; *et al.* Prevalence of celiac disease in at-risk and not-at-risk groups in the United States: A large multicenter study. *Arch. Intern. Med.* **2003**, *163*, 286–292.
5. Cataldo, F.; Montalto, G. Celiac disease in the developing countries: A new and challenging public health problem. *World J. Gastroenterol.* **2007**, *13*, 2153–2159.
6. Khoshoo, V.; Bhan, M.K.; Jain, R.; Phillips, A.D.; Walker-Smith, J.A.; Unsworth, D.J.; Stintzing, G. Coeliac disease as cause of protracted diarrhoea in Indian children. *Lancet* **1988**, *1*, 126–127.
7. Sood, A.; Midha, V.; Sood, N.; Malhotra, V. Adult celiac disease in northern India. *Indian J. Gastroenterol.* **2003**, *22*, 124–126.
8. Makharia, G.K.; Baba, C.S.; Khadgawat, R.; Lal, S.; Tevatia, M.S.; Madan, K.; Dattagupta, S. Celiac disease: Variations of presentations in adults. *Indian J. Gastroenterol.* **2007**, *26*, 162–166.
9. Bhattacharya, M.; Kapoor, S.; Dubey, A.P. Celiac disease presentation in a tertiary referral centre in India: Current scenario. *Indian J. Gastroenterol.* **2013**, *32*, 98–102.
10. Wu, J.; Xia, B.; von Blomberg, B.M.; Zhao, C.; Yang, X.W.; Crusius, J.B.; Peña, A.S. Coeliac disease: Emerging in China? *Gut* **2010**, *59*, 418–419.
11. Wang, X.Q.; Liu, W.; Xu, C.D.; Mei, H.; Gao, Y.; Peng, H.M.; Yuan, L.; Xu, J.J. Celiac disease in children with diarrhea in 4 cities in China. *J. Pediatr. Gastroenterol. Nutr.* **2011**, *53*, 368–370.
12. Watanabe, C.; Komoto, S.; Hokari, R.; Kurihara, C.; Okada, Y.; Hozumi, H.; Higashiyama, M.; Sakuraba, A.; Tomita, K.; Tsuzuki, Y.; *et al.* Prevalence of serum celiac antibody in patients with IBD in Japan. *J. Gastroenterol.* **2013**, doi:10.1007/s00535-013-0838-6.
13. Arshad, H.; Ahmad, Z. Histologic findings in biopsies/resection specimens from the small intestine with special emphasis on celiac disease: Experience from a developing country in South Asia. *Ann. Diagn. Pathol.* **2012**, *16*, 436–440.
14. Singh, P.; Shergill, S.; Makharia, G.K. Celiac disease in older adults. *J. Gastrointest. Liver Dis.* **2013**, *22*, 359–360.

15. Sood, A.; Midha, V.; Sood, N.; Kaushal, V.; Puri, H. Increasing incidence of celiac disease in India. *Am. J. Gastroenterol.* **2001**, *96*, 2804–2805.
16. Sharma, M.; Singh, P.; Agnihotri, A.; Das, P.; Mishra, A.; Verma, A.K.; Ahuja, A.; Sreenivas, V.; Khadgawat, R.; Gupta, S.D.; *et al.* Celiac disease: A disease with varied manifestations in adults and adolescents. *J. Dig. Dis.* **2013**, *14*, 518–525.
17. Sood, A.; Midha, V.; Sood, N.; Avasthi, G.; Sehgal, A. Prevalence of celiac disease among school children in Punjab, North India. *J. Gastroenterol. Hepatol.* **2006**, *21*, 1622–1625.
18. Makharia, G.K.; Verma, A.K.; Amarchand, R.; Bhatnagar, S.; Das, P.; Goswami, A.; Bhatia, V.; Ahuja, V.; Datta Gupta, S.; Anand, K. Prevalence of celiac disease in the northern part of India: A community based study. *J. Gastroenterol. Hepatol.* **2011**, *26*, 894–900.
19. Leffler, D.; Vanga, R.; Mukherjee, R. Mild enteropathy celiac disease: A wolf in sheep's clothing? *Clin. Gastroenterol. Hepatol.* **2013**, *11*, 259–261.
20. Zanini, B.; Caselani, F.; Magni, A.; Turini, D.; Ferraresi, A.; Lanzarotto, F.; Villanacci, V.; Carabellese, N.; Ricci, C.; Lanzini, A. Celiac disease with mild enteropathy is not mild disease. *Clin. Gastroenterol. Hepatol.* **2013**, *11*, 253–258.
21. Gee, S.J. On the celiac affection. *St. Bartholomew's Hosp. Rep.* **1888**, *24*, 17–20.
22. Haas, S.V. The value of the banana in the treatment of coeliac disease. *Am. J. Dis. Child.* **1924**, *24*, 421–423.
23. Yan, D.; Holt, P.R. Willem Dicke. Brilliant clinical observer and translational investigator. Discoverer of the toxic cause of celiac disease. *Clin. Transl. Sci.* **2009**, *2*, 446–448.
24. Dicke, W.K.; Weijers, H.A.; van de Kamer, J.H. Coeliac disease. II. The presence in wheat of a factor having a deleterious effect in cases of coeliac disease. *Acta Paediatr.* **1953**, *42*, 34–42.
25. Anjum, F.M.; Khan, M.R.; Din, A.; Saeed, M.; Pasha, I.; Arshad, M.U. Wheat gluten: High molecular weight glutenin subunits—Structure, genetics, and relation to dough elasticity. *J. Food Sci.* **2007**, *72*, R56–R63.
26. Wieser, H. Chemistry of gluten proteins. *Food Microbiol.* **2007**, *24*, 115–119.
27. Shewry, P.R.; Halford, N.G.; Belton, P.S.; Tatham, A.S. The structure and properties of gluten: An elastic protein from wheat grain. *Philos. Trans. R. Soc. Lond. B* **2002**, *357*, 133–142.
28. Kagnoff, M.F. Celiac disease: Pathogenesis of a model immunogenetic disease. *J. Clin. Investig.* **2007**, *11*, 41–49.
29. Hischenhuber, C.; Crevel, R.; Jarry, B.; Mäki, M.; Moneret-Vautrin, D.A.; Romano, A.; Troncone, R.; Ward, R. Review article: Safe amounts of gluten for patients with wheat allergy or coeliac disease. *Aliment. Pharmacol. Ther.* **2006**, *23*, 559–575.
30. Kupper, C. Dietary guidelines and implementation for celiac disease. *Gastroenterology* **2005**, *128*, S121–S127.
31. Catassi, C.; Fabiani, E.; Iacono, G.; D'Agate, C.; Francavilla, R.; Biagi, F.; Volta, U.; Accomando, S.; Picarelli, A.; de Vitis, I.; *et al.* A prospective, double-blind, placebo-controlled trial to establish a safe gluten threshold for patients with celiac disease. *Am. J. Clin. Nutr.* **2007**, *85*, 160–166.

32. Lanzini, A.; Lanzarotto, F.; Villanacci, V.; Mora, A.; Bertolazzi, S.; Turini, D.; Carella, G.; Malagoli, A.; Ferrante, G.; Cesana, B.M.; *et al.* Complete recovery of intestinal mucosa occurs very rarely in adult coeliac patients despite adherence to gluten-free diet. *Aliment. Pharmacol. Ther.* **2009**, *29*, 1299–1308.
33. Akobeng, A.K.; Thomas, A.G. Systematic review: Tolerable amount of gluten for people with coeliac disease. *Aliment. Pharmacol. Ther.* **2008**, *27*, 1044–1052.
34. Singh, G.P. Dr B.C. Dasgupta Memorial Oration. Green revolution and after: The public health perspective. *Indian J. Public Health* **2006**, *50*, 138–146.
35. Science in India. Green revolution: Caring for a continent. *Nature* **1984**, *308*, 598–599.
36. Gera, T.; Khetarpaul, N. Food consumption pattern and nutrient intake of Indian obese males. *Nutr. Health* **2000**, *14*, 205–216.
37. Shobana, R.; Snehalatha, C.; Latha, E.; Vijay, V.; Ramachandran, A. Dietary profile of urban south Indians and its relations with glycaemic status. *Diabetes Res. Clin. Pract.* **1998**, *42*, 181–186.
38. Mohan, V. Why are Indians more prone to diabetes? *J. Assoc. Physicians India* **2004**, *52*, 468–474.
39. Price, S. Understanding the importance to health of a balanced diet. *Nurs. Times* **2005**, *101*, 30–31.
40. Hall, N.J.; Rubin, G.; Charnock, A. Systematic review: Adherence to a gluten-free diet in adult patients with coeliac disease. *Aliment. Pharmacol. Ther.* **2009**, *30*, 315–330.
41. Haines, M.L.; Anderson, R.P.; Gibson, P.R. Systematic review: The evidence base for long-term management of coeliac disease. *Aliment. Pharmacol. Ther.* **2008**, *28*, 1042–1066.
42. García-Manzanares, A.; Lucendo, A.J. Nutritional and dietary aspects of celiac disease. *Nutr. Clin. Pract.* **2011**, *26*, 163–173.
43. Saturni, L.; Ferretti, G.; Bacchetti, T. The gluten-free diet: Safety and nutritional quality. *Nutrients* **2010**, *2*, 16–34.
44. See, J.; Murray, J.A. Gluten-free diet: The medical and nutrition management of celiac disease. *Nutr. Clin. Pract.* **2006**, *21*, 1–15.
45. Case, S. The gluten-free diet: How to provide effective education and resources. *Gastroenterology* **2005**, *128*, S128–S134.
46. Olsson, C.; Hörnell, A.; Ivarsson, A.; Sydner, Y.M. The everyday life of adolescent coeliacs: Issues of importance for compliance with the gluten-free diet. *J. Hum. Nutr. Diet.* **2008**, *21*, 359–367.
47. Nasr, I.; Leffler, D.A.; Ciclitira, P.J. Management of celiac disease. *Gastrointest. Endosc. Clin. N. Am.* **2012**, *22*, 695–704.
48. Niewinski, M.M. Advances in celiac disease and gluten-free diet. *J. Am. Diet. Assoc.* **2008**, *108*, 661–672.
49. Addolorato, G.; de Lorenzi, G.; Abenavoli, L.; Leggio, L.; Capristo, E.; Gasbarrini, G. Psychological support counselling improves gluten-free diet compliance in coeliac patients with affective disorders. *Aliment. Pharmacol. Ther.* **2004**, *20*, 777–782.
50. Fabiani, E.; Taccari, L.M.; Rätsch, I.M.; di Giuseppe, S.; Coppa, G.V.; Catassi, C. Compliance with gluten-free diet in adolescents with screening-detected celiac disease: A 5-year follow-up study. *J. Pediatr.* **2000**, *136*, 841–843.
51. Murray, J.; Watson, T.; Clearman, B.; Mitros, F. Effect of a gluten-free diet on gastrointestinal symptoms in celiac disease. *Am. J. Clin. Nutr.* **2004**, *79*, 669–673.

52. Zarkadas, M.; Cranney, A.; Case, S.; Molloy, M.; Switzer, C.; Graham, I.D.; Butzner, J.D.; Rashid, M.; Warren, R.E.; Burrows, V. The impact of a gluten-free diet on adults with coeliac disease: Results of a national survey. *J. Hum. Nutr. Diet.* **2006**, *19*, 41–49.
53. Lee, A.R.; Ng, D.L.; Zivin, J.; Green, P.H. Economic burden of a gluten-free diet. *J. Hum. Nutr. Diet.* **2007**, *20*, 423–430.
54. Stevens, L.; Rashid, M. Gluten-free and regular foods: A cost comparison. *Can. J. Diet. Pract. Res.* **2008**, *69*, 147–150.
55. Silvester, J.A.; Rashid, M. Long-term management of patients with celiac disease: Current practices of gastroenterologists in Canada. *Can. J. Gastroenterol.* **2010**, *24*, 499–509.
56. Leffler, D.A.; Edwards-George, J.; Dennis, M.; Schuppan, D.; Cook, F.; Franko, D.L.; Blom-Hoffman, J.; Kelly, C.P. Factors that influence adherence to a gluten-free diet in adults with celiac disease. *Dig. Dis. Sci.* **2008**, *53*, 1573–1581.
57. NIH Consensus Development Conference on Celiac Disease. NIH Consens State Sci Statements. Available online: http://consensus.nih.gov/2004/2004celiacdisease118html.htm (accessed on 21 November 2013).
58. Camarca, M.E.; Mozzillo, E.; Nugnes, R.; Zito, E.; Falco, M.; Fattorusso, V.; Mobilia, S.; Buono, P.; Valerio, G.; Troncone, R.; *et al.* Celiac disease in type 1 diabetes mellitus. *Ital. J. Pediatr.* **2012**, *38*, 10.
59. Franzese, A.; Lombardi, F.; Valerio, G.; Spagnuolo, M.I. Update on coeliac disease and type 1 diabetes mellitus in childhood. *J. Pediatr. Endocrinol. Metab.* **2007**, *20*, 1257–1264.
60. Scaramuzza, A.E.; Mantegazza, C.; Bosetti, A.; Zuccotti, G.V. Type 1 diabetes and celiac disease: The effects of gluten free diet on metabolic control. *World Diabetes* **2013**, *4*, 130–134.

4

Bone Mass and Mineral Metabolism Alterations in Adult Celiac Disease: Pathophysiology and Clinical Approach

Michele Di Stefano, Caterina Mengoli, Manuela Bergonzi and Gino Roberto Corazza *

1st Department of Internal Medicine, University of Pavia, IRCCS "S.Matteo" Hospital Foundation, Pavia 27100, Italy; E-Mails: m.distefano@unipv.it (M.S.); caterina.mengoli@libero.it (C.M.); manuela.bergonzi@libero.it (M.B.)

* Author to whom correspondence should be addressed; E-Mail: gr.corazza@smatteo.pv.it;

Abstract: Osteoporosis affects many patients with celiac disease (CD), representing the consequence of calcium malabsorption and persistent activation of mucosal inflammation. A slight increase of fracture risk is evident in this condition, particularly in those with overt malabsorption and in postmenopausal state. The adoption of a correct gluten-free diet (GFD) improves bone derangement, but is not able to normalize bone mass in all the patients. Biomarkers effective in the prediction of bone response to gluten-free diet are not yet available and the indications of guidelines are still imperfect and debated. In this review, the pathophysiology of bone loss is correlated to clinical aspects, defining an alternative proposal of management for this condition.

Keywords: celiac disease; osteoporosis; gluten-free diet; bone densitometry

---

1. Introduction

Osteoporosis is a condition characterized by low bone mass and micro-architectural deterioration of bone tissue resulting in enhanced bone fragility and an increase in fracture risk [1]. It affects more than 75 million people in developed countries, causing 8.9 million fractures annually worldwide. Osteoporotic fractures account for 2.8 million disability-adjusted life years annually: to make this even clearer, this index is higher than other conditions, such as breast cancer, gastric cancer and hypertension [2]. There is a general agreement in the literature that more than 75% of untreated adult celiac disease (CD) patients with an overt malabsorption syndrome at diagnosis suffer from a loss of bone mass [3–9], and this complication also affects about half the patients with subclinical CD, presenting with minimal, transient and apparently unrelated symptoms [3,9], or asymptomatic patients diagnosed because of their first-degree kinship [4].

Moreover, an increased prevalence of celiac disease in osteoporotic patients was reported [10–12] and, even if this result was not confirmed by others [13–15], all previous results show the importance of the problem from a clinical point of view. On the contrary, the value of active screening for CD in patients with otherwise unexplained bone loss is still under debate.

Accordingly, there is no doubt that CD is a condition at high risk for secondary osteoporosis, and the evaluation of bone mass and mineral metabolism is thus very important in the clinical management of these patients. In the last few years, while the mechanisms of bone derangement in CD have been extensively studied, less attention has been paid to the clinical management of this complication: there is in fact very little information available on the timing of the first bone mineral density (BMD) measurement, on follow-up frequency, even on the best treatment options.

2. Bone Damage and Mineral Metabolism Derangement in Celiac Disease

Intestinal malabsorption and inflammation contribute to the pathophysiology of bone damage in CD. Villous atrophy is responsible for alterations of intestinal absorption, and a negative calcium balance was shown in CD patients due to several mechanisms: malabsorption of calcium in untreated patients [16], partially reversible after gluten-free diet (GFD) [17]; the reduction of calcium intake [18] also due to a secondary lactose intolerance [19]; and the reduction of intestinal calcium absorption due to its binding to intraluminal unabsorbed fatty acids [16]. Hypocalcemia can induce a compensatory increase of serum levels of parathyroid hormone (PTH), in turn responsible for an increase of bone turnover [7,20]: in untreated CD, serum PTH correlates with markers of both bone synthesis, such as osteocalcin, as well as resorption, like telopeptide of type I collagen (ICTP) [5]. Bone resorption is faster than bone neoformation, resulting in net bone loss and a high turnover osteoporosis [21]. The increase of serum PTH enhances the activity of the renal enzyme 1-α-hydroxylase, which converts 25-vitamin D into 1,25 vitamin D, in order to improve calcium absorption at intestinal level. However, this effort is ineffective, mainly due to the lack in immature enterocytes of celiac mucosa of calbindin [22], a vitamin D-dependent calcium-binding protein, minimizing the role of vitamin D malabsorption [23]. Finally, high levels of 1,25 vitamin D might have the paradoxical effect of increasing bone resorption, as shown in patients with chronic renal failure [4]. Accordingly, vitamin D functions are rarely impaired in untreated CD, as hyperconversion of metabolite 25-vitamin D guarantees adequate levels of the active form 1,25 vitamin D.

Intestinal malabsorption could also lead to some deficits of other minerals, fat and water soluble vitamins that could affect normal bone metabolism. In particular, low levels of zinc were described in non-treated celiac patients [24], and related to low levels of insulin-like growth factor, that are subsequently responsible for derangement in bone metabolism, growth and immune function [25].

This complex network of events is present in both overt symptomatic and subclinical CD to be a disease that is below the threshold of clinical detection without signs or symptoms sufficient to trigger CD testing in routine practice—or it is silent, equivalent to asymptomatic CD patients, even if the extent of bone loss and the alterations of serum levels of indices of bone and mineral metabolism may be less severe than in CD patients with overt malabsorption [3].

More recently, much evidence has also suggested the role of both local and systemic inflammation in the pathophysiology of bone loss in CD, characterized by a chronic increase of both mucosal and serum pro-inflammatory cytokines, in particular TNFα, IL-1 and IL-6 [26,27]. IL-1 and TNFα stimulate osteoclastogenesis and bone resorption [28]; IL-6 has a pivotal role in bone resorption by recruiting osteoclast precursors and stimulating their differentiation [29]. In untreated CD patients, serum IL-6 levels inversely correlate with BMD [27] and directly with PTH and ICTP levels, a marker of bone resorption [30]. Recently, the existence of a complex cytokine imbalance in CD patients, affecting both osteoclast and osteoblast activity was shown: cultures of peripheral blood mononuclear cells of healthy donors with sera of untreated CD patients result in an increase in osteoclast number and IL-6 levels, together with an inhibition of IL-12 and IL-18 [31], two cytokines showing an *in vitro* inhibitory effect on osteoclastogenesis and osteoclast activity [32,33].

In the last 15 years, great attention has been given to the RANKL/RANK/osteoprotegerin pathway, that is today considered the main signaling system in bone metabolism. The receptor activator of nuclear factor κB ligand (RANKL) is expressed and secreted by osteoblasts; it binds RANK, located on the surface of osteoclast precursors, to induce the differentiation of these cells into mature osteoclasts, promoting bone resorption. Osteoprotegerin (OPG) is also secreted by osteoblasts; it acts as a decoy receptor for RANK and blocks RANK–RANKL interaction [34]. In CD patients, an increased level of OPG and RANKL was described, with an OPG/RANKL ratio significantly lower than controls. Moreover, the OPG/RANKL ratio was correlated with spine BMD [35] and with IL-6 levels [31].

The pathophysiological role of autoantibodies against OPG is also debated, as in a recent paper the presence of these antibodies was detected in a man with CD, high bone turnover and severe osteoporosis not responsive to GFD and to calcium and vitamin D supplementation [36]. This observation was not confirmed by a subsequent study on a large cohort of CD patients on GFD [37].

Further factors are linked to endocrine and reproductive disorders, commonly part of CD clinical presentation. In particular, early menopause and periods of amenorrhea could occur in women, due partly to malnutrition and partly to hormonal imbalance, and could worsen the severity of osteoporosis [38]. In men, hypogonadism was described, due to a reversible androgen resistance [39] and to hyperprolactinemia [40], and considered a possible adjunctive factor risk for osteoporosis [41]. Finally, CD is frequently associated with autoimmune thyroiditis and type I diabetes mellitus [42]: both these disorders are at high risk for osteoporosis [43,44].

2.1. Effect of GFD

Strict adherence to GFD allows BMD improvement but it is not able to normalize it in all cases. Mucosal recovery does not appear to be the only determining variable: in fact, with the same histological response, bone mass normalization is present in celiacs on GFD since early infancy [45] but not always in patients on GFD for the same length of time but diagnosed at a later age. In particular, normalization of BMD levels in childhood CD may be complete as early as after two years of GFD [46]. On the contrary, in adults, many cross-sectional studies demonstrated higher BMD levels in treated *vs.* untreated CD patients but still lower than in healthy volunteers [3–9,47–50]; also the prevalence of alterations of indices of bone and mineral metabolism is lower in treated *vs.* untreated patients [47,51,52]. These results were shown in patients on GFD for a median duration of 28.5 months [5], in patients on GFD from a mean of 3.6 years [47] and in a group of patients treated for a mean of 16 years, a very long period of GFD [52]. It is therefore evident that the early onset of bone damage, probably before achieving bone mass peak, is an important time point determining GFD-induced bone mass gain. Even longitudinal studies are of little help here, as the longest period of GFD evaluated was 5 years [53]. On the other hand, these studies have provided important information on the kinetic of bone mass recovery with the start of GFD and correlations with the modifications of bone-mineral metabolism parameters. Following a GFD with optimal compliance for a period of one year allows a significant improvement of BMD values, ranging from 5% [6] to 8% [3] according to different studies. These results were confirmed in a larger cohort of patients enrolled at diagnosis and restudied after one year of GFD [8]. In a two-year study, GFD improved not only bone mass but also serum levels of indices of bone and mineral metabolism. BMD improvement was more evident after two years than after one year of GFD, suggesting that a period longer than one year was necessary to point out intrinsic capacities of an individual patient to recover bone mass. Serum levels of propeptide of type I procollagen (PICP) at diagnosis proved to be a strong predictor of bone mass gain after two years, suggesting the possibility of selecting the group of patients with high levels of bone matrix formation activity that is more likely to readily respond to GFD [54]. In a three-year study, BMD increased in 92% of CD patients in GFD with a mean bone mass gain around 3%–4% per year. However, only 12% of patients showed a normalization of BMD. In particular, in a small group of patients, it was evident that relatively good bone mass gain was present during the first year, but was negligible in the subsequent study period [55]. These observations agree with a five-year study showing femoral and lumbar BMD values at five years similar to BMD values at one-year follow-up both in men and women, with the exception of trochanter values, which proved to be higher at five-year measurement than one-year values [53].

In summary, BMD values normalize only in children, when diagnosed early in infancy and if they follow a long-term GFD with optimal adherence. On the contrary, BMD values in adults show a good improvement in the first period, generally around two years, after the institution of a GFD; the improvement is then generally unsatisfactory and treatment with a mineral-active drug should probably be considered. Nevertheless, CD patients show a wide range of response to GFD and risk factors for osteoporosis include old age at diagnosis and the degree of osteopenia in late diagnosis, compliance to GFD, menstrual status, *i.e.*, late age at menarche, early menopause, periods of amenorrhea, low body mass index (BMI), low dietary calcium intake, inadequate physical activity and use of glucocorticoids [4,52,56,57]. What appears to emerge is that as age progresses and, in women as menopause approaches, the ability to recover bone mass seems to diminish, being greatest in childhood and lowest in peri- and postmenopausal women. In this latter subgroup of patients, waiting two or three years to determine the extent of GFD-induced bone mass gain could thus be incorrect and the start of treatment with a mineral-active drug should be earlier, probably at diagnosis.

The availability of predictive markers of GFD-induced bone mass gain could be a solution for this problem, but the mechanism responsible for the unsatisfactory improvement is not completely clear. A persistent reduction of fractional calcium absorption was shown in patients on GFD, besides the improvement of intestinal mucosa architecture [17], and in a subgroup of patients the persistence of a secondary hyperparathyroidism and a significant correlation between serum PTH levels and femoral BMD were shown [17]. The possible role of secondary hyperparathyroidism was suggested by other papers [20,58] but also disproved [59], and the proposed pathophysiological mechanisms for the persistent raise of serum PTH were residual villous atrophy leading to calcium malabsorption [20], a reduction of calcium intake [18], but also a slow reversal of parathyroid hyperplasia [60]. Partial adherence to GFD [55] and incomplete mucosal recovery [57] could also have a role in subgroups of treated patients.

Circulating factors secondary to persistent activation of the mucosal immune system could directly interfere with osteoclastogenesis and osteoblast activity. It was shown that in patients following GFD for a mean period of 40 months [31] the prevalence of bone damage is around 40%, and circulating levels of cytokines (IL-6, IL-1beta, TNF-alfa, TNF-beta, IL-12, IL-18, RANK-L, OPG) are significantly lower than in untreated patients, but significantly higher than in healthy volunteers. In particular, the osteoclastogenic activity of sera from patients on long-term GFD proved to be still significantly higher than sera of healthy volunteers and serum cytokine levels were not correlated to PTH levels [31]. An altered ratio between RANKL and OPG in untreated patients normalizes to healthy volunteer levels in patients on GFD [31,35]. Accordingly, the dietary treatment with GFD alone is not able to completely control the increased osteoclast differentiation and activity present in CD, as confirmed by a strong correlation between OPG/RANKL ratio and BMD [35], and the mechanism responsible for bone damage does not involve PTH. Finally, while a three-year period of GFD determines a significant decrease of IL 6, which is significantly inversely correlated at diagnosis with lumbar BMD, it cannot normalize IL-1β and IL-1 receptor antagonist serum levels [27].

Therefore, persistent inflammation in treated CD patients could have a role in the persistence of bone mass derangement. In particular, the predominant mechanism responsible for bone derangement seems different between short-term and long-term treated CD patients: in the period immediately after diagnosis, the malabsorption of calcium and the consequent hormonal and vitamin D alterations appear to be the prevalent pathophysiological mechanism, their correction allowing a satisfactory bone mass gain, comparable to the effect of administering mineral-active drugs in postmenopausal osteoporosis [61]. Unfortunately, the extent of the loss of bone mass in untreated CD is very often higher than the extent of the recovery induced just by GFD in the early stages of treatment and, once the GFD-induced metabolic surge that occurs in this phase is over, persistent bone loss seems due to the persistent activation of a local mechanism, related to chronic inflammation. Preliminary data from our group confirm this hypothesis, as an in-depth evaluation of hormonal and local factors suggests that high levels of OPG and low levels of PICP select the subgroup of CD patients with a persistent reduction of bone mass, despite strict adherence to GFD and architectural villi reconstitution [62]. If confirmed, these markers might be used to identify those patients who need mineral-active treatment associated with gluten-free diet.

3. Fracture Risk

BMD is only one of the factors that contribute to establishing the extent of fracture risk in osteoporotic patients. Other factors are related to bone mechanical characteristics, such as stiffness of cortical bone, but also to inadequacy of protectors from trauma (body mass, fat and muscle compartments) and to neuromuscular dysfunction [63].

Several studies pointed out the prevalence of fracture in celiac population, but with a very important heterogeneity in methods (study design, sample selection, fracture data collection) and cohorts studied (treated/untreated CD), making available data often inconsistent and difficult to interpret [64]. Most authors agree on the increased prevalence of fracture in CD patients [63,65–71] and a recent meta-analysis evaluating a total of 20,955 CD patients and 96,777 controls described a risk of fracture 43% greater in CD [72]. Data on fractures were collected by mailed questionnaires, by personal interviews or by medical records; consequently, results on peripheral fractures might be more easily estimated and axial fractures underestimated. Only a cross-sectional study explored the existence of asymptomatic vertebral fractures by spinal X-ray and did not find an increase of vertebral fractures in CD patients [68]. However, if CD patients are subdivided according to the clinical presentation, peripheral fracture risk proves to be higher than controls in patients with overt malabsorption symptom, while it is similar to the general population in subclinical and silent presentation [71]. These data were confirmed in a more recent case-control study, pointing out a higher peripheral fracture risk also in men and underlining again the importance of adherence to GFD [63]. However, to confirm what was said above with respect to pathophysiology, in a population-based study in Olmsted County, CD patients showed a fracture risk twice that of controls, and this figure persisted unchanged during GFD [66].

In general, however, large population-based studies should be interpreted with care, since, for example, in one study on the fracture risk in CD patients on a cohort of 1021 celiac patients, a possible misclassification of patients could have accounted for the negativity of results, as data were extracted from the National Patient Discharge Register, known for a low estimated validity of diagnosis of CD (78%) [73].

It is, finally, likely that, in addition to just BMD measurement, assessment of the physical characteristics of bone, such as its elasticity, can add something to our understanding of the mechanisms that favor fractures [74,75]. Unfortunately, no studies are available that correlate bone ultrasound densitometry parameters with fracture risk in CD patients.

4. Clinical Management

Only a limited number of international recommendations are available on the clinical management of osteoporosis in CD, probably due to the lack of sufficient data on patient follow-up and the role of the menopause. As already stated, there is no clinical or biochemical marker to select the subgroup of patients not responding to GFD alone with an improvement of bone mass and which will be characterized by a high risk of fractures; accordingly, we are not able, as yet, to optimize both treatment and timing of BMD follow-up measurement.

In 2000, the British Society of Gastroenterology published the guidelines for osteoporosis in CD [76]. General advice aimed at modifying lifestyle factor risk was provided, such as enhancing physical activity, stopping smoking, avoiding alcohol excess. Moreover, a daily calcium intake of 1500 mg, even by pharmacological supplementation, and vitamin D supplementation, if inadequate serum levels were evident, was suggested. Bone densitometry was recommended at diagnosis for all patients, to detect osteoporosis early and to obtain the greatest possible benefit from treatment, or at least at menopausal age for women and at the age of 55 years for men. Postmenopausal women with normal BMD should repeat densitometry after two years. Osteoporotic postmenopausal women and men over 55 years should be offered treatment and bone densitometry yearly to monitor treatment efficacy.

The subsequent awareness of an ultimately low absolute risk of fracture, even if higher than in the general population [77], determined strong criticism of the extensive use of bone densitometry at diagnosis, suggesting that BMD measurement should be restricted to patients with high short-term fracture risk, such as patients non-compliant with GFD or who failed to respond to dietary treatment, on glucocorticoid therapy, with untreated hypogonadism, older age, low BMI, and previous fragility fracture [78]. This led to reconsideration of the guidelines and the proposal of BMD measurement only in clinically non-responder patients, especially those with low BMI, in menopausal women and after 55 years for men [79]. In 2003, the American Gastroenterological Association guidelines on osteoporosis in gastrointestinal disease suggested that bone densitometry should be performed in adults with newly diagnosed celiac disease after one year of GFD, to allow for stabilization of bone density, implementation of GFD, calcium and vitamin D supplementation as needed, and, if necessary, bisphosphonates and hormonal therapy were strongly encouraged in osteoporotic patients [80].

A Canadian Position Statement on evaluation and management of skeletal health in CD was recently published [81]. BMD measurement was suggested at diagnosis only in adults with classic CD, and after one year of GFD in adults with asymptomatic or silent CD. The latter group of patients should be considered for earlier BMD evaluation in the presence of risk factors such as menopause, older age, history of fragility fracture, unexplained iron deficiency anemia, vitamin D deficiency/insufficiency, and high titers for CD serological markers. Indications for follow-up were also given: BMD should be re-evaluated after one year of GFD in the presence of osteopenia/osteoporosis at diagnosis, and after two years in cases of documentation of normal bone mass. The assessment of bone and mineral metabolism by dosing serum calcium, albumin, 1,25 dihydoxicolecalciferol and PTH levels should be repeated every six months until normalization.

Clinical application of the Canadian guidelines does not, however, seem to allow substantial resource savings, and is thus very similar to the earlier British proposal. In patients with asymptomatic or silent CD with the aforementioned risk factors, early prescription of bone densitometry is indicated, since anemia and vitamin D alterations show a very high prevalence also in this subgroup. Considering the prevalence of bone loss in patients with and without overt malabsorption symptoms, BMD measurement could provide more important information in asymptomatic than in clinically overt malabsorber patients: bone loss is highly prevalent in overt malabsorption, and these patients could undergo mineral-active therapy as of diagnosis; conversely, asymptomatic/silent patients should be screened for bone loss presence. Moreover, the most important risk factor at diagnosis seems to be the age of the patient, and patients well over the age of peak bone mass could be treated without measuring BMD, while those patients below or shortly after the age of the peak should undergo BMD measurement. This approach seems the most correct one in optimizing the use of bone densitometry, but the problem remains for the free dispensing of the mineral-active drug, which in Italy depends on the presence of a pathological fracture. Optimization of this phase could be achieved by performing a radiological study of the lumbar spine in patients most at risk, such as symptomatic subjects, peri- and postmenopausal women and men over the age of 55, in order to detect vertebral fractures, together with a complete case history for previous fractures. In Italy (Lombardia Region), the cost of lumbar and femoral densitometry is €88.66 (€44.33 for each segment), while the cost of a lumbar spine X-ray is only €34.80.

In conclusion, there is no general agreement on the correct timing of bone densitometry in celiac patients; screening at diagnosis seems to be not justified in all patients and the proposed alternative approach is explained in Figure 1.

Figure 1. Diagnostic and therapeutic approach to CD patients without a previous fracture.

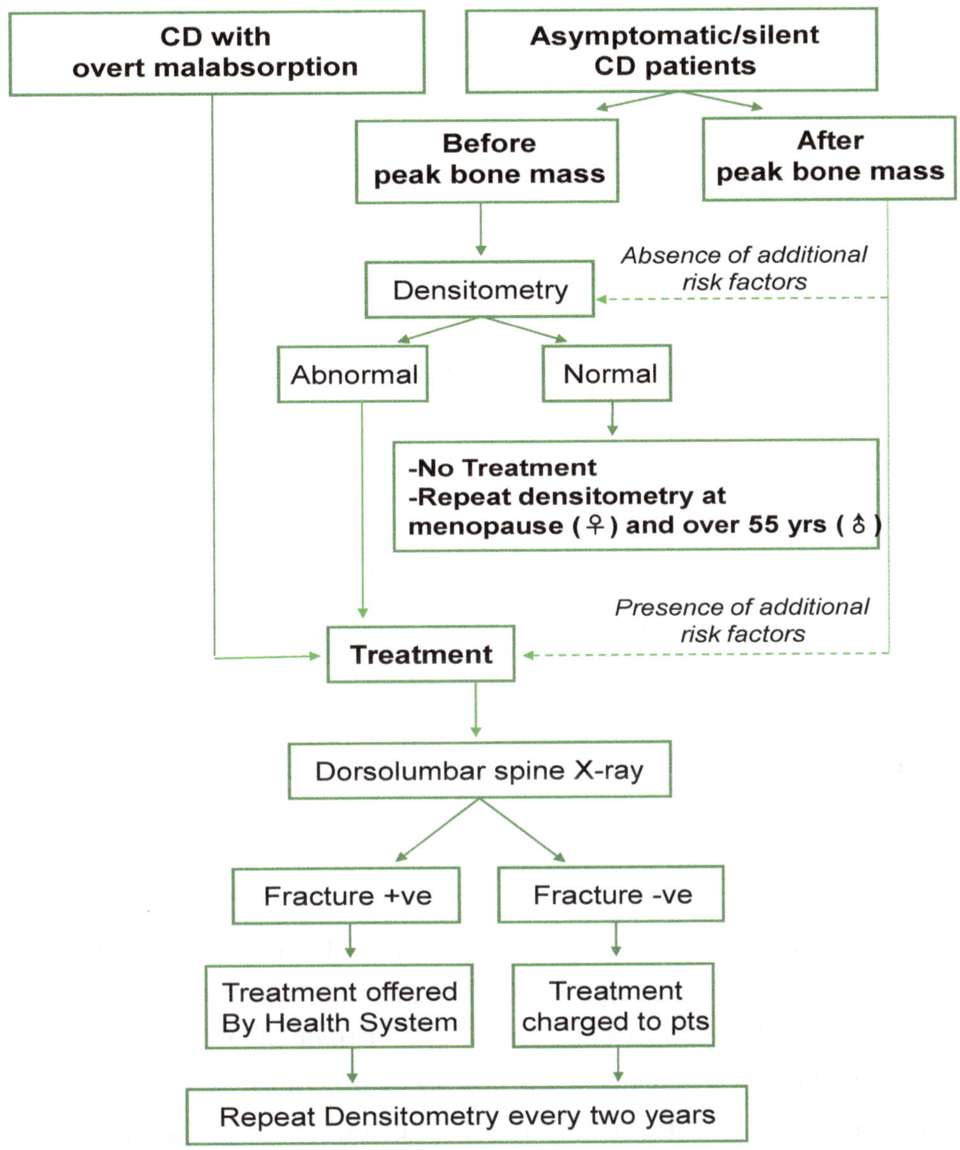

Treatment with a mineral-active drug in association to GFD, even without BMD measurement, should be prescribed to patients at high short-term risk of fracture, including symptomatic patients, asymptomatic patients in peri and postmenopausal period, men older than 55 years, low calcium intake, low BMI, poor compliance to GFD, or unresponsiveness to GFD following steroid therapy; in these cases, measure BMD after two years of treatment. To allow the free dispensing of the drug, patients should be screened for the presence of fracture and X-ray of the spine could be adequate to this aim. Young asymptomatic patients with a normal BMD should be re-evaluated at peri-menopausal period (female patients) or over 55 years (male patients).

As regards the choice of the drug for the treatment of osteoporosis in CD, there are no longitudinal studies dealing with this topic and we have no information on which to base our choice in the individual subgroups of patients. The current approach is clearly based on post-menopausal osteoporosis treatment with a choice between a weekly administration of alendronate and a monthly administration of ibandronate. The use of denosumab, a decoy receptor for RANKL able to reduce the activation of the osteoclast system, seems very interesting, also on the basis of the data obtained on the RANK/RANKL/OPG system. The results of the first studies are awaited in order to define the best strategy for the different types of CD patients.

5. Conclusions

In conclusion, in the pathophysiology of bone derangement in CD patients, both malabsorption and the persistent activation of inflammation at intestinal level are important, in a two-step model. Biomarkers with a predictive role of the normalization of BMD levels are needed and the evaluation of the RANK/RANKL/OPG system could offer some inputs on this topic.

References

1. Consensus development conference: Prophylaxis and treatment of osteoporosis. *Osteoporos. Int.* **1991**, *1*, 114–117.
2. WHO Scientific Group on the Assessment of Osteoporosis at Primary Health Care Levels. *Summary Meeting Report 2004*; World Health Organization: Brussels, Belgium, 2007; pp. 1–17.
3. Corazza, G.R.; Di Sario, A.; Cecchetti, A.; Jorizzo, R.A.; Di Stefano, M.; Minguzzi, L.; Brusco, G.; Bernardi, M.; Gasbarrini, G. Influence of pattern of clinical presentation and gluten-free diet on bone mass and metabolism in adult coeliac disease. *Bone* **1996**, *18*, 525–530.
4. Mazure, R.; Vazquez, H.; Gonzalez, D.; Mautalen, C.; Pedreira, S.; Boerr, L.; Bai, J.C. Bone mineral affectation in asymptomatic adult patients with celiac disease. *Am. J. Gastroenterol.* **1994**, *89*, 2130–2134.
5. Corazza, G.R.; di Sario, A.; Cecchetti, A.; Tarozzi, C.; Corrao, G.; Bernardi, M.; Gasbarrini, G. Bone mass and metabolism in patients with celiac disease. *Gastroenterology* **1995**, *109*, 122–128.
6. McFarlane, X.A.; Bhalla, A.K.; Robertson, D.A.F. Effect of gluten free diet on osteopenia in adults with newly diagnosed celiac disease. *Gut* **1996**, *39*, 180–184.
7. Keaveny, A.P.; Freaney, R.; McKenna, M.J.; Masterson, J.; O'Donoghue, D.P. Bone remodeling indices and secondary hyperparathyroidism in celiac disease. *Am. J. Gastroenterol.* **1996**, *91*, 1226–1231.
8. Valdimarsson, T.; Löfman, O.; Toss, G.; Ström, M. Reversal of osteopenia with diet in adult coeliac disease. *Gut* **1996**, *38*, 322–327.
9. Mustalahti, K.; Collin, P.; Sievänen, H.; Salmi, J.; Mäki, M. Osteopenia in patients with clinically silent coeliac disease warrants screening. *Lancet* **1999**, *354*, 744–745.

10. Duerksen, D.R.; Leslie, W.D. Positive celiac disease serology and reduced bone mineral density in adult women. *Can. J. Gastroenterol.* **2010**, *24*, 103–107.
11. Stenson, W.F.; Newberry, R.; Lorenz, R.; Baldus, C.; Civitelli, R. Increased prevalence of celiac disease and need for routine screening among patients with osteoporosis. *Arch. Intern. Med.* **2005**, *165*, 393–399.
12. Armagan, O.; Uz, T.; Tascioglu, F.; Colak, O.; Oner, C.; Akgun, Y. Serological screening for celiac disease in premenopausal women with idiopathic osteoporosis. *Clin. Rheumatol.* **2005**, *24*, 239–243.
13. Drummond, F.J.; Annis, P.; O'Sullivan, K.; Wynne, F.; Daly, M.; Shanahan, F.; Quane, K.A.; Molloy, M.G. Screening for asymptomatic celiac disease among patients referred for bone densitometry measurement. *Bone* **2003**, *33*, 970–974.
14. Mather, K.J.; Meddings, J.B.; Beck, P.L.; Scott, R.B.; Hanley, D.A. Prevalence of IgA-antiendomysial antibody in asymptomatic low bone mineral density. *Am. J. Gastroenterol.* **2001**, *96*, 120–125.
15. Karakan, T.; Ozyemisci-Taskiran, O.; Gunendi, Z.; Atalay, F.; Tuncer, C. Prevalence of IgA-antiendomysial antibody in a patient cohort with idiopathic low bone mineral density. *World J. Gastroenterol.* **2007**, *21*, 2978–2982.
16. Molteni, N.; Bardella, M.T.; Vezzoli, G.; Pozzoli, E.; Bianchi, P. Intestinal calcium absorption as shown by stable strontium test in celiac disease before and after gluten-free diet. *Am. J. Gastroenterol.* **1995**, *90*, 2025–2028.
17. Pazianas, M.; Butcher, G.P.; Subhani, J.M.; Finch, P.J.; Ang, L.; Collins, C.; Heaney, R.P.; Zaidi, M.; Maxwell, J.D. Calcium absorption and bone mineral density in celiacs after long term treatment with gluten-free diet and adequate calcium intake. *Osteoporos. Int.* **2005**, *16*, 56–63.
18. Kinsey, L.; Burden, S.T.; Bannermann, E. A dietary survey to determine if patients with celiac disease are meeting current healthy eating guidelines and how their diet compares to that of the british general population. *Eur. J. Clin. Nutr.* **2008**, *62*, 1333–1342.
19. Plotkin, G.R.; Isselbacher, K.J. Secondary disaccharidase deficiency in adult celiac disease (Nontropical Sprue) and other malabsorption states. *N. Engl. J. Med.* **1964**, *271*, 1033–1037.
20. Valdimarsson, T.; Toss, G.; Löfman, O.; Ström, M. Three years' follow-up of bone density in adult coeliac disease: Significance of secondary hyperparathyroidism. *Scand. J. Gastroenterol.* **2000**, *35*, 274–280.
21. Corazza, G.R.; di Stefano, M.; Maurino, E.; Bai, J.C. Bones in celiac disease: Diagnosis and treatment. *Best Pract. Res. Clin. Gastroenterol.* **2005**, *19*, 453–465.
22. Staun, M.; Jarnum, S. Measurement of the 10,000-molecular weight calcium-binding protein in small-intestinal biopsy specimens from patients with malabsorption syndromes. *Scand. J. Gastroenterol.* **1988**, *23*, 827–832.
23. Colston, K.W.; Mackay, A.G.; Finlayson, C.; Wu, J.C.; Maxwell, J.D. Localisation of Vitamin D receptor in normal human duodenum and in patients with coeliac disease. *Gut* **1994**, *35*, 1219–1225.
24. Valdimarsson, T.; Arnqvist, H.J.; Toss, G.; Järnerot, G.; Nyström, F.; Ström, M. Low circulating insulin-like growth factor i in coeliac disease and its relation to bone mineral density. *Scand. J. Gastroenterol.* **1999**, *34*, 904–908.

25. Jameson, S. Coeliac disease, insulin-like growth factor, bone mineral density, and zinc. *Scand. J. Gastroenterol.* **2000**, *35*, 894–896.
26. Kontakou, M.; Przemioslo, R.T.; Sturgess, R.P.; Limb, A.G.; Ciclitira, P.J. Expression of tumour necrosis factor-alpha, interleukin-6, and interleukin-2 mRNA in the jejunum of patients with coeliac disease. *Scand. J. Gastroenterol.* **1995**, *30*, 456–463.
27. Fornari, M.C.; Pedreira, S.; Niveloni, S.; González, D.; Diez, R.A.; Vázquez, H.; Mazure, R.; Sugai, E.; Smecuol, E.; Boerr, L.; *et al.* Pre- and post-treatment serum levels of cytokines IL-1beta, IL-6, and IL-1 receptor antagonist in celiac disease. Are they related to the associated osteopenia? *Am. J. Gastroenterol.* **1998**, *93*, 413–418.
28. Wei, S.; Kitaura, H.; Zhou, P.; Ross, F.P.; Teitelbaum, S.L. IL-1 mediates TNF-induced osteoclastogenesis. *J. Clin. Investig.* **2005**, *115*, 282–290.
29. Raisz, L.G. Local and systemic factors in the pathogenesis of osteoporosis. *N. Engl. J. Med.* **1988**, *318*, 818–828.
30. Di Stefano, M.; Sciarra, G.; Jorizzo, R.A.; Grillo, R.L.; Cecchetti, L.; Speziale, D.; Pichini, L.; Gasbarrini, G.; Corazza, G.R. Local and gonadal factors in the pathogenesis of coeliac bone loss. *Ital. J. Gastroenterol.* **1997**, *29*, 31.
31. Taranta, A.; Fortunati, D.; Longo, M.; Rucci, N.; Iacomino, E.; Aliberti, F.; Facciuto, E.; Migliaccio, S.; Bardella, M.T.; Dubini, A. Imbalance of Osteoclastogenesis-regulating Factors in Patients with Celiac Disease. *J. Bone Miner. Res.* **2004**, *19*, 1112–1121.
32. Horwood, N.J.; Elliott, J.; Martin, T.J.; Gillespie, M.T. IL-12 alone and in synergy with IL-18 inhibits osteoclast formation *in vitro*. *J. Immunol.* **2001**, *166*, 4915–4921.
33. Yamada, N.; Niwa, S.; Tsujimura, T.; Iwasaki, T.; Sugihara, A.; Futani, H.; Hayashi, S.; Okamura H.; Akedo, H.; Terada, N. Interleukin-18 and interleukin-12 synergistically inhibit osteoclastic bone-resorbing activity. *Bone* **2002**, *6*, 901–908.
34. Khosla, S. Minireview: The OPG/RANKL/RANK system. *Endocrinology* **2001**, *142*, 5050–5055.
35. Fiore, C.E.; Pennisi, P.; Ferro, G.; Ximenes, B.; Privitelli, L.; Mangiafico, R.A.; Santoro, F.; Parisi, N.; Lombardo, T. Altered osteoprotegerin/RANKL ratio and low bone mineral density in celiac patients on long-term treatment with gluten-free diet. *Horm. Metab. Res.* **2006**, *38*, 417–422.
36. Riches, P.L.; McRorie, E.; Fraser, W.D.; Determann, C.; van't Hof, R.; Ralston, S.H. Osteoporosis associated with neutralizing autoantibodies against osteoprotegerin. *N. Engl. J. Med.* **2009**, *361*, 1459–1465.
37. Larussa, T.; Suraci, E.; Nazionale, I.; Leone, I.; Montalcini, T.; Abenavoli, L.; Imeneo, M.; Pujia, A.; Luzza, F. No evidence of circulating autoantibodies against osteoprotegerin in patients with celiac disease. *World J. Gastroenterol.* **2012**, *18*, 1622–1627.
38. Ozgör, B.; Selimoğlu, M.A. Coeliac disease and reproductive disorders. *Scand. J. Gastroenterol.* **2010**, *45*, 395–402.
39. Green, J.R.; Goble, H.L.; Edwards, C.R.; Dawson, A.M. Reversible insensitivity to androgens in men with untreated gluten enteropathy. *Lancet* **1977**, *1*, 280–282.
40. Farthing, M.J.; Rees, L.H.; Dawson, A.M. Male gonadal function in coeliac disease: III. Pituitary regulation. *Clin. Endocrinol.* **1983**, *19*, 661–671.

41. Stazi, A.V.; Trecca, A.; Trinti, B. Osteoporosis in celiac disease and in endocrine and reproductive disorders. *World J. Gastroenterol.* **2008**, *14*, 498–505.
42. Di Sabatino, A.; Corazza, G.R. Coeliac disease. *Lancet* **2009**, *373*, 1480–1493.
43. Mosekilde, L.; Eriksen, E.F.; Charles, P. Effects of thyroid hormones on bone and mineral metabolism. *Endocrinol. Metab. Clin.* **1990**, *19*, 35–63.
44. Hofbauer, L.C.; Brueck, C.C.; Singh, S.K.; Dobnig, H. Osteoporosis in patients with diabetes mellitus. *J. Bone Miner. Res.* **2007**, *22*, 1317–1328.
45. Mora, S.; Barera, G.; Beccio, S.; Menni, L.; Proverbio, M.C.; Bianchi, C.; Chiumello, G. A prospective, longitudinal study of the long-term effect of treatment on bone density in children with celiac disease. *J. Pediatr.* **2001**, *139*, 516–521.
46. Mora, S.; Barera, G.; Ricotti, A.; Weber, G.; Bianchi, C.; Chiumello, G. Reversal of low bone density with a gluten-free diet in children and adolescents with celiac disease. *Am. J. Clin. Nutr.* **1998**, *67*, 477–481.
47. Bodé, S.; Hassager, C.; Gudmand-Høyer, E.; Christiansen, C. Body composition and calcium metabolism in adult treated coeliac disease. *Gut* **1991**, *32*, 1342–1345.
48. Valdimarsson, T.; Toss, G.; Ross, I.; Löfman, O.; Ström, M. Bone mineral density in coeliac disease. *Scand. J. Gastroenterol.* **1994**, *29*, 457–461.
49. Walters, J.R.; Banks, L.M.; Butcher, G.P.; Fowler, C.R. Detection of low bone mineral density by dual energy x-ray absorptiometry in unsuspected suboptimally treated coeliac disease. *Gut* **1995**, *37*, 220–224.
50. McFarlane, X.A.; Bhalla, A.K.; Reeves, D.E.; Morgan, L.M.; Robertson, D.A. Osteoporosis in treated adult coeliac disease. *Gut* **1995**, *36*, 710–714.
51. Ferretti, J.; Mazure, R.; Tanoue, P.; Marino, A.; Cointry, G.; Vazquez, H.; Niveloni, S.; Pedreira, S.; Mauriño, E.; Zanchetta, J.; *et al.* Analysis of the structure and strength of bones in celiac disease patients. *Am. J. Gastroenterol.* **2003**, *98*, 382–390.
52. González, D.; Mazure, R.; Mautalen, C.; Vazquez, H.; Bai, J. Body composition and bone mineral density in untreated and treated patients with celiac disease. *Bone* **1995**, *16*, 231–234.
53. Kemppainen, T.; Kröger, H.; Janatuinen, E.; Arnala, I.; Lamberg-Allardt, C.; Kärkkäinen, M.; Kosma, V.M.; Julkunen, R.; Jurvelin, J.; Alhava, E.; *et al.* Bone recovery after a gluten-free diet: A 5-year follow-up study. *Bone* **1999**, *25*, 355–360.
54. Corazza, G.R.; di Stefano, M.; Jorizzo, R.A.; Cecchetti, L.; Minguzzi, L.; Gasbarrini, G. Propeptide of Type I procollagen is predictive of posttreatment bone mass gain in adult celiac disease. *Gastroenterology* **1997**, *113*, 67–71.
55. Bai, J.C.; Gonzalez, D.; Mautalen, C.; Mazure, R.; Pedreira, S.; Vazquez, H.; Smecuol, E.; Siccardi, A.; Cataldi, M.; Niveloni, S.; *et al.* Long-term effect of gluten restriction on bone mineral density of patients with coeliac disease. *Aliment. Pharm. Ther.* **1997**, *11*, 157–164.
56. Pistorius, L.R.; Sweidan, W.H.; Purdie, D.W.; Steel, S.A.; Howey, S.; Bennett, J.R.; Sutton, D.R. Coeliac disease and bone mineral density in adult female patients. *Gut* **1995**, *37*, 639–642.
57. Kemppainen, T.; Kröger, H.;, Janatuinen, E.; Arnala, I.; Kosma, V.M.; Pikkarainen, P.; Julkunen, R.; Jurvelin, J.; Alhava, E.; Uusitupa, M. Osteoporosis in adult patients with celiac disease. *Bone* **1999**, *24*, 249–255.

58. Selby, P.L.; Davies, M.; Adams, J.E.; Mawer, E.B. Bone loss in celiac disease is related to secondary hyperparathyroidism. *J. Bone Miner. Res.* **1999**, *14*, 652–657.
59. Lemieux, B.; Boivin, M.; Brossard, J.H.; Lepage, R.; Picard, D.; Rousseau, L.; D'amour, P. Normal parathyroid function with decreased bone mineral density in treated celiac disease. *Can. J. Gastroenterol.* **2001**, *15*, 302–307.
60. Christensen, M.S.; Nielsen, H.E.; Torring, S. Hypercalcemia and parathyroid function after renal transplantation. *Acta Med. Scand.* **1977**, *201*, 35–39.
61. Liberman, U.A.; Weiss, S.R.; Bröll, J.; Minne, H.W.; Quan, H.; Bell, N.H.; Rodriguez-Portales, J.; Downs, R.W., Jr.; Dequeker, J.; Favus, M. Effect of oral alendronate on bone mineral density and the incidence of fractures in postmenopausal osteoporosis. *N. Engl. J. Med.* **1995**, *333*, 1437–1443.
62. Di Stefano, M.; Mengoli, C.; Tomarchio, O.; Bergonzi, M.; Pagani, E.; de Amici, M.; Ilardo, D.; Vattiato, C.; Biagi, F.; Zanaboni, A.; *et al.* Increased Osteoprotegerin and Decreased COOH-Terminal Propeptide of Type I Collagen Select Celiac Disease Patients on Long Term Gluten Free Diet with Persisting Low Bone Mass. In Proceedings of UEGW (21st United European Gastroenterology Week), Belin, Germany, 12–16 October 2013.
63. Sánchez, M.I.; Mohaidle, A.; Baistrocchi, A.; Matoso, D.; Vázquez, H.; González, A.; Mazure, R.; Maffei, E.; Ferrari, G.; Smecuol, E.; *et al.* Risk of fracture in celiac disease: Gender, dietary compliance, or both? *World J. Gastroenterol.* **2011**, *17*, 3035–3042.
64. Bianchi, M.L.; Bardella, M.T. Bone in celiac disease. *Osteoporos. Int.* **2008**, *19*, 1705–1716.
65. West, J.; Logan, R.F.; Card, T.R.; Smith, C.; Hubbard, R. Fracture risk in people with celiac disease: A population-based cohort study. *Gastroenterology* **2003**, *125*, 429–436.
66. Jafri, M.R.; Nordstrom, C.W.; Murray, J.A.; van Dyke, C.T.; Dierkhising, R.A.; Zinsmeister, A.R.; Melton, L.J., III. Long-term fracture risk in patients with celiac disease: A population-based study in Olmsted County, Minnesota. *Dig. Dis. Sci.* **2008**, *53*, 964–971.
67. Ludvigsson, J.F.; Michaelsson, K.; Ekbom, A.; Montgomery, S.M. Coeliac disease and the risk of fractures—A general population-based cohort study. *Aliment. Pharm. Ther.* **2007**, *25*, 273–285.
68. Vasquez, H.; Mazure, R.; Gonzalez, D.; Flores, D.; Pedreira, S.; Niveloni, S.; Smecuol, E.; Mauriño, E.; Bai, J.C. Risk of fractures in celiac disease patients: A cross-sectional, case-control study. *Am. J. Gastroenterol.* **2000**, *95*, 183–189.
69. Fickling, W.E.; McFarlane, X.A.; Bhalla, A.K.; Robertson, D.A. The clinical impact of metabolic bone disease in coeliac disease. *Postgrad. Med. J.* **2001**, *77*, 33–36.
70. Davie M.W.; Gaywood, I.; George, E.; Jones, P.W.; Masud, T.; Price, T.; Summers, G.D. Excess non-spine fractures in women over 50 years with celiac disease: A cross-sectional, questionnaire-based study. *Osteoporos. Int.* **2005**, *16*, 1150–1155.
71. Moreno, M.L.; Vazquez, H.; Mazure, R.; Smecuol, E.; Niveloni, S.; Pedreira, S.; Sugai, E.; Mauriño, E.; Gomez, J.C.; Bai, J.C. Stratification of bone fracture risk in patients with celiac disease. *Clin. Gastroenterol. Hepatol.* **2004**, *2*, 127–134.
72. Olmos, M.; Antelo, M.; Vazquez, H.; Smecuol, E.; Mauriño, E.; Bai, J.C. Systematic review and meta-analysis of observational studies on the prevalence of fractures in coeliac disease. *Dig. Liver Dis.* **2008**, *40*, 46–53.

73. Vestergaard, P.; Mosekilde, L. Fracture risk in patients with celiac disease, crohn's disease, and ulcerative colitis: A nationwide follow-up study of 16,416 patients in denmark. *Am. J. Epidemiol.* **2002**, *156*, 1–10.
74. Glüer, C.C. Quantitative ultrasound techniques for the assessment of osteoporosis: Expert agreement on current status. The international quantitative ultrasound consensus group. *J. Bone Miner. Res.* **1997**, *12*, 1280–1288.
75. Njeh, C.F.; Boivin, C.M.; Langton, C.M. The role of ultrasound in the assessment of oeteoporosis: A review. *Osteoporos. Int.* **1997**, *7*, 7–22.
76. Scott, E.M.; Gaywood, I.; Scott, B.B. Guidelines for osteoporosis in coeliac disease and inflammatory bowel disease. *Gut* **2000**, *46*, I1–I8.
77. Thomason, K.; West, J.; Logan, R.F.; Coupland, C.; Holmes, G.K. Fracture experience of patients with coeliac disease: A population based survey. *Gut* **2003**, *52*, 518–522.
78. Compston, J. Is fracture risk increased in patients with coeliac disease? *Gut* **2003**, *52*, 459–460.
79. Lewis, N.R.; Scott, B.B. Should patients with coeliac disease have their bone mineral density measured? *Eur. J. Gastroenterol. Hepatol.* **2005**, *17*, 1065–1070.
80. American Gastroenterological Association. American gastroenterological association medical position statement: Guidelines on osteoporosis in gastrointestinal diseases. *Gastroenterology* **2003**, *124*, 791–794.
81. Fouda, M.A.; Khan, A.A.; Sultan, M.S.; Rios, L.P.; McAssey, K.; Armstrong, D. Evaluation and management of skeletal health in celiac disease: Position statement. *Can. J. Gastroenterol.* **2012**, *26*, 819–829.

5

Oats in the Diet of Children with Celiac Disease: Preliminary Results of a Double-Blind, Randomized and Placebo-Controlled Multicenter Italian Study

Simona Gatti [1,*], Nicole Caporelli [1], Tiziana Galeazzi [1], Ruggiero Francavilla [2], Maria Barbato [3], Paola Roggero [4], Basilio Malamisura [5], Giuseppe Iacono [6], Andrea Budelli [7], Rosaria Gesuita [8], Carlo Catassi [1], Elena Lionetti [9]

Department of Pediatrics, Università Politecnica delle Marche, 60121 Ancona, Italy;
E-Mails: nicole.capo@hotmail.it (N.C.); t.galeazzi@univpm.it (T.G.); catassi@tin.it (C.C.)

2 Interdisciplinary Department of Medicine, University of Bari, 70124 Bari, Italy;
E-Mail: rfrancavilla@gmail.com

3 Department of Pediatrics, "Sapienza" University of Rome, 00161 Roma, Italy;
E-Mail: Maria.Barbato@uniroma1.it

4 Neonatal Intensive Care Unit, Department of Clinical Sciences and Community Health, Fondazione IRCCS Ca' Granda Ospedale Maggiore Policlinico, University of Milan, 20122 Milano, Italy;
E-Mail: paola.roggero@unimi.it

5 Department of Pediatrics, S. Maria dell'Olmo Hospital Cava de' Tirreni, 84013 Salerno, Italy;
E-Mail: basiliomalamisura@libero.it

6 Pediatric Gastroenterology Unit, "G. Di Cristina" Children Hospital, 90134 Palermo, Italy;
E-Mail: stoai@inwind.it

7 R&D Heinz Italia S.p.A, 04100 Latina, Italy; E-Mail: Andrea.Budelli@it.hjheinz.com

8 Department of Epidemiology, Biostatistics and Medical Information Technology, Università Politecnica delle Marche, 60121 Ancona, Italy; E-Mail: r.gesuita@univpm.it

9 Department of Pediatrics, Università di Catania, 95123, Catania, Italy;
E-Mail: elenalionetti@inwind.it

* Author to whom correspondence should be addressed; E-Mail: simona.gatti@hotmail.it;

Abstract: A gluten-free diet (GFD) is currently the only available treatment for patients with celiac disease (CD). Several clinical trials have demonstrated that most celiac patients can tolerate a medium-high quantity of oats without any negative clinical effects; however, the inclusion of oats in GFD is still a matter of debate. In this study, Italian children with CD were enrolled in a 15-month, randomized, double-blind, placebo-controlled multicenter trial. Participants were randomized in two groups following either A-B treatment (6 months of diet "A", 3 months of standard GFD, 6 months of diet "B"), or B-A treatment (6 months of diet "B", 3 months of standard GFD, 6 months of diet "A"). A and B diets included gluten-free (GF) products (flour, pasta, biscuits, cakes and crisp toasts) with either purified oats or placebo. Clinical data (Gastrointestinal Symptoms Rate Scale [GSRS] score) and intestinal permeability tests (IPT), were measured through the study period. Although the study is still blinded, no significant differences were found in GSRS score or the urinary lactulose/mannitol (L/M) ratio between the two groups after 6 months of treatment. These preliminary results suggest that the addition of non-contaminated oats from selected varieties in the treatment of children with CD does not determine changes in intestinal permeability and gastrointestinal symptoms.

Keywords: oats; celiac disease; gluten-free diet; intestinal permeability; gastrointestinal symptoms

---

1. Introduction

Celiac disease (CD) is an immune-mediated disorder, triggered in genetically susceptible individuals by ingested gluten, the alcohol-soluble complex present in wheat, rye, and barley. The clinical spectrum of CD is extremely variable, including (a) typical CD, with the classical features of intestinal malabsorption; (b) atypical CD (characterized by extra-intestinal manifestations); (c) silent CD, (occasionally found following serological screening in subjects who are asymptomatic); (d) potential CD, showing positivity of celiac serology associated with a normal (or nearly normal) intestinal mucosa at the small intestinal biopsy. The cornerstone of treatment is the lifelong exclusion of gluten-containing cereals from the diet, the gluten-free diet (GFD).

Oats were originally excluded from the diet of people with CD. However, evidence supporting the toxicity of oats for CD individuals was poor. More recently, several studies have shown that medium-high amounts of gluten-uncontaminated oats can be safely ingested by patients with CD. In 1995, Finnish investigators compared the effect of 50–70 g/day of oats to placebo in 92 adults with CD on a GFD at diagnosis or in follow-up. They found no difference in clinical and laboratory outcomes and, more importantly, there was no sign of histological damage after 12 months of an oat-containing GFD [1]. These data have been replicated in other studies conducted in adults and children affected with CD or dermatitis herpetiformis [2–11], thereby confirming the safety of oat-based products for CD patients, provided that gluten contamination is avoided in the production chain. Recent studies suggest that some oats varieties may show a degree of residual toxicity *in vitro*, suggesting that there are differences between oat varieties in relation to their safety/toxicity for people with CD [12–16].

Official recommendations acknowledge the safety of products containing purified oats, and several national associations for CD allow inclusion of oats in the diet of people with CD [17,18]. The European Commission Regulation No. 41/2009 has included oats among allowed ingredients when the gluten content does not exceed 20 parts per million (ppm). During the last years, thousands of CD patients have been consuming large amounts of oat-based products in Northern European countries and Canada without any reported major side effects.

Oat is not a staple food in the diet of Mediterranean populations. This is probably the main reason why an oats "resurrection" in the GFD has not raised immediate interest in Southern European countries. In Italy, products containing gluten-uncontaminated oats are not currently available. This situation will hopefully change in the near future; rich in soluble dietary fiber, vitamins and minerals, the inclusion of oats unquestionably improves the nutritional value and increases the palatability of the GFD, while expanding food choices and ultimately improving the quality of life for people with CD [17].

For these reasons, we undertook a prospective, multicenter investigation on the safety and acceptance of gluten-free (GF) oat-based products from selected oat varieties in the diet of Italian CD children in treatment with the GFD. Clinical monitoring during the study was based on: (a) score of intestinal symptoms, (b) serological CD markers (IgA class anti-transglutaminase antibody), and (c) results of the double sugar intestinal permeability test (IPT), as a marker of mucosal integrity of the small intestine. In this work, we present the preliminary clinical and intestinal permeability results of this multicenter, placebo-controlled and double-blind study.

2. Patients and Methods

2.1. Study Population

Children (age range: 4–14 years) with biopsy-proven diagnosis of CD, on a GFD for at least 2 years, were recruited in 7 different Pediatric Gastroenterology Services in Italy (Ancona, Bari, Catania, Monza, Palermo, Roma, Cava de' Tirreni). Patients who (1) have other chronic conditions (including type 1 diabetes or inflammatory bowel disease), or (2) did not adhere to the GFD (as demonstrated by elevation of serological markers at enrollment) or (3) were on a GFD for less than 2 years were excluded.

2.2. Study Design and Diets

The protocol of the study is shown in Figure 1.

Clinical data (gastrointestinal [GI] symptoms, growth data) and IPT by measurement of urinary lactulose/mannitol (L/M) ratio were monitored at 0, 3, 6, 9, 12 and 15 months. Serological (IgA-antitransglutaminase-TTG, IgG-deamidated gliadin peptide-DGP, and anti-avenin antibodies) and biochemical data were measured at 0, 6, 9, and 15 months. An accurate food diary was completed in the 3 days preceding each visit at 3, 6, 12 and 15 months. Symptoms and/or side effects related to the ingestion of the products under investigation were promptly recorded and the decision to continue or withdraw from the study protocol was made after discussion with the children and their families.

In this preliminary report, we describe the GI symptoms and IPT findings after 6 months of participation in this study.

Figure 1. Flow-chart of the multicenter trial (t0: baseline, t3: 3-month follow-up, t6: 6-month follow-up, t9: 9-month follow-up, t12: 12-month follow-up, t15: 15-month follow-up; GSRS: Gastrointestinal Symptoms Rate Scale, IgA tTG: IgA class anti-transglutaminase antibody, IgG DGP: IgG class deamidated gliadin peptides antibody).

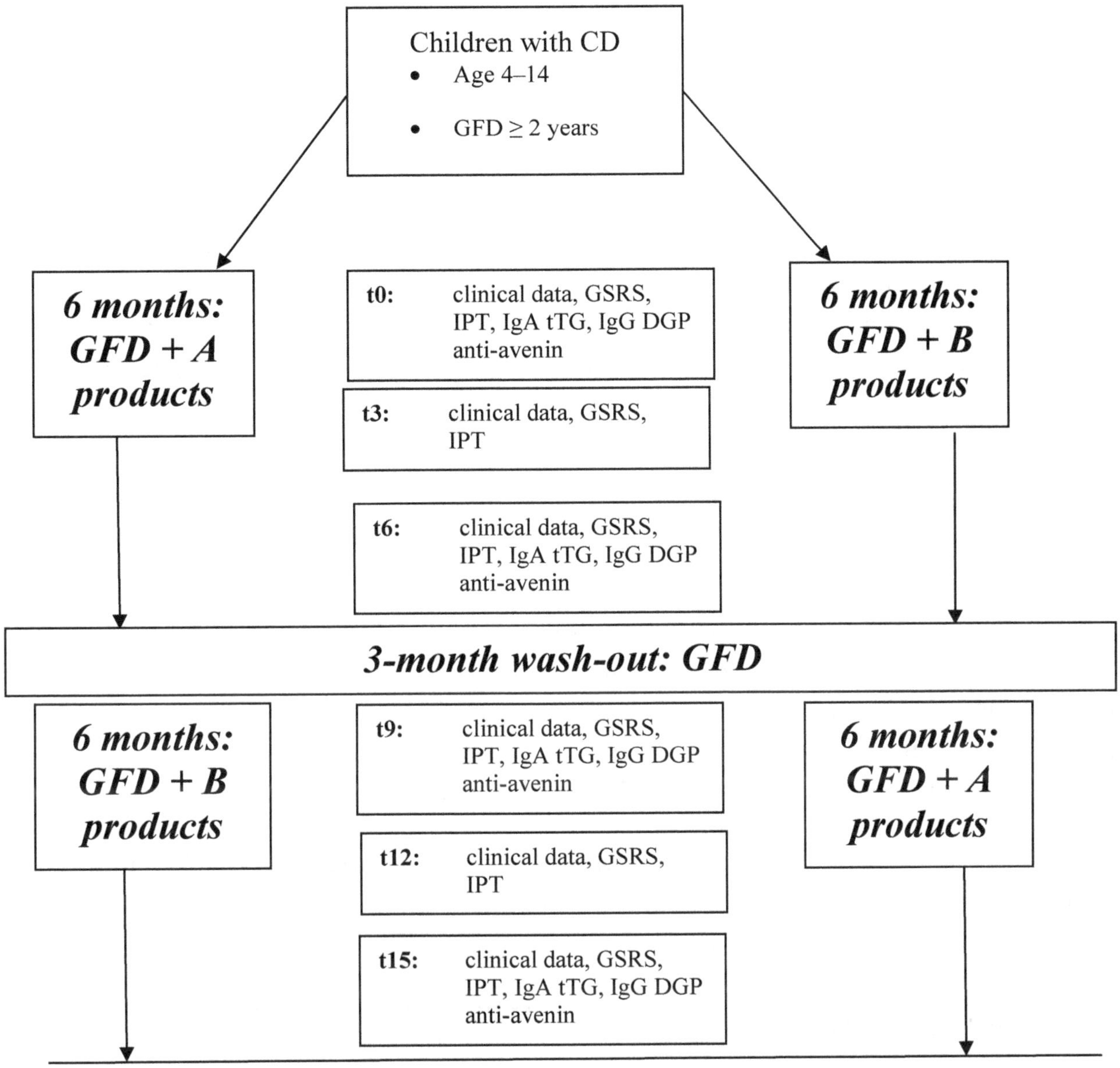

2.3. Methods

The occurrence of GI symptoms was monitored through the Gastrointestinal Symptoms Rate Scale (GSRS) at 0, 3, 6, 9, 12 and 15 months.

The IPT was performed as previously described [19]. After an overnight fast and bladder emptying, an oral solution containing 5 g of lactulose and 2 g of mannitol was administered. Urine was collected during the following 5 h. An aliquot was preserved at −20 °C with sodium azide. Urinary excretion of each sugar was assessed using a high performance anion-exchange Chromatography (Dionex DX-500). The ratio of recovered to ingested sugar was reported as ratio of lactulose% to mannitol% (L/M). According to our own reference values, a urinary L/M ratio > 0.08 was considered abnormal (data not published). All IPTs were performed in the Laboratory of the Department of Pediatrics, Università Politecnica delle Marche, Ancona.

2.4. Ethics

Patients and families received appropriate information and informed consent was obtained. The protocol was approved by the Ethical Committee of Università Politecnica delle Marche, Ancona. The trial was registered on www.clinicaltrials.gov (identifier: NCT00808301).

2.5. Statistical Analysis

Statistical analyses were performed using GraphPad Prism version 5 (GraphPad Software, San Diego, CA, USA). Non-parametric tests were used because variables were not normally distributed and did not have equal variance. Results are presented as median (interquartile range [IQR]). Differences between groups were assessed by the Mann-Whitney U test. The Wilcoxon matched pairs test was used to calculate the differences for pair data. A p value < 0.05 was considered significant.

3. Results

Overall, 306 children (group A-B: 154, group B-A: 152) were enrolled in the study (median age = 9.62, IQR = 7.23–11.9 years). Patients' enrollment was concluded in March 2013. Fifty-five out of 154 patients enrolled in group A-B (35.7%) and 42/152 patients in group B-A (27.6%) dropped out from the study within the first 6 months of treatment (p = 0.14). One hundred-seventy one children received at least 6 months of treatment, 75 patients received A treatment (group A), and 96 received B treatment (group B). Clinical and biochemical data from these subgroups were considered for the purpose of this preliminary analysis.

Table 1 summarizes clinical and demographic characteristics of the study-group at enrollment.

Table 1. Clinical and demographic features of children in group A and B at enrollment. M = males, F = females, IQR = interquartile range.

	Group A (*N* = 75)	**Group B (*N* = 96)**	***p***
Gender distribution (M:F)	1:2.5	1:1.9	0.50
Age at diagnosis Median (IQR)	3.48 (1.98–6.36)	2.84 (1.83–6.03)	0.38
Age at enrollment Median (IQR)	8.76 (7.07–11.38)	9.35 (7.24–12.01)	0.54
Duration of diet Median (IQR)	4.25 (2.11–6.04)	4.49 (1.25–6.55)	0.06
GSRS score at enrollment Median (IQR)	3 (0–5.25)	2 (0–4.5)	0.36
L/M at enrollment Median (IQR)	0.055 (0.030–0.083)	0.052 (0.026–0.088)	0.62

In both groups, a significant decrease in gastrointestinal symptoms was recorded through the 6-months period (Figure 2), with no differences detected comparing the delta-GSRS score (Δ-GSRS score) between the 2 groups (Figure 3).

Figure 2. GSRS score in group A and B at enrollment and after 6 months (median and IQR): in both groups a significant reduction in GI symptoms was observed.

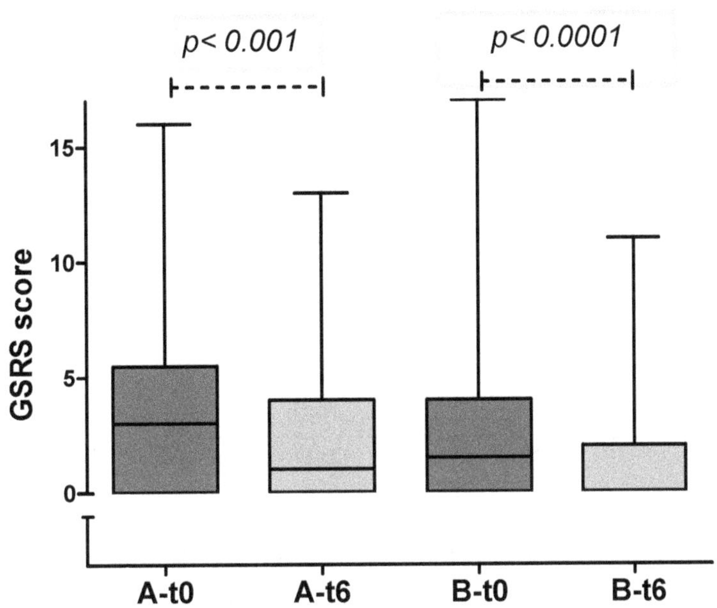

Figure 3. Change in GSRS score (Δ-GSRS score, median and IQR) between t6 and t0 in the 2 groups.

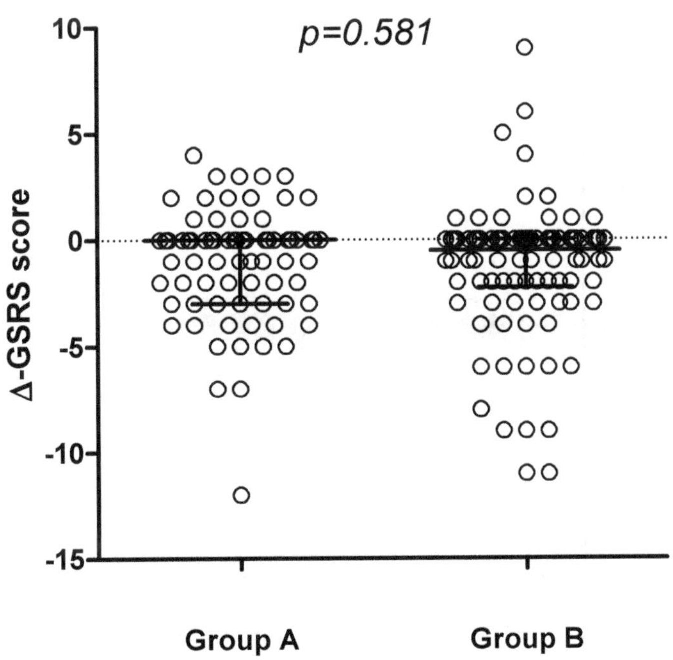

In both A and B groups, there was no significant change in urinary L/M ratio after 3 (data not shown) and 6 months of treatment (Figure 4).

Figure 4. Urinary L/M ratio in group A and B at t0 and t6 (median, IQR): in both groups no significant difference was observed after 6 months of treatment.

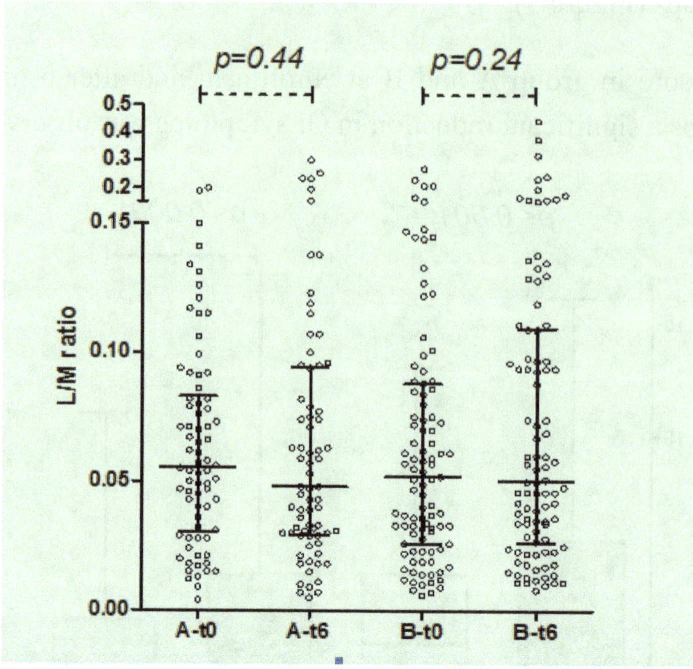

Furthermore, comparing the 6-month change in urinary L/M ratio (Δ-L/M), no difference was found between groups A and B, suggesting no relevant impact of a 6-month period of either oats or placebo-added GFD on the intestinal permeability test (Figure 5).

Figure 5. Comparison between t6 and t0 urinary L/M values in groups A and B (Δ t6-t0, median and IQR).

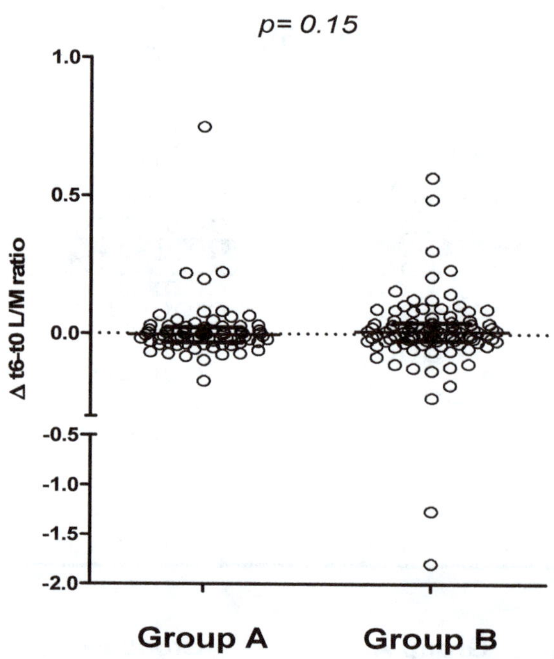

The 6-month Δ L/M value did not show a significant trend according to the different age groups (corresponding to different amount of oats or placebo) (Figure 6a,b).

Figure 6. Changes in L/M values (median, IQR) according to the 3 age classes, in groups A and B, respectively.

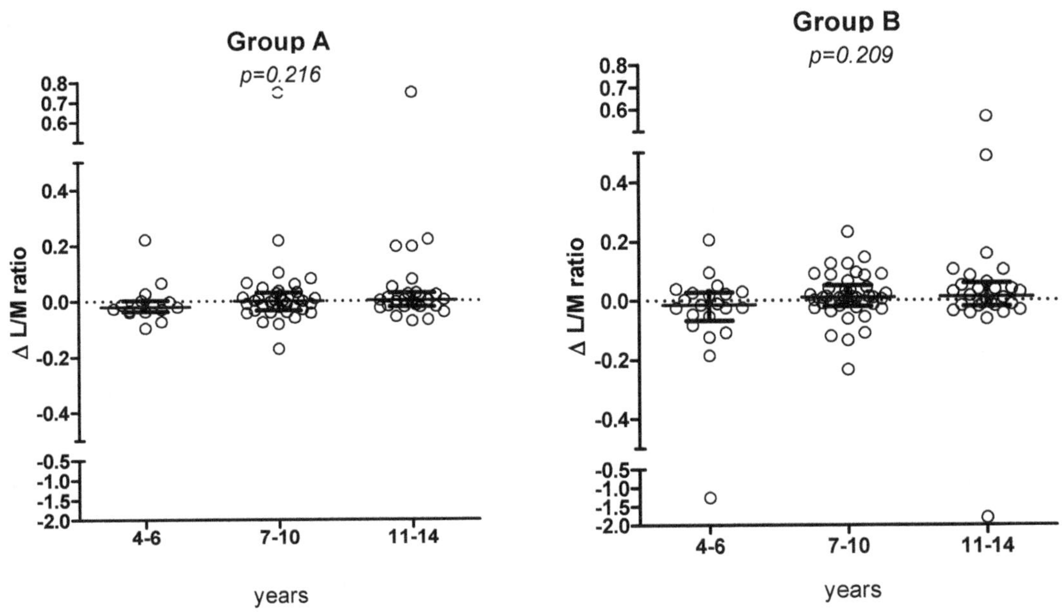

4. Discussion

In a large group of CD children that had not previously consumed oats, we found that the prolonged intake of a considerable amount of daily oats did not determine any relevant change in terms of clinical symptoms and intestinal permeability, even though the results were analyzed in a blind fashion.

Gastrointestinal symptoms were evaluated using the GSRS, that is an interview-based rating scale consisting of 15 items, validated and widely used for assessment of GI symptoms both in adults and children [20–24]. In both groups, there was a significant reduction in GI symptoms during the 6-month period of observation. Such a finding could simply reflect the effect of "being enrolled in a trial." The addition of non-contaminated oats from selected varieties in one of the two groups apparently had no impact on this clinical trend. Dyspeptic symptoms (described in other studies as related to the high amount of fiber in oats) were not recorded in our population. Although the number of dropouts was not significantly different in group A and B during the first 6 months of dietary intervention, the final analysis of this study, including reasons for withdrawal, will clarify the possible impact of oats ingestion on GI symptoms.

Besides a few exceptional cases reported in the literature [25], previous studies showed that the prolonged administration of oats does not induce any mucosal change at the intestinal level. Since performing repeated follow-up small intestinal biopsies was deemed unethical in our study, we evaluated the mucosal integrity by a non-invasive procedure, *i.e.*, the IPT. The integrity of the intestinal barrier can be evaluated by the IPT, by quantifying the amount of orally administered substances recovered in urine. Mannitol (monosaccharide) and lactulose (disaccharide) are largely used as permeability probes due to their different intestinal permeability index. Mannitol is absorbed through enterocyte membrane's pores (transcellular pathway), while lactulose is absorbed through tight junctions (paracellular pathway). Ratio between the percentage of lactulose and mannitol excretion represents the permeability index that reflects the intestinal epithelium integrity. The non-invasive functional IPT is a sensitive tool for both triage of active celiac disease, as well as for monitoring celiac patients on a GFD [26]. In patients with active CD, a sugar "paradox" pathway is usually observed: the amount of urinary recovered mannitol is decreased due to the small intestine reduced absorptive surface (villous atrophy), while urinary recovered lactulose is increased because of damage of the TJs and consequent widening of paracellular spaces. For these reasons, an increased excretion disaccharide/monosaccharide ratio is the usual finding associated with CD damage of the small intestinal mucosa. In adults with CD, the IPT has been shown to be more sensitive than serological methods in monitoring patients during follow-up and detecting minimal changes related to gluten ingestion [27,28]. Conversely, the same test was not a reliable instrument to detect asymptomatic CD subjects in a mass screening project [29]. Furthermore, IPT did not perform optimally in two recent trials of larazotide acetate in measuring changes in intestinal permeability after a 14-day [30] or 6-week [31] gluten challenge.

In our study, IPT was chosen as a non-invasive surrogate measure to detect minimal damages of the small intestinal mucosa at different time points. Thus far, no study has been performed to investigate the effects of prolonged oats ingestion on the intestinal permeability test in patients with CD. We did not find significant changes in urinary L/M ratio either in group A or B. This finding is further supported by the comparison of the Δ L/M in the two groups, again failing to show any difference between groups. However, the final results of our large study will give more information about the possible effect of oats ingestion on the results of the intestinal permeability. More data will also be available on the correlation between permeability indexes and serological CD markers.

The daily amount of suggested intake of oats products was calculated to guarantee medium-high amounts of oats (up to 40 g/day for older children). Although it was not possible to analyze the data according to the amount of ingested oats, the evaluation of the IPT results in the three age groups (corresponding to the different quantity of study products suggested) again showed no significant differences between groups. Overall, the lack of changes in intestinal permeability suggests that the varieties of gluten-uncontaminated oats chosen for production of these oat-based items are safe. The sample analyzed for the purpose of this analysis represents more than 50% of the enrolled study group. However, this analysis has not considered the original cross-over design of the protocol. Such a limitation implies caution in the interpretation of the results.

5. Conclusions

The preliminary results of this investigation suggest that the oats varieties used for producing the gluten-uncontaminated products used in this study are safe when administered for a 6-month period of time. These preliminary conclusions are based on both clinical data and the results of a non-invasive test for intestinal mucosa barrier function (IPT). The final analysis of the data collected in this study will provide conclusive data on the safety and the acceptance of these oat-based products in Italian children in treatment with the GFD.

Acknowledgments

The intervention trial "Oats products in the treatment of Coeliac Disesase in children" is sponsored by Heinz Italia S.p.A. (Latina, Italy). The authors wish to express their gratitude to all the members of the Italian Working Group on "Oats for Children with Celiac Disease, including: Michela Grilli (Department of Pediatrics, Università Politecnica delle Marche, Ancona); Lisa Tonelli (Department of Pediatrics, Università Politecnica delle Marche, Ancona); Claudia Fontana (Interdisciplinary Department of Medicine, University of Bari, Bari); Chiara Di Camillo (Department of Pediatrics, "Sapienza" University of Rome, Roma); Stefania Leoni (Department of Pediatrics, "Sapienza" University of Rome, Roma); Roberto Panceri (Department of Pediatrics, Ospedale di Monza, Monza); Tiziana Passaro (Department of Pediatrics, S. Maria dell'Olmo Hospital Cava de' Tirreni , Salerno); Sara Manferdelli (R&D Heinz Italia S.p.A, Latina); Alessia Grinzato (R&D Heinz Italia S.p.A, Latina); Flavia Carle (Department of Epidemiology, Biostatistics and Medical Information Technology, Università Politecnica delle Marche, Ancona); Mario La Rosa (Department of Pediatrics, Università di Catania, Catania).

References

1. Janatuinen, E.K.; Pikkarainen, P.H.; Kamppainen, T.A.; Kosma, V.M.; Jarvinen, R.M.; Uusitupa, M.I.; Julkunen, R.J. A comparison of diets with and without oats in adults with celiac disease. *N. Engl. J. Med.* **1995**, *333*, 1033–1037.
2. Srinivasan, U.; Leonard, N.; Jones, E.; Kasarda, D.D.; Weir, D.G.; O'Farrelly, C.; Feighery, C. Absence of oats toxicity in adult coeliac disease. *BMJ* **1996**, *313*, 1300–1301.
3. Hardman, C.M.; Gariogh, J.J.; Leonard, J.N.; Thomas, H.J.; Walker, M.M.; Lortan, J.E.; Lister, A.; Fry, L. Absence of toxicity of oats in patients with dermatitis herpetiformis. *N. Engl. J. Med.* **1997**, *337*, 1884–1887.
4. Reunala, T.; Collin, P.; Holm, K.; Pikkarainen, P.; Miettinen, A.; Vuolteenaho, N.; Mäki, M. Tolerance to oats in dermatitis herpetiformis. *Gut* **1998**, *43*, 490–493.
5. Hoffenberg, E.J.; Haas, J.; Drescher, A.; Bamhurst, R.; Osberg, I.; Bao, F. A trial of oats in children with newly diagnosed celiac disease. *J. Pediatr.* **2000**, *137*, 361–366.
6. Janatuinen, E.K.; Kemppainen, T.H.; Julkunen, R.J.; Kosma, V.M.; Maki, M.; Heikkinen, M.; Uusitupa, M.I. No harm from five year ingestion of oats in coeliac disease. *Gut* **2002**, *50*, 332–335.
7. Storsrud, S.; Olsson, M.; Arvidsson Lenner, M.; Nilsson, L.A.; Nilsson, O.; Kilander, A. Adult coeliac patients do tolerate large amounts of oats. *Eur. J. Clin. Nutr.* **2003**, *57*, 163–169.
8. Högberg, L.; Laurin, P.; Falth-Magnusson, K.; Grant, C.; Grodzinsky, E.; Jansson, G.; Ascher, H.; Browaldh, L.; Hammersjö, J.A.; Lindberg, E.; *et al.* Oats to children with newly diagnosed coeliac disease: A randomised double blind study. *Gut* **2004**, *53*, 649–654.

9. Holm, K.; Maki, M.; Vuolteenaho, N.; Mustalahti, K.; Ashorn, M.; Ruuska, T.; Kaukinen, K. Oats in the treatment of childhood coeliac disease: A 2-year controlled trial and a long-term clinical follow-up study. *Aliment. Pharmacol. Ther.* **2006**, *23*, 1463–1472.
10. Sey, M.S.; Parfitt, J.; Gregor, J. Prospective study of clinical and histological safety of pure and uncontaminated Canadian oats in the management of celiac disease. *J. Parenter. Enteral. Nutr.* **2011**, *35*, 459–464.
11. Cooper, S.E.; Kennedy, N.P.; Mohamed, B.M.; Abuzakouk, M.; Dunne, J.; Byrne, G.; McDonald, G.; Davies, A.; Edwards, C.; Kelly, J.; *et al.* Immunological indicators of coeliac disease activity are not altered by long-term oats challenge. *Clin. Exp. Immunol.* **2013**, *171*, 313–318.
12. Silano, M.; Di Benedetto, R.; Maialetti, F.; De Vincenzi, A.; Calcaterra, R.; Cornell, H.J.; De Vincenzi, M. Avenins from different cultivars of oats elicit response by coeliac peripheral lymphocytes. *Scand. J. Gastroenterol.* **2007**, *42*, 1302–1305.
13. Ballabio, C.; Uberti, F.; Manferdelli, S.; Vacca, E.; Boggini, G.; Redaelli, R.; Catassi, C.; Lionetti, E.; Penãs, E.; Restani, P. Molecular characterisation of 36 oat varieties and *in vitro* assessment of their suitability for coeliacs' diet. *J. Cereal Sci.* **2011**, *54*, 110–115.
14. Comino, I.; Real, A.; de Lorenzo, L.; Cornell, H.; López-Casado, M.Á.; Barro, F.; Lorite, P.; Torres, M.I.; Cebolla, A.; Sousa, C. Diversity in oat potential immunogenicity: Basis for the selection of oat varieties with no toxicity in coeliac disease. *Gut* **2011**, *60*, 915–922.
15. Real, A.; Comino, I.; de Lorenzo, L.; Merchán, F.; Gil-Humanes, J.; Giménez, M.J.; López-Casado, M.Á.; Torres, M.I.; Cebolla, Á.; Sousa, C.; *et al.* Molecular and immunological characterization of gluten proteins isolated from oat cultivars that differ in toxicity for celiac disease. *PLoS One* **2012**, *7*, e48365.
16. Mujico, J.R.; Mitea, C.; Gilissen, L.J.W.J.; de Ru, A.; van Veelen, P.; Smulders, M.J.M.; Koning, F. Natural variation in avenin epitopes among oat varieties: Implications for celiac disease. *J. Cereal Sci.* **2011**, *54*, 8–12.
17. Rashid, M.; Butzner, D.; Burrows, V.; Zarkadas, M.; Case, S.; Molloy, M.; Warren, R.; Pulido, O.; Switzer, C. Consumption of pure oats by individuals with celiac disease: A position statement by the Canadian Celiac Association. *Can. J. Gastroenterol.* **2007**, *21*, 649–651.
18. American Dietetic Association. Evidence-based nutrition practice guidelines on celiac disease. Available online: http://www.guideline.gov/content (accessed on 17 November 2013).
19. Generoso, M.; De Rosa, M.; De Rosa, R.; De Magistris, L.; Secondulfo, M.; Fiandra, R.; Carratù, R.; Cartenì, M.J. Cellobiose and lactulose coupled with mannitol and determined using ion-exchange chromatography with pulsed amperometric detection, are reliable probes for investigation of intestinal permeability. *J. Chromatogr. B Analyt. Technol. Biomed. Life Sci.* **2003**, *783*, 349–357.
20. Dimenas, E.; Glise, H.; Hallerback, B.; Hernqvist, H.; Svedlund, J.; Wiklund, I. Well-being and gastrointestinal symptoms among patients referred to endoscopy owing to suspected duodenal ulcer. *Scand. J. Gastroenterol.* **1995**, *30*, 1046–1052.
21. Dimenas, E.; Carlsson, G.; Glise, H.; Israelsson, B.; Wiklund, I. Relevance of norm values as part of the documentation of quality of life instruments for use in upper gastrointestinal disease. *Scand. J. Gastroenterol. Suppl.* **1996**, *221*, 8–13.

22. Lohiniemi, S.; Mäki, M.; Kaukinen, K.; Laippala, P.; Collin, P. Gastrointestinal symptoms rating scale in coeliac disease patients on wheat starch-based gluten-free diets. *Scand. J. Gastroenterol.* **2000**, *35*, 947–949.
23. Hallert, C.; Grännö, C.; Grant, C.; Hultén, S.; Midhagen, G.; Ström, M.; Svensson, H.; Valdimarsson, T.; Wickström, T. Quality of life of adult coeliac patients treated for 10 years. *Scand. J. Gastroenterol.* **1998**, *33*, 933–938.
24. Thomson, M.; Fritscher-Ravens, A.; Hall, S.; Afzal, N.; Ashwood, P.; Swain, C.P. Endoluminal gastroplication in children with significant gastro-oesophageal reflux disease. *Gut* **2004**, *53*, 1745–1750.
25. Arentz-Hansen, H.; Fleckenstein, B.; Molberg, Ø.; Scott, H.; Koning, F.; Jung, G.; Roepstorff, P.; Lundin, K.E.; Sollid, L.M. The molecular basis for oat intolerance in patients with celiac disease. *PLoS Med.* **2004**, *1*, e1.
26. Vogelsang, H.; Schwarzenhofer, M.; Oberhuber, G. Changes in gastrointestinal permeability in celiac disease. *Dig. Dis.* **1998**, *16*, 333–336.
27. Duerksen, D.R.; Wilhelm-Boyles, C.; Parry, D.M. Intestinal permeability in long-term follow-up of patients with celiac disease on a gluten-free diet. *Dig. Dis. Sci.* **2005**, *50*, 85–90.
28. Vilela, E.G.; Ferrari, M.L.; de Gama Torres, H.O.; Martins, F.P.; Goulart, E.M.; Lima, A.S.; da Cunha, A.S. Intestinal permeability and antigliadin antibody test for monitoring adult patients with celiac disease. *Dig. Dis. Sci.* **2007**, *52*, 1304–1309.
29. Catassi, C.; Fabiani, E.; Rätsch, I.M.; Bonucci, A.; Dotti, M.; Coppa, G.V.; Giorgi, P.L. Is the sugar intestinal permeability test a reliable investigation for coeliac disease screening? *Gut* **1997**, *40*, 215–217.
30. Kelly, C.P.; Green, P.H.; Murray, J.A.; Dimarino, A.; Colatrella, A.; Leffler, D.A.; Alexander, T.; Arsenescu, R.; Leon, F.; Jiang, J.G.; *et al.* Larazotide Acetate in patients with celiac disease undergoing a gluten-challenge: A randomized placebo-controlled study. *Aliment. Pharmacol. Ther.* **2013**, 37, 252–262.
31. Leffler, D.A.; Kelly, C.P.; Abdallah, H.Z.; Colatrella, A.M.; Harris, L.A.; Leon, F.; Arterburn, L.A.; Paterson, B.M.; Lan, Z.H.; Murray, J.A. A randomized, double-blind study of larazotide acetate to prevent the activation of celiac disease during gluten challenge. *Am. J. Gastroenterol.* **2012**, *107*, 1554–1562.

6

The Clinical Response to Gluten Challenge

Maaike J. Bruins

DSM Biotechnology Center, Alexander Fleminglaan 1, Delft 2613AX, The Netherlands;
E-Mail: maaike.bruins@dsm.com

Abstract: The aim of this review was to identify, evaluate and summarize all relevant studies reporting on the clinical response to gluten challenge by adult or pediatric patients with suspected or diagnosed coeliac disease (CD) on a gluten-free diet. We evaluated the effect of gluten challenge on changes in symptoms, intestinal mucosa histology, and serum antibodies. A systematic electronic search was performed for studies published as of 1966 using PubMed and Scopus databases. In the reviewed studies, doses ranged from 0.2 to 30 g/day of wheat gluten or comprised a gluten-containing diet. The onset of symptoms upon gluten intake varied largely from days to months and did not parallel serum antibody or histological changes. Within 3 months of gluten challenge, 70%–100% of pediatric CD patients became positive for AGA-IgA and EMA-IgA antibodies and 50%–70% for AGA-IgG. A limited number of trials suggest that no more than half of adult patients developed positive AGA-IgA, EMA-IgA, tTG-IgA or DGP-IgA/IgG titers. Approximately 50%–100% of pediatric and adult patients experienced mucosal relapse of gluten provocation within 3 months, which was preceded by increased mucosal intra-epithelial lymphocytes within several days of challenge. A 3-month high-dose gluten challenge should be suitable to diagnose the majority of CD patients. In some cases prolonged challenge may be needed to verify diagnosis. Combination testing for antibodies and mucosal histology may fasten the diagnosis.

Keywords: gluten challenge; coeliac disease; diagnosis

---

1. Introduction

Significant health complications may occur when coeliac patients remain on a normal gluten-containing diet. Diagnosis of coeliac disease (CD) should accurately be established before starting a person on a livelong gluten-free diet. In children and adults, diagnostic testing includes blood HLA-DQ2 and HLA-DQ8 testing, histological examination of small-intestinal biopsies and serum CD-specific antibodies [1–7]. The diagnosis is confirmed by decline in antibody levels after the exclusion of gluten from the diet. Clinical improvement and histological remission are also supportive clinical endpoint to confirm the disease. Gluten challenge is not necessary, except under unusual circumstances [4] where doubt exists about the initial diagnosis; for example, when the patient is on a gluten-free diet or presents with antibodies or complaints but, nonetheless, normal histology. Moreover, failure to respond to a gluten-free diet may raise doubt regarding the initial diagnosis. Examination of mucosal biopsy, however, involves a potential risk of misdiagnosis since it is subject to large method variability [8,9] and moderate-to-poor inter- and intra-observer reproducibility has been shown [10–12]. Unfortunately, histological findings in CD are characteristic but not specific as several disorders can produce comparable histopathological changes [13]. Over recent years, more reliable, specific and sensitive serological diagnostic tests and markers have become available. Small bowel histology remains the gold standard for diagnosis. Symptomatic relapse is not sufficient for a diagnosis of coeliac disease in isolation. Particularly in children in whom the initial biopsy was performed before two years of age, a gluten challenge may be necessary because of the risk of misdiagnosis due to confusion with other causes of enteropathy at this age [3]. In patients suspected of CD and following a gluten-free diet, diagnosis may be confirmed by reintroduction of gluten into the diet or by an oral gluten challenge followed by clinical relapse [3,4,7,14].

Currently, the monitoring of parameters during a gluten challenge is largely empirical, particularly in those patients who remain asymptomatic, and the optimum duration and dose of a gluten challenge has not been established yet. Some guidelines propose a gluten diet/challenge until relapse, even for up to 2 years or longer if patients remain symptom free. The ESPGHAN guidelines recommend that daily gluten intake during gluten challenge should contain at least the normal amount of gluten intake for children (approximately 15 g/day) [4,15]. There is considerable inter-individual variability of clinical presentation among patients with CD [16,17] but also in clinical response time to gluten intake [17]. The large variability and lack of predictability in the response time and severity to gluten complicate defining recommendations regarding the duration and dose of necessary gluten challenge in the diagnostic setting as well as the clinical trial setting.

A standardized approach regarding the amount and duration of dietary gluten necessary to provoke a clinical response in children and adults could provide guidance to physicians and investigators. Therefore, the aim of this article was to perform a review of the literature reporting on the course of the clinical symptoms, serum CD autoantibodies, and intestinal histological changes in response to a gluten challenge in children and adults with diagnosed or suspected CD.

2. Method

The data sources used for this systematic review of references published between 1966 and July 2013 included PubMed and Scopus. Only publications in English were included. We included studies that evaluated the effect of oral gluten challenge in individuals with CD on clinical parameters, *i.e.*, CD-specific antibodies, histology of small bowel mucosa biopsies, symptoms, and urinary sugar absorption test. We reviewed the studies that described the effect of a gluten challenge on clinical relapse in order to confirm diagnosis of CD in children or adults with diagnosed and/or suspected CD. We also extracted valuable information of patients receiving a gluten challenge in the placebo arm of clinical trials testing CD-related therapies. Gluten challenge studies with the aim to determine the safe threshold of prolonged exposure to trace amounts of gluten were beyond the scope of this paper. Studies reporting on positive anti-gliadin antibodies (AGA), anti-endomysial antibodies (EMA), anti-tissue transglutaminase antibodies (tTG), and anti-deaminated gliadin peptide antibodies (DGP) were included. Anti-reticulin antibodies were not reviewed as this test has nowadays been replaced by the more reliable AGA test. While AGA antibodies have been in use for several decades. However, there is a wide variability in their diagnostic accuracy and both AGA-IgA and AGA-IgG have sensitivities and specificities inferior to tTG-IgA and DGP-IgA and are no longer included in the routine testing strategy for CD [5]. Positivity for CD-specific antibodies was defined as concentrations above the assay cutoff value, which varied among assays used in the different studies. The definition of abnormal mucosa histology of small bowel biopsies also varied depending on the biopsy rating scores used (e.g., villous height to crypt depth ratio, Marsh scores). Clinical symptoms in most studies comprised CD-specific symptoms including vomiting, abdominal pain or distension, obstipation, diarrhea, fatty or loose stool, anorexia, weight loss, and growth failure. Only in the summary table we specified whether symptoms constituted mild, moderate or severe symptoms. Studies that were excluded were studies investigating a single-dose gluten challenge, studies investigating oat challenge, rectal gluten challenge, transamidated, hydrolyzed or digested gluten, gluten-specific peptides, and *ex-vivo* studies. Since gluten intake at baseline is likely to influence the response to a gluten challenge, we excluded studies in which patients were on a normal gluten-containing diet or had positive baseline autoantibodies at start. Trials were categorized into trials enrolling pediatric or adult patients with mean age below 18 years or 18 years and older, respectively. Moreover, less patients suspected of having CD can be expected to respond to gluten than patients with a confirmed diagnosis of CD. Therefore, we classified trials according to "confirmed diagnosis based on a biopsy in the past", or "diagnosed based on inadequate grounds" referring to as "suspected CD". If possibly, results were reported separately for subgroups of patients with diagnosed and suspected CD in one study. When the amount of dietary gluten in bread was not reported [18–20], we estimated the gluten content, assuming that a slice of bread weighs 25–30 g and contains 8–11 g/100 g of protein [15,21], which corresponds to approximately 2–3 g of gluten [7,22]. In some studies the gluten dose was expressed per kg of body weight. If body weight was not given, estimates were based on WHO child growth charts [23].

3. Results

Table 1 gives an overview of the included studies. In total, the following studies were identified that investigated the clinical effect of dietary gluten challenge; 16 trials with pediatric patients with biopsy-diagnosed CD, 13 trials with pediatric patients with suspected CD, 11 trials with biopsy-diagnosed adult CD patients and 3 with adolescent or adult patients suspected of having CD. Of the eleven trials with diagnosed adult patients, five reported on the clinical response to a placebo as part of a clinical intervention study [24–29]. In the studies included, a gluten challenge consisted of a gluten-containing diet, wheat-derived food products, wheat flour, or wheat gluten powder. The gluten doses ranged from 0.2 to 30 g/day and duration from 1 day to 8 years.

3.1. CD-Specific Symptoms in Pediatric Patients with Diagnosed or Suspected CD

The response rates and onset of symptoms throughout the course of gluten challenge in the different studies was highly variable (Table 1); when a gluten-containing diet was given to children with diagnosed CD, 4% of them developed symptoms within 1–2 of weeks [30]. At least 10 g/day of gluten caused symptoms in 13% of children within 12 h [31], 33% of children within 4 weeks of gluten challenge [32], and 60% of children within 3-months of challenge [33]. When given a gluten-containing diet or 3–15 g/day of gluten, 32% of children experienced symptoms within 4–5 months [34]. Smaller amounts of about 2 g/day of gluten caused symptoms in 4% children on the fourth day and in 25% of children after 6 months [18].

In children with suspected CD, a gluten-containing diet induced symptoms in about 26%–33% of children within between a few days to 13 months of gluten challenge [35,36], a gluten challenge of at least 10 g/day caused symptoms in approximately 24%–42% of children from 4 weeks to several [32,37–39] months of challenge, only few patients reported severe symptoms during gluten challenge [38]. A gluten-containing diet providing 5 to 15 g/day of gliadin caused symptoms in 59% of children within 45 days of challenge [40]. About 32% of adolescents with diagnosed or suspected CD who received at least 10 g/day of gluten for 2.4 months to 2 years experienced abdominal symptoms at the time of appearance of antireticulin-IgA [41]. In 70% of the cases, the mucosa relapsed before any symptoms had occurred [41]. Lower doses of 0.2–4.3 g/day of gluten, surprisingly triggered symptoms in 79% and 96% of children within 4 and 15 weeks, respectively [42]. No correlation was observed between time of appearance of symptoms and positive antibodies.

Summarizing, in most studies only few children with diagnosed or suspected CD respond by symptoms to a low or high gluten dose during the first 2 weeks. During prolonged low or high dose gluten challenge 24%–42% of children may experience symptoms, although in three studies higher response rates were reported of 60% [33,40], and even 96% [42]. Large variability exists in time of onset of symptoms during gluten challenge: symptoms appear almost immediately in some children while some do not develop symptoms until several months of challenge or develop no symptoms at all. Symptoms are generally mild to moderate. Some studies indicated that clinical symptoms are a very unreliable indicator of antibody response and mucosal relapse [34,41,42].

Table 1. The effect of a gluten challenge in pediatric or adult patients on response rate of clinical symptoms, serology, and histology parameters.

Author (year)	Age Group and Age	Diagnosed/ Suspected CD	Time on Gluten-Free Diet	Gluten Type and Dose	Duration of Challenge	CD-Symptoms	CD-Antibodies	Mucosal Immunohistology	Sugar Absorption Test
Mayer *et al.* (1989) [31]	Children 3.5^{Mdn} (1.8–9.6) years	Diagnosed by biopsy ($n = 37$)	≥1 year, 17^{Mdn} month	10 g/day gluten either as biscuit or as powder	60^{Mdn} (14–205) days	Acute symptoms in 13% (4/32) within 12 h and symptoms in 0% (0/31) within ~7 months	Increased AGA-IgA and IgG in 65% (20/31) within 15 days	Worsening histology score by Whitehead in 68% (21/31) at 2 month, 84% at 3 month, and 97% within 2 years	Decreased blood xylose within 15 days, remained low up to 150 day
Packer *et al.* (1978) [33]	Children 9.9^{M} (3.0–15.3) years	Diagnosed by biopsy (n =32)	6.5^{M} years (0.25–11.0)	≥10 g/day as 4 slices white bread	Up to 3 month	Symptoms in 60% (19/32) within 3 months		Increase in villous atrophy in 78% (25/32) within 3 months	
Hamilton *et al.* (1972) [18]	Children $7.2^{M} \pm 1.5^{SD}$ years	Diagnosed by biopsy ($n = 23$)	3.8^{M} years	2.25 g/day as wheat gluten followed by 1 slice/day of bread or equivalent flour (~2–3 g of gluten [1])	6 days 6 days–15 months	Symptoms in 4% (1/23) at 4 day, in 8% (1/12) at 1 month, in 25% (3/12) at 6 months		Mucosal lesions in 7% (1/13) within 6 days, 92% (11/12) within 1 year, and 100% within 15 months	
Mavromichalis *et al.* (1976) [43]	Children 6.5^{M} years	Diagnosed by biopsy ($n = 23$)	6.5^{M} year (1.5–10) ($n = 11$ on gluten-free diet)	20 g/day as gluten-containing diet	4–9 weeks			Worsening histology score (III or IV on scale I–IV) in 100% (11/11) within 4–9 weeks Increased IEL in 100% (11/11) within 4–9 weeks	

Table 1. *Cont.*

Hansson *et al.* (1997) [44]	Children 4^{Mdn} (1–18) years	Diagnosed by biopsy (ESPGAN) (*n* = 57)	(*n* = 20 on gluten-free diet)	gluten-containing diet (dose not mentioned)	2 weeks	Positive -AGA-IgA in 30% (6/20) within 2 weeks and 75% (21/28) within 12 weeks -AGA-IgG 15% (3/20) within 2 weeks and 71% (20/28) within 12 weeks -EMA-IgA 35% (7/20) within 2 weeks and 71% (20/28) within 12 weeks -AGA-IgA cells in peripheral blood in 75% (15/20) within 2 weeks and 86% (24/28) within 12 weeks	Increased IEL density in 25% (5/20) within 12 weeks
Hansson *et al.* (2002) [20]	Children 4^{Mdn} (1–16) years	Diagnosed by biopsy (ESPGAN) (*n* = 57)	(*n* = 21 on gluten-free diet and *n* = 38 on gluten-containing diet	2–3 slices/day of white bread (~4–9 g/day [1] of gluten)	12 weeks	Positive -AGA-IgA in 78% (31/40) within 2 weeks, 89% (41/46) within 12 weeks -EMA-IgA in 45% (18/40) within 2 weeks, 91% (42/46) within 12 weeks -tTG-IgA in 45% (18/40) within 2 weeks, 89% (41/46) within 12 weeks	Increased IEL density in 16% (6/38) within 12 weeks
Schaad *et al.* (1981) [45]	Children 8.1^{M} (3.1–13.1) years	Diagnosed	1.5–10 years	1 g raw cooked gluten/kg/day (~25 g gluten/day [1,2])	30 days		Increased IEL in 100% (22/22) at 30 day
Scott *et al.* (1980) [19]	Children 5.8^{Mdn} (2.9–8.8) years	Diagnosed by biopsy (*n* = 10)	-	One 20 g-slice/day of bread (~2 g/day [1] gluten) followed by gluten-containing diet	1 month of bread followed by gluten-containing diet up to 11 month		Mucosal relapse in 100% (10/10) within 2–11 months (7 $months^{Mdn}$) Increased IEL within 2–11 months

Table 1. *Cont.*

Bürginn-Wolff *et al.* (1991) [46]	Children 4 months–18 years	Diagnosed by biopsy ($n = 135$)	-	Gluten-containing diet (dose not mentioned)	Up to 15 year		Positive AGA-IgA in 97% (28/29) within 3 months, 85% (73/86) within 1 year, and 49% within ≥3 years EMA-IgA 65% (13/20) within 3 months, 84% (49/58) within 1 year, and 93% within ≥3 years	Abnormal mucosa in 72% (31/43) within 1 month, 94% (31/33) within 7–10 months, 95% (18/19) within 20 months
Ascher *et al.* (1990) [30]	Children 1.4 [Mdn] (0.5–16.5) years	Diagnosed by biopsy (ESPGAN) ($n = 45$)	1 year	Gluten-containing diet (dose not mentioned)	3–31 months	Strong symptoms in 4% (2/45) within 1–2 weeks	Positive AGA-IgA in 90% (38/42) of not-IgA deficient patients within 10 months	
Bodé *et al.* (1983) [47]	Children 2.8[Mdn] (0.3–15.5) years	Diagnosed by biopsy (ESPGAN) ($n = 14$)	≥1 year	≥10 g/day (type not mentioned)	3 months–2 years		Positive AGA-IgG in 79% (11/14) within 3 months–2 years AGA-IgA in 57% (8/14) within 3 months–2 years	
Danielsson *et al.* (1990) [48]	Children ~2[M] (1–5.6) years	Diagnosed by biopsy ($n = 67$)	0.9–1.4 years	10 g/day as gluten-containing diet	0.5–4.4 years			Abnormal histology score (II–IV on scale I–IV) in 96% (64/67) within 2 years
Berg *et al* (1997) [34]	Children ~1 year	Diagnosed by biopsy ($n = 34$)	1–1.5 years	Gluten-containing diet or 3–15 g/day of gluten		Symptoms in 32% (11/34) within 4–5 months		Abnormal histology in 100% (23/23) in patients without symptoms within 4–5 months

Table 1. *Cont.*

Troncone *et al.* (1994) [37]	Children 7.3^{M} (4.9–9.8) years	Suspected (n = 6) and diagnosed by biopsy (n = 9)	6 years^{Mdn} (3–8)	10 g/day as biscuits or pasta	30^{Mdn} days (14 days–6 months)	Symptoms in 42% (5/12) within 6 months	Positive AGA-IgA in ~AGA-IgA in ~50% at 2 weeks, ~25% at 1 month, ~50% at 2 month, ~70% at 3 month, 57% within 6 months AGA-IgG in ~10% at 1 month, ~25% at 2 month, ~50% at 3 month, 29% within 6 months EMA-IgA in ~77% (10/13) at 1 month, 93% within 6 months		Increased urinary cellulose/mannitol ratio in 86% (12/14) within 3 months
Korponay-Szabó *et al.* (1997) [38]	Children 5.1^{Mdn} (1.9–15.3) years	Suspected (n = 67) and diagnosed by biopsy (ESPGAN) (n = 90)	Not reported	5–10 g/day as purified gluten	6 weeks–2 years	-Mild symptoms in 34.3% (46/134) -Severe symptoms in 2.9% (4/134) of patients with histological relapse within 6 weeks–2 years	Positive EMA-IgA or -IgG in 66% at 3 month, 90% at 6 month, and 88% (134/153) within 21 months	Abnormal histology score (scale I-III by Fontaine and Navarro) in 88% (134/153) within 2 years. Relapse time (A + B) 5^{Mdn} month (1.8–26.5) and (C) 6^{Mdn} month (1.4–25.3)	
Rolles *et al.* (1976) [32]	Children 5.7^{M} (1.5–15) years	Suspected (n = 35)	4.2^{M} (1–10) years	20 g/day as gluten powder	4–13 weeks	Mild to severe symptoms in 29% (10/35) within 4–13 weeks		Abnormal histology score (scale 3 or 4 on 0–4) in 51% (18/35) within 4–13 weeks	
Lancaster *et al.* (1976) [49]	Children 11.5^{M} (5–16.5) years	Suspected (n = 16)	6.9^{M} (1.5–13) years	10 g/day as wheat protein	Up to 24 month			Decrease in Vh in 62% (10/16) within 3 months, in 81% (13/16) within 3–24 months Increased in IEL density in 100% (13/13) within 3 months	

Table 1. *Cont.*

Laurin *et al.* (2002) [42]	Children 3.8^{Mdn} (2.7–8.8) years	Suspected ($n = 25$)	≥1 year	1.4^{Mdn} g/day (0.2–4.3) as gluten-containing diet	13^{Mdn} week (5 week–1 year)	Symptoms in 79% within 4 weeks, 96% (23/24) within 15 weeks	Positive -AGA-IgA in 25% (5/20) within 4 weeks, 75% within 8 weeks -AGA-IgG in 0% (0/19) within 4 weeks, 5% (5/20) within 8 weeks -EMA-IgA in 65% (13/20) within 4 weeks, 75% within 8 weeks -EMA-IgG in 16% (3/19) within 4 weeks, 25% (5/20) within 8 weeks	-Abnormal histology score (3 or 4 on scale 0–4 by Marsh) in 91% (21/23) within 1 year -Increased IEL count in 96% (22/23) within 1 year
Laurin *et al.* (2003) [50]	Children 3.8^{Mdn} (2.7–8.8) years	Suspected ($n = 25$)	≥1 year	1.4^{Mdn} g/day (0.2–4.3) as gluten-containing diet	Up to 3 month		Positive -AGA-IgA in 90% (16/18) within 8 weeks -EMA-IgA in 90% within 8 weeks	
Valletta *et al.* (1990) [40]	Children 3.8^{M} (2.7–8.8) years	Suspected ($n = 17$)	0.4–8 years	Gluten-containing diet with 5, 10, 15 g/day gliadin at age 1–3, 3–5, and 5–10 years, respectively	20–45 days	-Symptoms in 59% (10/17) -Food refusal in 100% (17/17) within 45 days	Positive -AGA-IgA in 94% (16/17) within 15–35 days -EMA-IgA in 90% within 2 months	-Worsening histology in 94% (16/17) within 25–45 days -Increased IEL score in 100% (17/17) within 25–45 days
Jansson *et al.* (2001) [51]	Children 2.7^{M} ± 1^{SD} years	Suspected ($n = 54$)	≥1 year	Gluten powder 0–4 weeks: 0.2 g/kg/day (~2.6 g/day [1,3]) (A) 0.5 g/kg/day (~6.5 g/day [1,3]) (B) 4–8 weeks: 0.5 g/kg/day (~6.5 g/day) (A and B)	4–8 weeks		A and B: Positive -AGA-IgA in 76% (38/50) at 2 week, 88% at 4 week, 94% at 8 week no difference between A and B -EMA-IgA in 59% (32/54) at 2 week, 65% at 4 week, 67% at 8 week no difference between A and B	A and B: Worsening histology score (≥3 increase on scale 4–16) in 94% (51/54) at 4 week and 100% at 8 week

Table 1. *Cont.*

Wauters *et al.* (1991) [39]	Children 5.6^{M} (2–16) years	Suspected (n = 17)	46^{M} months (10–168)	Gluten powder: 750 mg/kg bw/day (~14 g/day [4]) with max 20 g/day	3 months	Symptoms in 24% (4/17) within 3 months	Positive -AGA-IgA in 90% (9/10) within 6 weeks, and 100% (7/7) within 12 weeks -AGA-IgG in 90% (9/10) within 6 weeks, and 100% (7/7) within 12 weeks	Villous atrophy in 59% (10/17) within 12 weeks	
Savilahti *et al.* (1983) [35]	Children 1.6^{M} years	Suspected (n = 19)	0.7–2.3 years	Gluten-containing diet (dose not mentioned)	0.1–1.1 year	Symptoms in 26% (5/19) within 0.1–1.1 year	Positive AGA-IgA in 73% (11/15) within 0.1–1.1 year	Abnormal mucosa in 95% (18/19) within 0.1–1.1 year	
Rolles *et al.* (1975) [52]	Children 0.5–5.7 years	Suspected (n = 16)	0.1–5 years	20 g/day as gluten powder	Up to 1.5 year	Symptoms in 33% (5/15) within 28 days		Histology score (3 or 4 on scale 0–4) in 80% (4/5) within 1.5 years	Decreased blood xylose in 40% (6/15) within 1 day, 67% (10/15) within 2–7 days, and 100% (15/15) within 14–28 days
Bonamico *et al.* (2005) [36]	Children and adolescents 9.2^{M} (5.4–19) years	Suspected (n = 24)		Three gluten-containing meals/day (n = 24)	up to 2 month	Symptoms after *in vivo* challenge in 33% (8/24) within few days–2 months	Positive EMA-IgA in 63% (15/24) within 2 months	Abnormal histology score (3 on scale 0–3 by Marsh) in 87% (13/15) within 2 months	
Mäki *et al.* (1989) [41]	Adolescents 16.6^{M} (14.3–22.1) years	Suspected (n = 9) and diagnosed by biopsy (ESPGAN) (n = 20)	~8^{M} years (3.0–16.0)	≥10 g/day as gluten-containing diet	Up to 2 year	Symptoms in 32% (7/22) anti-reticulin positives within 2.4–24 months	Positive -AGA-IgA in 79% (23/29) within 2.4–24 months -AGA-IgG in 62% (18/29) within 2.4–24 months	Lower Vh in 85% (23/27) within 2.4–24 months. 15% (4/27) did not relapse in 2 years	

Table 1. *Cont.*

Lancaster-Smith *et al.* (1975) [53]	Adults	Diagnosed by biopsy ($n = 11$)	4.3 (1–15) years	25 g as single gluten dose ($n = 8$) or 10 or 20 g/day as gluten-containing diet ($n = 4$)	Single-dose (A) 7 days (B)			A: Increased IEL in 24–48 h B: Increased IEL in 100% within 1 week	
Lähdeaho *et al.* (2011) [54]	Adults: 49^{Mdn} (21–68) years	Diagnosed by biopsy ($n = 21$)	11^{Mdn} (2–34) years	1–3 g/day (biscuits) (A) 3–5 g/day (biscuits) (B)	12 weeks	A: Symptoms in 64% (7/11) within 3 months B: Symptoms in 80% (8/10) within 3 months	A: Positive tTG-IgA in 36% (4/11) within 12 weeks B: Positive tTG-IgA in 50% (5/10) within 12 weeks	A: decreased Vh/Cd in 64% (7/11) within 12 weeks A: Increased IEL in 55% (6/11) patients within 12 weeks B: decreased Vh/Cd ratio in 70% (7/10) within 12 weeks B: Increased IEL in 80% (8/10) patients within 12 weeks	
Leffler *et al.* (2012) [24]	Adults $43^{M} \pm 14^{SD}$ years	Diagnosed by biopsy ($n = 20$)	5 years	3 or 7.6 g/day (bread)	2 weeks	Increased symptom severity at 3 day, 1 and 2 week	Positive -tTG-IgA in 25% (5/20) within 2 weeks (increase to 50% 2 weeks post-challenge) -DGP-IgA/IgG in 30% (6/20) within 2 weeks	Abnormal histology score (3 or 4 on scale 0–4 by Marsh) in 68% (13/19) within 2 weeks Increased IEL within 2 weeks	Increase in urinary lactulose:mannitol ratio within 2 weeks
Montgomory (1988) [55]	Adults 40^{M} (17–74) years	Diagnosed by biopsy ($n = 13$ on GFD)	13^{Mdm} (6–27) months	2.5–5 g/day	14 months		Positive AGA-IgA in 17% (11/13) within 3–14 months	Increased Vh within 14 months: no effect Increased IEL within 14 months	

Table 1. *Cont.*

Brottveit (2011) [56]	Adults 41^M (16–65) years	Diagnosed by biopsy (*n* = 13 on GFD)	13.9 (0.8–31.6) years	40 g/day (four slices bread)	3 days			Abnormal histology score (3 or 4 on scale 0–4 by Marsh) in 23% (4/13) within 3 days	
Daveson (2011) [57]	Adults 44^M (25–58) years	Diagnosed by biopsy (*n* = 10 on GFD in control group)	≥6 months	16 g/day (two slices bread)	5 days			Abnormal histology score (3 or 4 on scale 0–4 by Marsh) in 70% (7/10) within 1 week Increased IEL at 1 week	
Cornell *et al*. (2005) [25]	Adults 18–70 year	Diagnosed by biopsy (*n* = 21 on placebo)	Not reported	3 Cracker biscuits (~1.3 g/day gluten)	2 weeks	>5 Episodes of moderate-to-severe symptoms in 33% (7/21) on placebo within 2 weeks challenge and the following 10 week	Positive tTGA >5 U/mL in 19% (4/21) within 2 weeks and 3–15 weeks post-challenge	-Increased lymphocyte score in 83% (5/6) at 2 week -Increased epithelial stunting in 50% (3/6) at 2 week	
Tye-Din *et al*. (2010) [26]	Adults 41^Mdn (21–67) years	Diagnosed by biopsy (*n* = 10 on placebo)	≥8 weeks	16 g/day Wheat flour slurry	3 days	Symptoms increased within 1 week, 75% of symptoms were mild	No positive tTGA and DGP-IgA/IgG at 6 day		
Kelly *et al*. (2013) [27]	Adults 18–65 years	Diagnosed by biopsy (*n* = 44 on placebo)	≥6 weeks	2.7 g/day Gluten powder (3 × daily 0.9 g)	6 weeks	Symptoms increased in 80% within 6 weeks. Plateau at 3 week	Positive tTG-IgA > 10 U/mL in 30% (13/44) at 6 week		Increase in urinary lactulose:mannitol ratio. Plateau at 4 week

Table 1. *Cont.*

Leffler *et al.* (2012b) [28]	Adults 18–72 years	Diagnosed by biopsy (*n* = 14 on placebo)	≥6 weeks	2.4 g/day Gluten powder (3 × daily 0.8 g)	2 weeks	Symptoms increased in 50% within 2 weeks	No positive tTG-IgA at 2 week		Increase in urinary lactulose:mannitol ratio at 2 week
Tack *et al.* 2010 [58]	Adults 55^{Mdn} (20–68) years	Diagnosed by biopsy (*n* = 7 on placebo)	7.5 (2–40) years	7 g/day (5 toasts)	2 weeks	Symptoms increased in 43% (3/7) within 2 weeks	Positive -tTG-IgA in 14% (1/7) -AGA-IgA in 14% (1/7) -AGA-IgG in 14% (1/7) No positive EMA-IgA within 2 weeks	-Increased tTG-IgA deposits in 71% (5/7) -Abnormal histology score (3 or 4 on scale 0–4 by Marsh) in 23% (2/7) Within 2 weeks	
Kumar *et al.* (1979) [59]	Adolescents 16.1^{M} (14–21) years Adults: 37.7^{M} (17–59) years	Suspected (*n* = 28)	Adolescents: 6.4^{M} (1–14) years Adults: 2.8^{M} (0.75–7) years	≥4 Slices bread (~10 g/day gluten)	Adolescents 4–17.5 weeks (23^{Mdn}) Adults: median 4–25.5 weeks (11.5^{Mdn})	Adolescents: Symptoms in 67% (6/9) within 1 h–2 weeks, no symptoms in 33% within 1 year Adults: Symptoms in 84% (16/19) within 4 days–3 months, no symptoms in 16% within 1 year		Adolescents: Decreased Vh in 56% (5/9) within 8 weeks, 100% within 10 momths Increased IEL in 100% within 10 months Adults: Decreased Vh in 95% (18/19) within 7 weeks, still 95% within 1 year Increased IEL in 95% within 7 weeks	
Wahab (2001) [60]	Adults 40^{M} (16–74) years	Suspected (*n* = 37)		30 g/day on top of GCD	2 months	Symptoms in 55% (17/38) within 3 months	Positive AGA-IgA in 22% (8/37) within 2 months Positive EMA-IgA in 17% (4/23)within 2 months	Abnormal histology score (2, 3 or 4 on scale 0–4 by Marsh) in 32% (12/38) at 2 month	
Kaukinen *et al.* (2005) [61]	Adults 45^{M} (19–70) years	Suspected (*n* = 21)	Not reported	≥15 g/day (5 Slices of bread)	6 months			-Increased tTG-IgA deposits in 24% (5/21)	

Abbreviations: CD: Coeliac Disease, Vh: villous height, Cd: crypt depth, M: mean; Mdn: median; SD: standard deviation. [1] Assumption made as described in the Methods. [2] Assuming an 8-years old child weighs 25 kg. [3] Assuming a 2.7-years old child weighs 13 kg. [4] Assuming a 5.6-year old child weighs 19 kg.

3.2. CD-Specific Symptoms in Adults with Diagnosed or Suspected CD

In three studies, effects were reported of gluten challenge on symptoms in diagnosed or suspected adult or adolescent CD patients [54,59,62]. In five clinical trials [25–28,58], the effects of gluten challenge given to diagnosed adult patients in the placebo arm were reported. Reintroduction of a gluten-containing diet induced gastrointestinal symptoms in 77% of patients suspected of CD between 1 and 8 months of challenge and CD was confirmed in 40% of these patients [62]. The diagnosis CD was nevertheless confirmed in 65% of the 33% patients who did not develop symptoms. Symptoms occurred in 67% of patients with confirmed diagnosis of CD. When diagnosed or suspected CD patients received 7 to 10 g/day of gluten, 43% [58] and 67% [59] reported symptoms within two weeks of challenge. Within 3 months 84% had experienced symptoms [59]. Most symptoms occurred after one week of challenge [59]. After a 2-week and 6-week challenge period with about 2.5 g/day of gluten three times daily, about 50% of patients [28] and 80% of patients [27] reported complaints, respectively. The severity of symptoms increased after 2 weeks [27,28] reaching a plateau at 3 weeks [27]. When diagnosed CD patients received a low (1–3 g/day) or a high (3–5 g/day) dose of gluten, 64% and 80% of them, respectively, reported symptoms within 3 months [54]. A 2-week challenge of ~1.3 g/day of gluten triggered symptoms in 66% of patients the following 12 weeks; about 33% had more than five episodes of moderate to severe symptoms [25].

In summary, the number of adult patients reporting symptoms as well as the severity of symptoms may increase throughout gluten challenge. Within 3 months of gluten challenge, about 64%–80% of adult patients can be expected to experience symptoms. A proportion of patients with CD may never develop symptoms during gluten challenge. The onset of symptoms is rather unpredictable. The appearance of symptoms during gluten challenge is no indicator of CD.

3.3. Antibodies in Pediatric Patients with Diagnosed or Suspected CD

3.3.1. AGA-IgA and AGA-IgG Antibodies

Figure 1 illustrates the time course of children with diagnosed or suspected CD responding to a gluten challenge by positive AGA-IgA antibodies.

The proportion of children with diagnosed or suspected CD responding to gluten challenge by AGA-IgA antibodies varied widely. After 2 weeks, about 30% to 78% of children had responded to a challenge providing 3 to 15 g/day of gluten [20,31,44,63,64]. After 2 to 3 months of challenge with 4 to 14 g/day of gluten, about 70%–100% of children showed positive AGA-IgA antibodies in their serum [20,44,46,63,64]. No clear dose-response effect was observed between the different studies. In two studies with a low dose of gluten (0.2–4.3 g/day), the percentage of children responding by AGA-IgA was 90% [50] or 75% after 2 months [42]. Within 10 months to 1 year, 73%–90% of children had developed AGA-IgA antibodies [30,35,46]. Interestingly, the percentage of CD children with AGA-IgA was highest (97%) after a gluten consumption period of about 1 to 3 months and decreases thereafter to 85% at 1 year, and 49% after 3 years or more of gluten intake [46].

Figure 1. Percentage of pediatric patients with diagnosed or suspected coeliac disease (CD) showing an anti-gliadin antibodies (AGA)-IgA response to gluten over time.

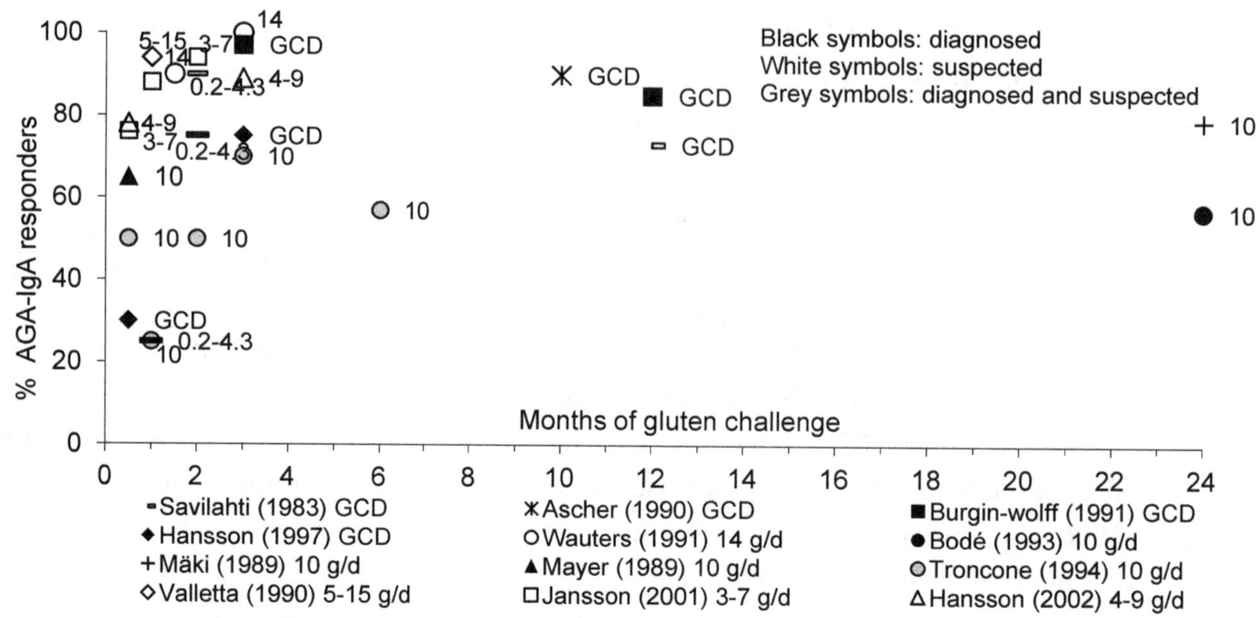

Figure 2 shows the proportion of diagnosed or suspected CD children responding with positive AGA-IgG antibodies to a gluten challenge.

Figure 2. Percentage of pediatric patients with diagnosed or suspected CD showing an AGA-IgG response to gluten over time.

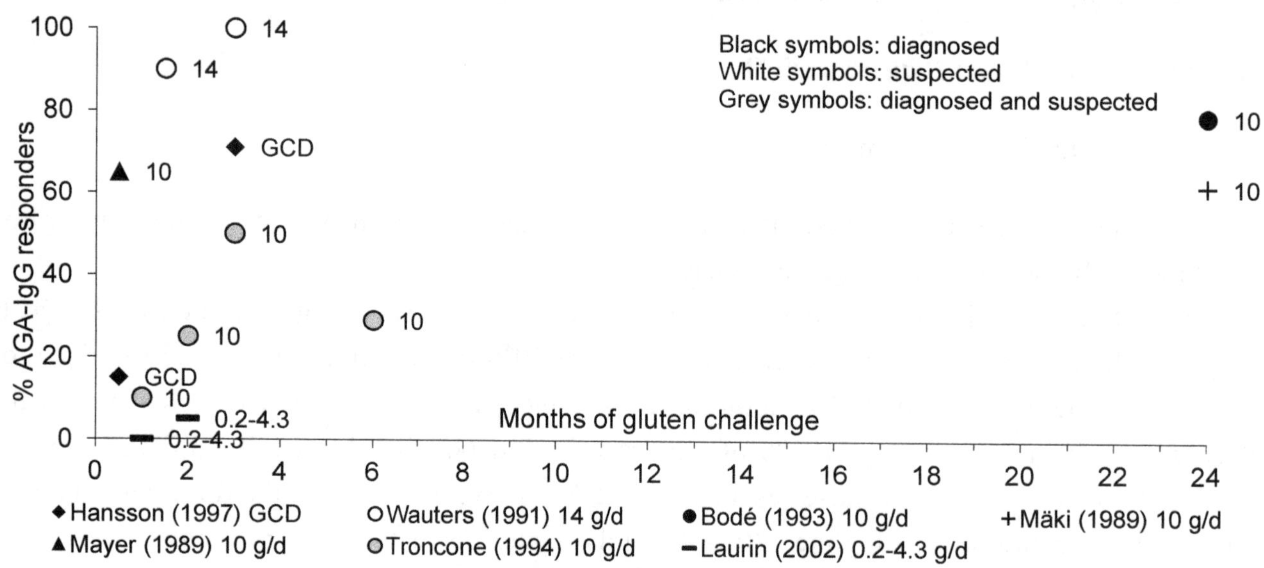

Whereas most studies showed less children responding by AGA-IgG than by AGA-IgA throughout the course of gluten challenge [41,42,44,63], two studies showed similar response rates by AGA-IgA and AGA-IgG [31,39]. When children with CD were given a gluten-containing diet or 10 to 14 g/day of gluten, AGA-IgG rose significantly in 15% [44] or 65% [31] of children within 2 weeks and in 71%–100% of children within 3 months of challenge [39,44]. In two studies in which children received 10 g/day [63] or 0.2–4.3 g/day [42] of gluten, only 25% and 5% of children had responded by AGA-IgA after 2 months of gluten challenge, respectively.

3.3.2. EMA-IgA Antibodies

Figure 3 summarizes the proportion of children with diagnosed or suspected CD developing positive EMA-IgA during gluten challenge.

Figure 3. Percentage of pediatric patients with diagnosed or suspected CD showing an anti-endomysial antibodies (EMA)-IgA response to gluten over time.

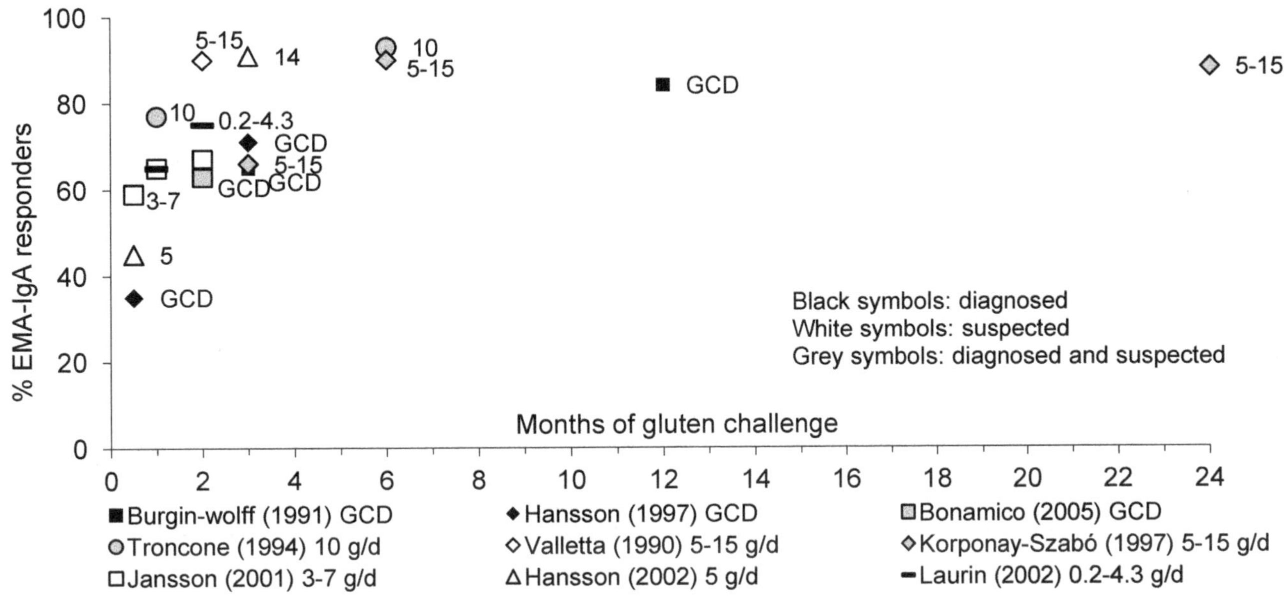

In a number of trials with children with diagnosed or suspected CD, results on serum EMA-IgA levels were reported during gluten challenge doses from 0.2 to 15 g/day of gluten or a gluten-containing diet. After 2 weeks of challenge, 35% to 59% of children showed positive EMA-IgA antibodies [20,36,40,42,44,46,63–65], 65% to 77% of children after 1 month [42,51,63], between 63% and 100% of children became EMA-IgA positive between 2 and 3 months [20,36,38,40,42,44,46,51], while 84% to 93% of children had become positive from 6 months to 3 years of challenge [38,46,63]. Even small gluten amounts caused relapse by EMA-IgA [42]. There was no clear difference in time to EMA-IgA positivity between the different gluten doses.

3.3.3. tTG-IgA Antibodies

In one study, diagnosed CD children received 4–9 g/day of gluten [20]; positive tTG-IgA levels were detected in 45% and 89% of children within 2 and 12 weeks, respectively.

3.3.4. Antibodies in Pediatric Patients: Summary

In summary, the time it takes for children to relapse by antibodies with a gluten challenge is variable. Moderate-to-high gluten challenge doses given to children with diagnosed or suspected CD increased

AGA-IgA, AGA-IgG and EMA-IgA to positive levels within the first few weeks. Within 3 months of challenge, the majority of children had developed AGA-IgA, AGA-IgG, EMA-IgA or tTG-IgA antibodies. Only few children relapsed by AGA-IgA, AGA-IgG and EMA-IgA after 1 year. No clear difference in relapse rate to gluten was observed between children with diagnosed and suspected CD. Conversion of AGA-IgA positive to negative tests has been reported to occur in some patients.

3.4. Antibodies in Adult Patients with Diagnosed or Suspected CD

3.4.1. AGA-IgA and EMA-IgA Antibodies

In four trials, AGA-IgA antibody titers in gluten-challenged adult patients with suspected or diagnosed CD were reported [26,29,55,60]. The AGA-IgA titers increased in 14% of diagnosed patients in the placebo arm after a 2-week 7 g/day gluten challenge [58] and in 85% of diagnosed patients receiving 2.5–5 g/day of gluten for up to 14 months [55]. Increased AGA-IgA was observed in 22% of borderline patients receiving 30 g/day on top of a normal diet for up to 2 months [60], None of the diagnosed CD patients receiving 16 or 7 g/day of gluten developed positive EMA-IgA antibodies within 2 weeks [29,58]. In borderline patients, 17% became EMA-IgA positive after a 2-month very high-dose gluten challenge [60].

3.4.2. tTG-IgA and DGP-IgA/IgG Antibodies

Figure 4 shows diagnosed adult CD patients responding by tTG-IgA throughout gluten challenge.

Figure 4. Percentage of adult patients with diagnosed CD showing a tTG-IgA response to gluten over time.

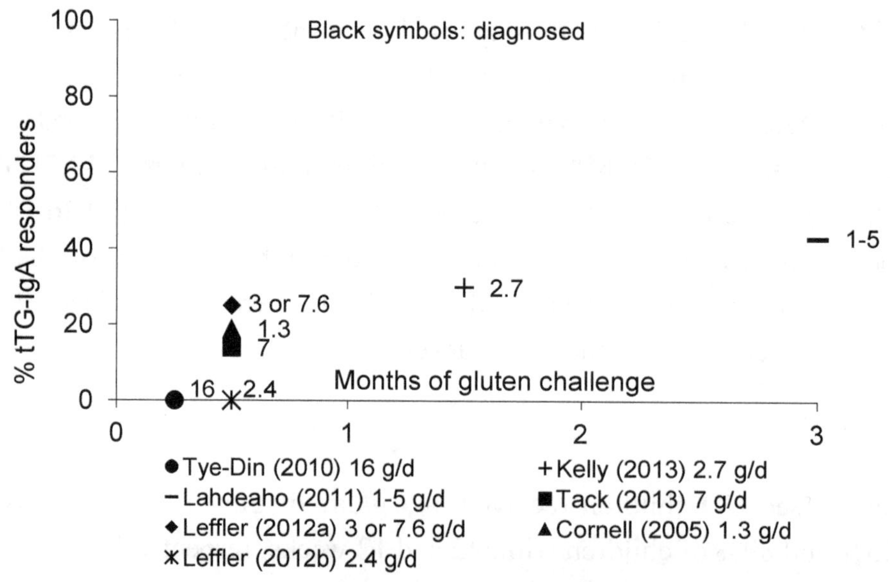

The effects of gluten challenge on tTG-IgA titers in diagnosed adult CD patients were reported either [24–29] or not [54] as part of a clinical trial. No positive tTG-IgA antibodies were observed at day 6 post-challenge in any of the diagnosed CD patients receiving 16 g of gluten for 3 days [26]. After a 2-week challenge with a dose from 1.3 to 7.6 g/day of gluten, tTG-IgA increased in

0% to 25% of adult diagnosed CD patients [24,25,28,29]. Longer gluten challenge form 6 weeks to 3 months increased the proportion of tTG-IgA-positive patients to 30%–43% [27,54]. A 3-day gluten challenge of 16 g/day did not increase DGP-IgA/IgG titers at day 6 [26], but 3 or 7.5 g/day induced positive DGP-IgA/IgG titers in 30% of diagnosed patients within two weeks and 45% the following two weeks [24].

3.4.3. Antibodies in Adult Patients: Summary

In summary, few diagnosed CD patients responded by AGA-IgA, EMA-IgA, tTG-IgA, or DGP-IgA/IgG antibodies after 2 weeks of gluten challenge. Within 6 weeks to 3 months of gluten challenge, still no more than 50% of patients became positive for these antibodies.

3.5. Mucosal Immunohistology in Pediatric Patients with Diagnosed or Suspected CD

3.5.1. Mucosal IEL

When children with diagnosed or suspected CD received 5 to 25 g/day of gluten, 91% to 100% of them developed increased mucosal IEL within 1 to 2 months [40,42,43,45,50]. Within 3 months of gluten challenge with 10 g/day, all children with suspected CD showed increased mucosal IEL counts [49]. In one study less children, 16% to 25%, responded with increased IEL within 3 months of about 6 g/day of gluten challenge [20,44]. The authors of one study found that the gluten intake dose strongly correlated with the degree of inflammation in the biopsy, as expressed by IEL [42]. A gluten challenge increased IEL in mucosal biopsies before histological changes occurred.

3.5.2. Mucosal Histology

Figure 5 gives an overview of children with diagnosed or suspected CD developing changes in mucosal morphology throughout gluten challenge.

The proportion of children with diagnosed or suspected CD having abnormal mucosal histology gradually increased during the course of gluten challenge. Only 7% of children with diagnosed CD developed mucosal lesions after 1 week when a gluten challenge of 2–3 g/day of gluten was given [18]. However, when doses of 3 to 20 g/day of gluten were given, the proportion of children developing an abnormal small bowel mucosal histology scores within 1 month ranged from 72% to 100% [43,46,64]. Mucosal relapse rates after 2 to 3 months of challenge ranged between 51% and 100% [31–33,36,39,49,64]. After 5 months to 2 years of gluten challenge, the majority of children have relapsed by mucosal abnormalities, with relapse rates of 79% to 100% reported in the different studies [18,19,31,33,34,41,42,46,48,49,52]. After 1 year low-dose gluten challenge (0.2 to 4.3 g/day gluten), the proportion of children showing abnormal small bowel mucosal histology scores did not differ from those receiving a higher dose challenge (5 g/day or higher). For some children it took 2 or even 8 years to relapse on gluten [48]. As expected, the intestinal mucosa relapse rate was higher in diagnosed than in suspected patients: within 3 months of gluten intake, respectively, about 60% and 80% had relapsed.

Figure 5. Percentage of pediatric patients with diagnosed or suspected CD showing histological response to gluten over time.

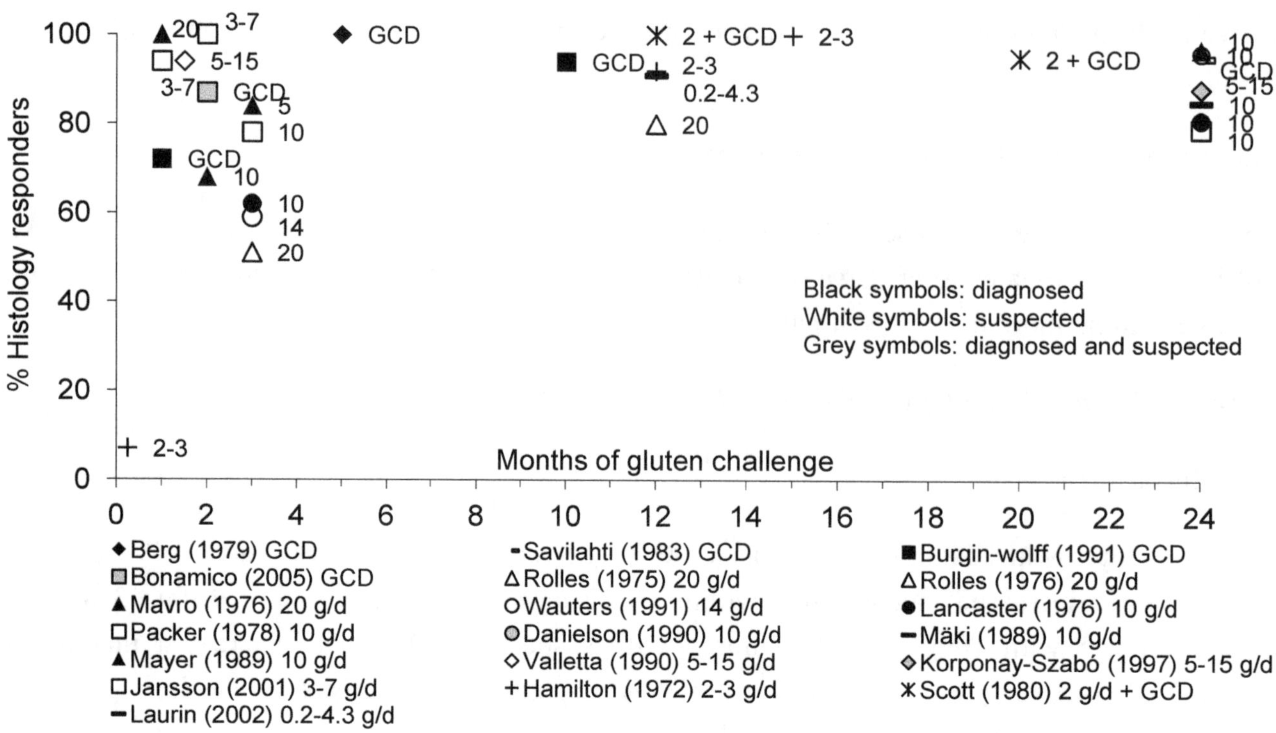

3.5.3. Mucosal Immunohistology: Summary

In summary, within 1 month of gluten exposure, mucosal IEL counts were increased in almost all children with diagnosed or suspected CD. The percentage of children developing moderate to severe mucosal histological abnormalities within 2 to 3 months of gluten challenge ranged between 51%–100%. When child patients are biopsied after one week of challenge, only a minority show morphological relapse. The majority of children will have relapsed after 2 to 3 months of challenge, and only few children relapse thereafter.

3.6. Mucosal Immunohistology in Adult Patients with Diagnosed or Suspected CD

3.6.1. Mucosal IEL

A single 25-g gluten challenge given to adult patients with proven CD increased IEL in the mucosal biopsy as soon as 24–48 h following challenge [49]. A one-week 10 to 20 g gluten-containing diet increased IEL density in the mucosal biopsy of all patients [49,57]. Lower gluten doses (3–7.6 g/day) also increased mucosal IEL of patients within 2 weeks [24]. Gluten challenges of 10–25 g/day increased mucosal IEL counts in 95% to 100% of adult or adolescent patients with diagnosed or suspected CD within 1 to 2 months [59], and 3 to 14-months [55,59]. Increased IEL were found in 55% and 80% of diagnosed CD patients receiving, respectively, 1–3 g/day and 3–5 g/day of gluten for 3 months [54].

3.6.2. Mucosal Histology

Figure 6 illustrates the proportion of adult diagnosed or suspected CD patients responding by abnormal small bowel mucosal histology throughout a gluten challenge.

Figure 6. Percentage of adult patients with diagnosed or suspected CD showing histological response to gluten over time.

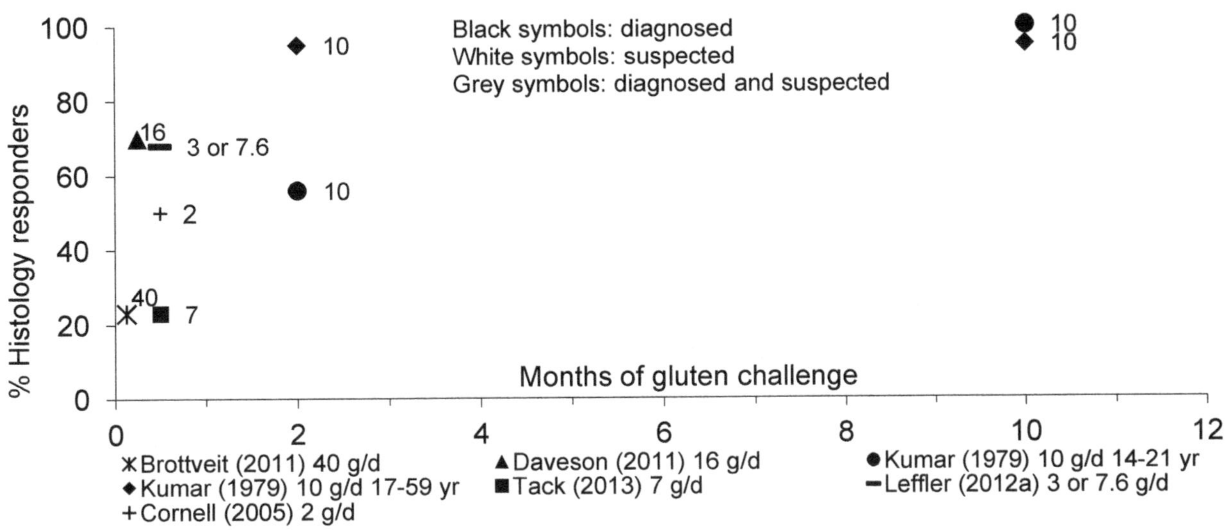

Increased biopsy Marsh scores were observed in 23% of diagnosed CD patients receiving 40 g/day of gluten for 3 days [56], and in 70% of diagnosed CD patients receiving 16 g/day of gluten for 5 days [57]. Gluten doses between 1 and 7 g/day induced abnormal histology scores in 23% to 68% of adult diagnosed CD patients within 2 weeks [24,25,29], and 67% of patients within 3 months [54]. In adolescents and adult patients with suspected CD, 10 g/day of gluten triggered mucosal relapse in 56% and 95% of them within 2 months, and 95% and 100% of them within 1 year, respectively [59]. Less patients with borderline CD may respond to gluten; 32% showed abnormal histology scores within 2 months of high-dose gluten challenge [60].

3.6.3. Mucosal tTGA-IgA Deposits

A gluten challenge of at least 15 g/day for 6 months induced positive tTGA-specific mucosal IgA deposits in 24% of suspected CD patients [61].

3.6.4. Mucosal Immunohistology: Summary

In summary, the results of gluten challenge on mucosal histology in adult patients are variable. More than two weeks of high-dose gluten challenge may be required to induce small intestinal mucosal morphology changes in the majority of patients. However, IEL can appear as early as 1 to 2 days after gluten challenge with increased counts in all patients after 4 weeks. Mucosal tTGA-IgA deposits is another marker appearing in the majority of patients within 2 weeks of challenge.

4. Discussion

4.1. Strength and Weaknesses

To our knowledge, this is the first review giving an overview of gluten challenge studies in patients suffering from CD or suspected of having CD and the consequences on symptoms, mucosal damage and CD-specific antibodies. In this review, we excluded studies with patients who were on a regular gluten diet at the time of challenge, as their response to gluten may be lower and not representative for patients on a gluten-free diet. This review has, however, several limitations. The gluten challenges used in all studies were wheat-derived and hence, findings relate to wheat gluten. There is very limited data looking at the effect of barley hordein or rye secalin on CD outcomes in the published literature (e.g., [66,67]), but evidence exists that these prolamins induce effects different to wheat gluten, at least at an immunologic level. Moreover, the quoted gluten amounts in the publications were mostly estimates and probably not accurate. In a few studies, gluten amounts were analyzed by R5 ELISA probably providing better estimates. Although several studies looked at the effect of gluten challenge in pediatric patients, the number of studies with adult patients is limited. The clinical response to gluten is most likely larger in diagnosed CD patients than in patients suspected of having CD in whom part may not have CD. Nevertheless, the results for both groups were combined in the figures. Furthermore, the participants in the different studies convey a heterogeneous group with respect to age, gluten dose, and time on a gluten-free diet, and criteria for diagnosis and are therefore difficult to compare. Also methodologies for measurement of antibodies, biopsies, and histology were different including the cutoff levels used to define antibody or histological positivity. Another limitation is that in most studies in the seventies to nineties, AGA-IgA and AGA-IgG antibodies were most commonly measured. However, particularly AGA-IgA has a poor sensitivity compared to newer antibodies such as EMA-IgA, tTG-IgA, and DGP-IgA/IgG which may have resulted in an underestimation of the patients responding to gluten by positive AGA-IgA titers.

4.2. Occurrence of Symptoms in Response to Gluten

Until recently, no proper guidelines for categorizing symptoms were available, making it difficult to compare the symptoms reported in the different studies. Moreover, symptoms in response to gluten are not CD-specific as approximately half of non-coeliac patients also show exacerbation of symptoms during gluten challenge [62]. Gastrointestinal symptoms are not specific for CD. The predictive value of symptoms after gluten re-introduction or gluten challenge is very low [34,38,39,41,62]. In one study the positive predictive value of symptoms for having CD was 52% [62]. In diagnosed adult patients, the symptom response rate seems to range somewhere between 65% and 85% [26,59] and most symptoms seem to occur within 1 to 2 weeks [26,59]. Less children (24%–42%) than adults (64%–80%) reported symptoms throughout prolonged gluten challenge but this may strongly depend on the methodology used in the different studies.

In summary, symptoms upon gluten challenge are hard to predict and have low positive predictive value. Recently, a validated disease-specific symptom index for coeliac disease was developed, but it remains to be established whether this can be used as an independent outcome measure for the monitoring of coeliac disease [68].

4.3. Occurrence of Antibodies in Response to Gluten

The CD-specific antibody and mucosal response is more predictable than the appearance of symptoms. Nevertheless, considerable variation between patients exists in the time to serological relapse on gluten [17]. On average, about 70%–100% of diagnosed pediatric CD patients given a moderate to high-dose gluten challenge will have responded by AGA-IgA, EMA-IgA, and tTG-IgA antibodies within 3 months of moderate-to-high gluten intake. Less children responded to gluten by AGA-IgG than by AGA-IgA. Compared to diagnosed patients, slightly less patients suspected of CD developed positive antibodies, but the majority had responded by 3 months. Also low dose prolonged gluten challenge caused serological or histological relapse in children with (suspected) CD [25,69]. In these studies, mucosal changes to gluten correlated with the gluten dose given, suggesting a dose-dependent response to gluten. Histological relapse occurred faster in children receiving a larger gluten dose in children with diagnosed CD [51,70], also suggesting a dose-response effect. Therefore, when testing serological antibodies during gluten challenge of approximately 15 g/day on a 3 to 6 monthly basis as recommended by the current ESPGHAN recommendations [4], most cases of CD should be detected. While the majority relapses in three months, for a few patients it may take longer to relapse, and in rare cases it may take years to relapse. Conversion to antibody negativity during prolonged gluten intake has been reported, suggesting that in rare cases gluten tolerance may develop [46,71].

In adult patients, the few available studies suggest that no more than half of the patients develop positive serum antibodies (AGA-IgA, EMA-IgA, tTG-IgA, and DGP-IgA/IgG) in response to a 6-week to 3-month gluten challenge. The few available studies suggest that the AGA-IgA and EMA-IgA response rates of adult CD patients to high-dose gluten challenge was very low. This suggests a lower response in diagnosed adult than pediatric patients. Whether this lower antibody responsiveness to gluten in adults is due to a longer period of gluten withdrawal remains to be established.

4.4. Occurrence of Histological Changes in Response to Gluten

About 50% to 100% of children with diagnosed or suspected CD developed moderate to severe mucosal histological abnormalities within 2 to 3 months of gluten challenge. Comparable response rates were reported for adult patients. As can be expected, the average 3-month relapse rate in patients with diagnosed CD was generally higher than those with suspected CD. Some patients may still show histological relapse on gluten challenge continuing up to 1 or 2 years.

The earliest stages of gluten challenge include increased density of IEL in the mucosa, crypt hyperplasia, and finally, the development of villous atrophy [72], which was confirmed by the reviewed data. The gluten challenge studies showed that mucosal IEL infiltrates respond fast to gluten (days to weeks) whereas the CD-associated antibodies and mucosal morphological deterioration appeared later within weeks to years. In some studies, relapse by abnormal histology of the small bowel biopsy paralleled positive antibodies [38,40,41,51]. In other studies, antibodies and primarily AGA-IgA preceded the worsening of mucosal histology [30,31,39,46] whereas in one study the mucosal changes preceded serum EMA-IgA positivity during gluten challenge [36]. The AGA-IgA antibodies may appear earlier than EMA-IgA during gluten challenge [37,46]. Both in adults and children, symptoms were unpredictable and did not coincide with histological or serological relapse.

Within one month of gluten challenge, serological and histological relapse does not occur in all cases during challenge [31,32]. In contrast, increased mucosal IEL were reported in almost all diagnosed pediatric and adult patients within 1 month of gluten challenge [43,45,49,53]. High IEL counts in the mucosa are therefore a fast and sensitive marker of responsiveness to gluten although not specific for CD [42,73–75]. In addition, mucosal tTG-IgA deposits are considered to appear rapidly in response to gluten and are both a sensitive and specific marker of early stage CD present in biopsy samples with normal mucosal architecture [61,76]. Although not reviewed in this paper, tetramer staining of gluten-specific T-cells may be supportive in the diagnosis of CD due to the fast appearance after start of a gluten challenge [77].

5. Conclusions

To diagnose pediatric patients with suspected CD on a gluten-free diet, a moderate-to-high dose gluten challenge for up to 3 months should be sufficient to induce changes in mucosal histology and antibodies in the majority of patients. In adults on a gluten-free diet, histological and serological relapse rates to gluten may be slower and prolonged challenge may be considered if no relapse is observed. Moreover, testing for combinations of conventional and new early markers with high sensitivity and specificity will significantly shorten the time of gluten challenge to diagnose CD.

Acknowledgments

The author is an employee of DSM Biotechnology Center (Delft, The Netherlands). The author would like to acknowledge Sheryl Roumen (DSM Biotechnology Center) who substantially contributed to searching the literature and compiling the data.

References

1. Coeliac Disease: Recognition and Assessment of Coeliac Disease, 2009. Available online: http://www.nice.org.uk/nicemedia/pdf/cg86fullguideline.pdf (accessed on 7 August 2013).
2. Richey, R.; Howdle, P.; Shaw, E.; Stokes, T.; Guideline Development Group. Recognition and assessment of coeliac disease in children and adults: Summary of NICE guidance. *BMJ* **2009**, *338*, b1684.
3. Walker-Smith, J.A.; Guandalini, S.; Schmitz, J.; Shmerling, D.H.; Visakopi, J.L. Revised criteria for diagnosis of coeliac disease. Report of Working Group of European Society of Paediatric Gastroenterology and Nutrition. *Arch. Dis. Child* **1990**, *65*, 909–911.
4. Husby, S.; Koletzko, S.; Korponay-Szabo, I.R.; Mearin, M.L.; Phillips, A.; Shamir, R.; Troncone, R.; Giersiepen, K.; Branski, D.; Catassi, C.; *et al.* European society for pediatric gastroenterology, hepatology, and nutrition guidelines for the diagnosis of coeliac disease. *J. Pediatr. Gastroenterol. Nutr.* **2012**, *54*, 136–160.

5. Rubio-Tapia, A.; Hill, I.D.; Kelly, C.P.; Calderwood, A.H.; Murray, J.A.; American College of Gastroenterology. ACG clinical guidelines: Diagnosis and management of celiac disease. *Am. J. Gastroenterol.* **2013**, *108*, 656–676.
6. Hill, I.D.; Dirks, M.H.; Liptak, G.S.; Colletti, R.B.; Fasano, A.; Guandalini, S.; Hoffenberg, E.J.; Horvath, K.; Murray, J.A.; Pivor, M.; *et al.* Guideline for the diagnosis and treatment of celiac disease in children: Recommendations of the North American society for pediatric gastroenterology, hepatology and nutrition. *J. Pediatr. Gastroenterol. Nutr.* **2005**, *40*, 1–19.
7. Murch, S.; Jenkins, H.; Auth, M.; Bremner, R.; Butt, A.; France, S.; Furman, M.; Gillett, P.; Kiparissi, F.; Lawson, M.; *et al.* Joint BSPGHAN and Coeliac UK guidelines for the diagnosis and management of coeliac disease in children. *Arch. Dis. Child* **2013**, *98*, 806–811.
8. Catassi, C.; Fasano, A. Is this really celiac disease? Pitfalls in diagnosis. *Curr. Gastroenterol. Rep.* **2008**, *10*, 466–472.
9. Ravelli, A.; Bolognini, S.; Gambarotti, M.; Villanacci, V. Variability of histologic lesions in relation to biopsy site in gluten-sensitive enteropathy. *Am. J. Gastroenterol.* **2005**, *100*, 177–185.
10. Corazza, G.R.; Villanacci, V.; Zambelli, C.; Milione, M.; Luinetti, O.; Vindigni, C.; Chioda, C.; Albarello, L.; Bartolini, D.; Donato, F. Comparison of the interobserver reproducibility with different histologic criteria used in celiac disease. *Clin. Gastroenterol. Hepatol.* **2007**, *5*, 838–843.
11. Corazza, G.R.; Villanacci, V. Coeliac disease. *J. Clin. Pathol.* **2005**, *58*, 573–574.
12. Weile, B.; Hansen, B.F.; Hagerstrand, I.; Hansen, J.P.; Krasilnikoff, P.A. Interobserver variation in diagnosing coeliac disease. A joint study by Danish and Swedish pathologists. *APMIS* **2000**, *108*, 380–384.
13. Freeman, H.J. Refractory celiac disease and sprue-like intestinal disease. *World J. Gastroenterol.* **2008**, *14*, 828–830.
14. Guidelines for the Management of Patients with Coeliac Disease. British Society of Gastroenterology. Available online: www.bsg.org.uk (accessed on 8 April 2013).
15. United States Department of Agriculture, Agricultural Research Service. USDA National Nutrient Database for Standard Reference, Release 26. Available online: http://ndb.nal.usda.gov/ (accessed on 24 October 2013).
16. Setty, M.; Hormaza, L.; Guandalini, S. Celiac disease: Risk assessment, diagnosis, and monitoring. *Mol. Diagn. Ther.* **2008**, *12*, 289–298.
17. Akobeng, A.K.; Thomas, A.G. Systematic review: Tolerable amount of gluten for people with coeliac disease. *Aliment. Pharmacol. Ther.* **2008**, *27*, 1044–1052.
18. Hamilton, J.R.; McNeill, L.K. Childhood celiac disease: Response of treated patients to a small uniform daily dose of wheat gluten. *J. Pediatr.* **1972**, *81*, 885–893.
19. Scott, H.; Ek, J.; Baklien, K.; Brandtzaeg, P. Immunoglobulin-producing cells in jejunal mucosa of children with coeliac disease on a gluten-free diet and after gluten challenge. *Scand. J. Gastroenterol.* **1980**, *15*, 81–88.
20. Hansson, T.; Dahlbom, I.; Rogberg, S.; Dannaeus, A.; Hopfl, P.; Gut, H.; Kraaz, W.; Klareskog, L. Recombinant human tissue transglutaminase for diagnosis and follow-up of childhood coeliac disease. *Pediatr. Res.* **2002**, *51*, 700–705.

21. Dutch Food Composition Database Online Version 2013/4.0. Available online: http://www.rivm.nl/en/Topics/Topics/D/Dutch_Food_Composition_Database (accessed on 24 October 2013).
22. Van Overbeek, F.M.; Uil-Dieterman, I.G.; Mol, I.W.; Köhler-Brands, L.; Heymans, H.S.; Mulder, C.J. The daily gluten intake in relatives of patients with coeliac disease compared with that of the general Dutch population. *Eur. J. Gastroenterol. Hepatol.* **1997**, *9*, 1097–1099.
23. World Health Organisation. The WHO Child Growth Standards. Available online: http://www.who.int/childgrowth/en/ (accessed on 7 August 2013).
24. Leffler, D.; Schuppan, D.; Pallav, K.; Najarian, R.; Goldsmith, J.D.; Hansen, J.; Kabbani, T.; Dennis, M.; Kelly, C.P. Kinetics of the histological, serological and symptomatic responses to gluten challenge in adults with coeliac disease. *Gut* **2012**, *62*, 996–1004.
25. Cornell, H.J.; Macrae, F.A.; Melny, J.; Pizzey, C.J.; Cook, F.; Mason, S.; Bhathal, P.S.; Stelmasiak, T. Enzyme therapy for management of coeliac disease. *Anon. Scand. J. Gastroenterol.* **2005**, *40*, 1304–1312.
26. Tye-Din, J.A.; Anderson, R.P.; Ffrench, R.A.; Brown, G.J.; Hodsman, P.; Siegel, M.; Botwick, W.; Shreeniwas, R. The effects of ALV003 pre-digestion of gluten on immune response and symptoms in celiac disease *in vivo*. *Clin. Immunol.* **2010**, *134*, 289–295.
27. Kelly, C.P.; Green, P.H.; Murray, J.A.; Dimarino, A.; Colatrella, A.; Leffler, D.A.; Alexander, T.; Arsenescu, R.; Leon, F.; Jiang, J.G.; *et al.* Larazotide acetate in patients with coeliac disease undergoing a gluten challenge: A randomised placebo-controlled study. *Aliment. Pharmacol. Ther.* **2013**, *37*, 252–262.
28. Leffler, D.A.; Kelly, C.P.; Abdallah, H.Z.; Colatrella, A.M.; Harris, L.A.; Leon, F.; Arterburn, L.A.; Paterson, B.M.; Lan, Z.H.; Murray, J.A. A randomized, double-blind study of larazotide acetate to prevent the activation of celiac disease during gluten challenge. *Am. J. Gastroenterol.* **2012**, *107*, 1554–1562.
29. Tack, G.J.; van de Water, J.M.; Bruins, M.J.; Kooy-Winkelaar, E.M.; van Bergen, J.; Bonnet, P.; Vreugdenhil, A.C.; Korponay-Szabo, I.; Edens, L.; von Blomberg, B.M.; *et al.* Consumption of gluten with gluten-degrading enzyme by celiac patients: A pilot-study. *World J. Gastroenterol.* **2013**, *19*, 5837–5847.
30. Ascher, H.; Lanner, A.; Kristiansson, B. A new laboratory kit for anti-gliadin IgA at diagnosis and follow-up of childhood celiac disease. *J. Pediatr. Gastroenterol. Nutr.* **1990**, *10*, 443–450.
31. Mayer, M.; Greco, L.; Troncone, R.; Grimaldi, M.; Pansa, G. Early prediction of relapse during gluten challenge in childhood celiac disease. *J. Pediatr. Gastroenterol. Nutr.* **1989**, *8*, 474–479.
32. Rolles, C.J.; McNeish, A.S. Standardised approach to gluten challenge in diagnosing childhood coeliac disease. *Br. Med. J.* **1976**, *1*, 1309–1311.
33. Packer, S.M.; Charlton, V.; Keeling, J.W. Gluten challenge in treated coeliac disease. *Arch. Dis. Child* **1978**, *53*, 449–455.
34. Berg, N.O.; Lindberg, T. Incidence of coeliac disease and transient gluten intolerance in children in a Swedish urban community. *Acta Paediatr. Scand.* **1979**, *68*, 397–400.
35. Savilahti, E.; Viander, M.; Perkkio, M.; Vainio, E.; Kalimo, K.; Reunala, T. IgA antigliadin antibodies: A marker of mucosal damage in childhood coeliac disease. *Lancet* **1983**, *1*, 320–322.

36. Bonamico, M.; Sabbatella, L.; di Tola, M.; Vetrano, S.; Ferri, M.; Nenna, R.; Mariani, P.; Picarelli, A. Antiendomysial antibody detection in biopsy culture allows avoidance of gluten challenge in celiac children. *J. Pediatr. Gastroenterol. Nutr.* **2005**, *40*, 165–169.
37. Troncone, R.; Auricchio, R.; Granata, V. Issues related to gluten-free diet in coeliac disease. *Curr. Opin. Clin. Nutr. Metab. Care* **2008**, *11*, 329–333.
38. Korponay-Szabo, I.R.; Kovacs, J.B.; Lorincz, M.; Gorácz, G.; Szabados, K.; Balogh, M. Prospective significance of antiendomysium antibody positivity in subsequently verified celiac disease. *J. Pediatr. Gastroenterol. Nutr.* **1997**, *25*, 56–63.
39. Wauters, E.A.K.; Jansen, J.; Houwen, R.H.; Veenstra, J.; Ockhuizen, T. Serum IgG and IgA anti-gliadin antibodies as markers of mucosal damage in children with suspected celiac disease upon gluten challenge. *J. Pediatr. Gastroenterol. Nutr.* **1991**, *13*, 192–196.
40. Valletta, E.A.; Trevisiol, D.; Mastella, G. IgA anti-gliadin antibodies in the monitoring of gluten challenge in celiac disease. *J. Pediatr. Gastroenterol. Nutr.* **1990**, *10*, 169–173.
41. Maki, M.; Lahdeaho, M.L.; Hallstrom, O.; Viander, M.; Visakorpi, J.K. Postpubertal gluten challenge in coeliac disease. *Arch. Dis. Child* **1989**, *64*, 1604–1607.
42. Laurin, P.; Wolving, M.; Fälth-Magnusson, K. Even small amounts of gluten cause relapse in children with celiac disease. *J. Pediatr. Gastroenterol. Nutr.* **2002**, *34*, 26–30.
43. Mavromichalis, J.; Brueton, M.J.; McNeish, A.S.; Anderson, C.M. Evaluation of the intraepithelial lymphocyte count in the jejunum in childhood enteropathies. *Gut* **1976**, *17*, 600–603.
44. Hansson, T.; Dannaeus, A.; Kraaz, W.; Sjöberg, O.; Klareskog, L. Production of antibodies to gliadin by peripheral blood lymphocytes in children with celiac disease: The use of an enzyme-linked immunospot technique for screening and follow-up. *Pediatr. Res.* **1997**, *41*, 554–559.
45. Schaad, U.B.; Gaze, H.; Hadorn, B. Intraepithelial lymphocytes before and after gluten challenge in children with celiac disease. *Am. J. Dis. Child* **1981**, *135*, 272–273.
46. Burgin-Wolff, A.; Gaze, H.; Hadziselimovic, F.; Huber, H.; Lentze, M.J.; Nusslé, D.; Reymond-Berthet, C. Antigliadin and antiendomysium antibody determination for coeliac disease. *Arch. Dis. Child* **1991**, *66*, 941–947.
47. Bode, S.; Weile, B.; Krasilnikoff, P.A.; Gudmand-Høyer, E. The diagnostic value of the gliadin antibody test in celiac disease in children: A prospective study. *J. Pediatr. Gastroenterol. Nutr.* **1993**, *17*, 260–264.
48. Danielsson, L.; Stenhammar, L.; Astrom, E. Is gluten challenge necessary for the diagnosis of coeliac disease in young children? *Scand. J. Gastroenterol.* **1990**, *25*, 957–960.
49. Lancaster Smith, M.; Packer, S.; Kumar, P.J.; Harries, J.T. Cellular infiltrate of the jejunum after re introduction of dietary gluten in children with treated coeliac disease. *J. Clin. Pathol.* **1976**, *29*, 587–591.
50. Laurin, P.; Fälth-Magnusson, K.; Sundqvist, T. Increase in nitric oxide urinary products during gluten challenge in children with coeliac disease. *Scand. J. Gastroenterol.* **2003**, *38*, 55–60.
51. Jansson, U.H.; Gudjonsdottir, A.H.; Ryd, W.; Kristiansson, B. Two different doses of gluten show a dose-dependent response of enteropathy but not of serological markers during gluten challenge in children with coeliac disease. *Acta Paediatr.* **2001**, *90*, 255–259.
52. Rolles, C.J.; Anderson, M.; McNeish, A.S. Confirming persistence of gluten intolerance in children diagnosed as having coeliac disease in infancy. *Arch. Dis. Child* **1975**, *50*, 259–263.

53. Lancaster-Smith, M.; Kumar, P.J.; Dawson, A.M. The cellular infiltrate of the jejunum in adult coeliac disease and dermatitis herpetiformis following the reintroduction of dietary gluten. *Gut* **1975**, *16*, 683–688.
54. Lahdeaho, M.L.; Maki, M.; Laurila, K.; Huhtala, H.; Kaukinen, K. Small-bowel mucosal changes and antibody responses after low- and moderate-dose gluten challenge in celiac disease. *BMC Gastroenterol.* **2011**, *11*, 129.
55. Montgomery, A.M.; Goka, A.K.; Kumar, P.J.; Farthing, M.J.; Clark, M.L. Low gluten diet in the treatment of adult coeliac disease: Effect on jejunal morphology and serum anti-gluten antibodies. *Gut* **1988**, *29*, 1564–1568.
56. Brottveit, M.; Raki, M.; Bergseng, E.; Fallang, L.E.; Simonsen, B.; Løvik, A.; Larsen, S.; Løberg, E.M.; Jahnsen, F.L.; Sollid, L.M.; *et al.* Assessing possible celiac disease by an HLA-DQ2-gliadin Tetramer Test. *Am. J. Gastroenterol.* **2011**, *106*, 1318–1324.
57. Daveson, A.J.; Jones, D.M.; Gaze, S.; McSorley, H.; Clouston, A.; Pascoe, A.; Cooke, S.; Speare, R.; Macdonald, G.A.; Anderson, R.; *et al.* Effect of hookworm infection on wheat challenge in celiac disease—A randomised double-blinded placebo controlled trial. *PLoS One* **2011**, *6*, e17366.
58. Tack, G.J.; van de Water, J.M.; Kooy-Winkelaar, E.M.; van Bergen, J.; Meijer, G.A.; von Blomberg, B.M.; Schreurs, M.W.; Bruins, M.J.; Edens, L.; Mulder, C.J.; *et al.* 379 Can prolyl endoprotease enzyme treatment mitigate the toxic effect of gluten in coeliac patients? *Gastroenterology* **2010**, *138*, S54.
59. Kumar, P.J.; O'Donoghue, D.P.; Stenson, K.; Dawson, A.M. Reintroduction of gluten in adults and children with treated coeliac disease. *Gut* **1979**, *20*, 743–749.
60. Wahab, P.J.; Crusius, J.B.A.; Meijer, J.W.; Mulder, C.J. Gluten challenge in borderline gluten-sensitive enteropathy. *Am. J. Gastroenterol.* **2001**, *96*, 1464–1469.
61. Kaukinen, K.; Peraaho, M.; Collin, P.; Partanen, J.; Woolley, N.; Kaartinen, T.; Nuutinen, T.; Halttunen, T.; Mäki, M.; Korponay-Szabo, I. Small-bowel mucosal transglutaminase 2-specific IgA deposits in coeliac disease without villous atrophy: A prospective and randomized clinical study. *Scand. J. Gastroenterol.* **2005**, *40*, 564–572.
62. Campanella, J.; Biagi, F.; Bianchi, P.I.; Zanellati, G.; Marchese, A.; Corazza, G.R. Clinical response to gluten withdrawal is not an indicator of coeliac disease. *Scand. J. Gastroenterol.* **2008**, *43*, 1311–1314.
63. Troncone, R.; Caputo, N.; Micillo, M.; Maiuri, L.; Poggi, V. Immunologic and intestinal permeability tests as predictors of relapse during gluten challenge in childhood coeliac disease. *Scand. J. Gastroenterol.* **1994**, *29*, 144–147.
64. Jansson, U.H.; Kristiansson, B.; Magnusson, P.; Larsson, L.; Albertsson-Wikland, K.; Bjarnason, R. The decrease of IGF-I, IGF-binding protein-3 and bone alkaline phosphatase isoforms during gluten challenge correlates with small intestinal inflammation in children with coeliac disease. *Eur. J. Endocrinol.* **2001**, *144*, 417–423.
65. Korponay-Szabo, I.; Kovacs, J.; Lorincz, M.; Körmendy, M.; Sashegyi, J. New cases of celiac disease detected by anti-endomysial antibody test in families of gluten-sensitive patients and among children examined for non-specific gastrointestinal complaints. *Orv. Hetil.* **1993**, *134*, 15–20.

66. Baker, P.G.; Read, A.E. Oats and barley toxicity in coeliac patients. *Postgrad. Med. J.* **1976**, *52*, 264–268.
67. Anand, B.S.; Piris, J.; Truelove, S.C. The role of various cereals in coeliac disease. *Q. J. Med.* **1978**, *47*, 101–110.
68. Leffler, D.A.; Dennis, M.; Edwards George, J.; Jamma, S.; Cook, E.F.; Schuppan, D.; Kelly, C.P. A validated disease-specific symptom index for adults with celiac disease. *Clin. Gastroenterol. Hepatol.* **2009**, *7*, 1328–1334.e3.
69. Anderson, R.P.; van Heel, D.A.; Tye-Din, J.A.; Barnardo, M.; Salio, M.; Jewell, D.P.; Hill, A.V.S. T cells in peripheral blood after gluten challenge in coeliac disease. *Gut* **2005**, *54*, 1217–1223.
70. Catassi, C.; Rossini, M.; Ratsch, I.M.; Bearzi, I.; Santinelli, A.; Castagnani, R.; Pisani, E.; Coppa, G.V.; Giorgi, P.L. Dose dependent effects of protracted ingestion of small amounts of gliadin in coeliac disease children: A clinical and jejunal morphometric study. *Gut* **1993**, *34*, 1515–1519.
71. Hadziselimovic, F.; Bürgin-Wolff, A. P0429: Indication of gluten tolerance development in patients with coeliac disease. *J. Pediatr. Gastroenterol. Nutr.* **2004**, *39*, S218–S219.
72. Murray, J.A. The widening spectrum of celiac disease. *Am. J. Clin. Nutr.* **1999**, *69*, 354–365.
73. Chang, F.; Mahadeva, U.; Deere, H. Pathological and clinical significance of increased intraepithelial lymphocytes (IELs) in small bowel mucosa. *APMIS* **2005**, *113*, 385–399.
74. Collin, P.; Wahab, P.J.; Murray, J.A. Intraepithelial lymphocytes and coeliac disease. *Best Pract. Res. Clin. Gastroenterol.* **2005**, *19*, 341–350.
75. Ferguson, A.; Arranz, E.; O'Mahony, S. Clinical and pathological spectrum of coeliac disease—Active, silent, latent, potential. *Gut* **1993**, *34*, 150–151.
76. Koskinen, O.; Collin, P.; Korponay-Szabo, I.; Salmi, T.; Iltanen, S.; Haimila, K.; Partanen, J.; Mäki, M.; Kaukinen, K. Gluten-dependent small bowel mucosal transglutaminase 2-specific IgA deposits in overt and mild enteropathy coeliac disease. *J. Pediatr. Gastroenterol. Nutr.* **2008**. *47*, 436–442.
77. Raki, M.; Fallang, L.E.; Brottveit, M.; Bergseng, E.; Quarsten, H.; Lundin, K.E.; Sollid, L.M. Tetramer visualization of gut-homing gluten-specific T cells in the peripheral blood of celiac disease patients. *Proc. Natl. Acad. Sci. USA* **2007**, *104*, 2831–2836.

7

Non-Celiac Gluten Sensitivity: The New Frontier of Gluten Related Disorders

Carlo Catassi [1], Julio C. Bai [2], Bruno Bonaz [3], Gerd Bouma [4], Antonio Calabrò [5], Antonio Carroccio [6], Gemma Castillejo [7], Carolina Ciacci [8], Fernanda Cristofori [9], Jernej Dolinsek [10], Ruggiero Francavilla [9], Luca Elli [11], Peter Green [12], Wolfgang Holtmeier [13], Peter Koehler [14], Sibylle Koletzko [15], Christof Meinhold [16], David Sanders [17], Michael Schumann [18], Detlef Schuppan [19,20], Reiner Ullrich [18], Andreas Vécsei [21], Umberto Volta [22], Victor Zevallos [19], Anna Sapone [23] and Alessio Fasano [24,*]

1 Department of Pediatrics, Università Politecnica delle Marche, Ancona 60121, Italy; E-Mail: catassi@tin.it

2 Departamento de Medicina, Hospital de Gastroenterología "Dr. Carlos Bonorino Udaondo", Buenos Aires 1264, Argentina; E-Mail: jbai@intramed.net

3 Department of Gastroenterology and Liver Diseases, CHU Grenoble 38043, France; E-Mail: bbonaz@chu-grenoble.fr

4 Department of Gastroenterology and Hepatology, Vrije Universiteit Medical Center, Amsterdam 1081 HV, The Netherlands; E-Mail: g.bouma@vumc.nl

5 Gastroenterology Unit, Department of Experimental and Clinical Biomedical Sciences, University of Florence, Florence 50134, Italy; E-Mail: a.calabro@dfc.unifi.it

6 Department of Internal Medicine, "Giovanni Paolo II" Hospital, Sciacca (AG) and University of Palermo, Sciacca 92019, Italy; E-Mail: acarroccio@hotmail.com

7 Pediatric Gastroenterology Unit, Hospital Universitari de Sant Joan de Reus, Universitat Rovira i Virgili, Tarragona 43204, Spain; E-Mail: gcv@tinet.cat

8 Department of Medicine and Surgery, University of Salerno, Baronissi Campus, Salerno 84081, Italy; E-Mail: cciacci@unisa.it

9 Interdisciplinary Department of Medicine, University of Bari, Bari 70124, Italy; E-Mails: fernandacristofori@gmail.com (F.C.); rfrancavilla@gmail.com (R.F.)

10 Gastroenterology Unit, Department of Pediatrics, University Medical Centre Maribor, Maribor 2000, Slovenia; E-Mail: jernej.dolinsek@ukc-mb.si

11 Centro Prevenzione e Diagnosi Malattia Celiaca Fondazione IRCCS Ca Granda, Milan 20122, Italy; E-Mail: lucelli@yahoo.com

12 Department of Medicine, Celiac Disease Center, Columbia University Medical Center, New York, NY 10032, USA; E-Mail: pg11@columbia.edu

13 Division of Gastroenterology and Internal Medicine, Hospital Porz am Rhein, Köln 51149, Germany; E-Mail: w.holtmeier@khporz.de

[14] German Research Center for Food Chemistry, Leibniz Institute, Freising 85354, Germany; E-Mail: peter.koehler@tum.de
[15] Division of Pediatric Gastroenterology and Hepatology, Dr. von Hauner Children's Hospital, University of Munich Medical Center, Munich 80337, Germany; E-Mail: sybille.koletzko@med.uni-muenchen.de
[16] Practice of Nutrition Therapy Meinhold & Team, Köln 50674, Germany; E-Mail: praxis@christof-meinhold.de
[17] Department of Gastroenterology and Hepatology, Royal Hallamshire Hospital and University of Sheffield Medical School, Sheffield S10 2JF, UK; E-Mail: david.sanders@sth.nhs.uk
[18] Department of Gastroenterology, Rheumatology and Infectiology, Charité University Medicine, Berlin 10203, Germany; E-Mails: michael.schumann@charite.de (M.S.); reiner.ullrich@charite.de (R.U.)
[19] Department of Medicine I, University Medical Center, Johannes Gutenberg University Mainz, Mainz 55131, Germany; E-Mails: dschuppa@bidmc.harvard.edu (D.S.); zevallos@uni-mainz.de (V.Z.)
[20] Division of Gastroenterology and Celiac Center, Beth Israel Deaconess Medical Center and Harvard Medical School, Boston, MA 02215, USA
[21] St. Anna Children's Hospital, Vienna 1090, Austria; E-Mail: andreas.vecsei@stanna.at
[22] Department of Medical and Surgical Sciences, University of Bologna, Bologna 40138, Italy; E-Mail: uvolt@yahoo.com
[23] Department of Gastroenterology, Second University of Naples, Naples 80136, Italy; E-Mail: annasapone@yahoo.it
[24] Pediatric Gastroenterology and Nutrition, MassGeneral Hospital for Children, Boston, MA 02129, USA

* Author to whom correspondence should be addressed; E-Mail: afasano@partners.org; Tel.: +1-617-726-1450.

Received: 20 August 2013; in revised form: 17 September 2013 / Accepted: 18 September 2013 / Published: 26 September 2013

Abstract: Non Celiac Gluten sensitivity (NCGS) was originally described in the 1980s and recently a "re-discovered" disorder characterized by intestinal and extra-intestinal symptoms related to the ingestion of gluten-containing food, in subjects that are not affected with either celiac disease (CD) or wheat allergy (WA). Although NCGS frequency is still unclear, epidemiological data have been generated that can help establishing the magnitude of the problem. Clinical studies further defined the identity of NCGS and its implications in human disease. An overlap between the irritable bowel syndrome (IBS) and NCGS has been detected, requiring even more stringent diagnostic criteria. Several studies suggested a relationship between NCGS and neuropsychiatric disorders, particularly autism and schizophrenia. The first case reports of NCGS in children have been described.

Lack of biomarkers is still a major limitation of clinical studies, making it difficult to differentiate NCGS from other gluten related disorders. Recent studies raised the possibility that, beside gluten, wheat amylase-trypsin inhibitors and low-fermentable, poorly-absorbed, short-chain carbohydrates can contribute to symptoms (at least those related to IBS) experienced by NCGS patients. In this paper we report the major advances and current trends on NCGS.

Keywords: gluten sensitivity; celiac disease; wheat allergy; gluten-related disorders; gluten-free diet

---

1. Introduction

Gluten sensitivity (GS) was originally described in the 1980s [1] and a recently "re-discovered" syndrome entity, characterized by intestinal and extra-intestinal symptoms related to the ingestion of gluten-containing food, in subjects that are not affected with either celiac disease (CD) or wheat allergy (WA). Following the landmark work by Sapone and coworkers, describing the clinical and diagnostic features of GS in the year 2010 [2], a rapidly increasing number of papers have been published by many independent groups, confirming that GS should definitely be included in the spectrum of gluten-related disorders. However, many aspects of GS epidemiology, pathophysiology, clinical spectrum, and treatment are still unclear. Given the recent increase of the gluten-free market worldwide, partially sustained by individuals who claim a medical necessity to undertake a gluten-free diet (GFD), there is a need of "separating the wheat from the chaff" [3]. This goal will be achieved by (a) proper scientific information, (b) shared definitions, and (c) prospective, multi-center studies addressing the many unsolved issues on GS. In order to develop a consensus on new nomenclature and classification of gluten-related disorders, a panel of experts first met in London, in February 2011. The panel proposed a series of definitions and developed a diagnostic algorithm that has been recently published [4].

After the 2011 London Meeting, many new papers have been published on GS. Although its frequency in the general population is still unclear, epidemiological data have been generated that can help establish the magnitude of the problem. Clinical studies further defined the identity of GS and its possible implications in human disease. An overlap between the irritable bowel syndrome (IBS) and GS has been suspected, requiring even more stringent diagnostic criteria. The first case reports of GS in children have been described. Lack of biomarkers is still a major limitation of clinical studies, making the differential diagnosis with other gluten related disorders, as well conditions independent to gluten exposure, difficult.

Evaluation and discussion of this new information was the aim of a Second Expert Meeting on GS that was held in Munich, November 30–December 2, 2012. In this paper we report the major advances and current trends on GS, as presented and debated at the Munich meeting.

2. Nomenclature

At least three papers have recently addressed the issue of defining gluten-related disorders [4–6]. Interestingly, one of these [4] ranks among the most frequently downloaded paper of the publishing journal (*BMC Medicine*), particularly by physicians, internists or general pediatricians, and directors of diagnostic labs. There is a general agreement that the term "gluten-related disorders" is the umbrella-term to be used for describing all conditions related to ingestion of gluten-containing food. CD is a chronic small intestinal, immune-mediated, enteropathy precipitated by exposure to dietary gluten and related prolamines in genetically predisposed individuals, characterized by specific autoantibodies against tissue transglutaminase 2 (anti-TG2) and endomysium (EMA). WA is an adverse immunologic reaction to wheat proteins. In the pathogenesis of WA, wheat specific IgE antibodies play a central role, however non-IgE-mediated WA does exist [7], and this form may be difficult to distinguish from GS.

GS, which this review will focus on primarily, is a condition in which symptoms are triggered by gluten ingestion, in the absence of celiac-specific antibodies and of classical celiac villous atrophy, with variable Human Leukocyte Antigen (HLA) status and variable presence of first generation anti-gliadin antibodies (AGA). The "labeling" of this disorder was a matter of debate among the panel experts. In order to avoid confusion with CD, sometimes defined as gluten-sensitive enteropathy, "non celiac gluten sensitivity" (NCGS) appeared as an improved definition. Doubtless this is still too vague a terminology, simply reflecting the poor knowledge of the pathophysiology of this condition. As triggering cereal proteins could include fractions other than gluten (see Section 10 below) some panelists were in favor of "non-celiac wheat (protein) sensitivity", a terminology that would however conflict with the possibility that other gluten-containing cereals (rye, barley) may be offensive for the "gluten sensitive" patient. Bearing these limitations in mind, the experts' panel agreed that this entity can provisionally be defined as NCGS, a definition requiring refinement in the future.

3. Epidemiology

The overall prevalence of NCGS in the general population is still unknown, mainly because many patients are currently self-diagnosed and start a GFD without medical advice or consultation. However, new data confirm that this is not an uncommon disorder at all. In a region of New Zealand, 5% of children reported non-CD-related avoidance of gluten-containing food [8]. Gluten avoidance was associated with improvement of nonspecific behavioral and gastrointestinal complaints [9]. It remains to be elucidated how many children reporting gluten avoidance were indeed affected by NCGS, as the vast majority of the children involved in this study were not tested for CD nor underwent to an intestinal biopsy. In a US study performed on 7762 unselected persons aged six years or older who participated in the National Health and Nutrition Examination Survey (NHANES) 2009–2010, Digiacomo *et al.* found a 0.55% prevalence of persons on a self-reported GFD. The prevalence was higher in females and older participants [10]. Many of the NHANES subjects on a GFD could indeed be affected by NCGS, however this is likely to be an underestimate as (a) the possible relationship between gastro-intestinal symptoms and gluten intake was not systematically explored in this population sample, and (b) the NHANES survey was conducted before NCGS was described in the medical literature.

The analysis of the epidemiology of IBS provides an indirect estimate of intestinal NCGS frequency. According to recent population-based surveys performed in Northern Europe, the prevalence of IBS in the general adult population is 16%–25% [11,12]. In a selected (and, therefore, probably biased) series of adults with IBS, the frequency of NCGS, documented by a double-blind, placebo-controlled challenge, was 28% [13]. In the large study performed by Carroccio *et al.*, 276 out of 920 (30%) subjects with IBS-like symptoms, according to the Rome II criteria, suffered from wheat sensitivity or multiple food hypersensitivity, including wheat sensitivity [14]. Should a consistent proportion of IBS patients be affected with NCGS, the prevalence of NCGS in the general population could well be higher than CD (1%).

Although risk factors for NCGS have not yet been identified, the disorder seems to be more common in females and in young/middle age adults. The prevalence of NCGS in children is still unknown.

4. Clinical Picture and Natural History

NCGS is characterized by symptoms that usually occur soon after gluten ingestion, disappear with gluten withdrawal and relapse following gluten challenge, within hours or few days. The "classical" presentation of NCGS is a combination of IBS-like symptoms, including abdominal pain, bloating, bowel habit abnormalities (either diarrhea or constipation), and systemic manifestations such as "foggy mind", headache, fatigue, joint and muscle pain, leg or arm numbness, dermatitis (eczema or skin rash), depression, and anemia [2,15]. When seen at the specialty clinic, many NCGS patients already report the causal relationship between the ingestion of gluten-containing food and worsening of symptoms. In children, NCGS manifests with typical gastrointestinal symptoms, such as abdominal pain and chronic diarrhea, while the extra-intestinal manifestations seem to be less frequent, the most common extra-intestinal symptom being tiredness [16].

During the last decade, several studies suggested a relationship between NCGS and neuropsychiatric disorders (see following paragraphs).

While it is undisputable that in some cases the positive effect of gluten withdrawal can be explained by a placebo effect, this is not the case in true NCGS. In a double-blind randomized placebo-controlled study design, Biesiekierski *et al.* found that IBS-like symptoms of NCGS were more frequent in the gluten-treated group (68%) than in subjects on placebo (40%) [13]. Furthermore a recent study found no significant differences between CD and NCGS patients regarding personality traits, level of somatization, quality of life, anxiety, and depressive symptoms. The somatization level was low in both diseases. Additionally, symptom increase after a gluten challenge was not related to personality in NCGS patients [17].

No major complication of untreated NCGS has so far been described; especially autoimmune comorbidity, as observed in CD, has not been reported so far. However, natural history data on NCGS are still lacking. Therefore it is difficult to draw firm conclusions on the outcome of this condition.

5. NCGS and IBS: A Complex Relationship

The complex relationship between IBS and dietary proteins has been recently reviewed [18]. Patients with CD often report symptoms compatible with IBS persisting after treatment with the GFD.

In a recent meta-analysis the pooled prevalence of IBS-type symptoms in patients with treated CD was 38.0% (95% CI, 27.0%–50.0%). The pooled odds ratio (OR) for IBS-type symptoms was higher in patients with CD than in controls (5.60; 95% CI, 3.23–9.70). In patients who were non-adherent with a GFD, the pooled OR for IBS-like symptoms, compared with those who were strictly adherent, was 2.69 (95% CI, 0.75–9.56) [19].

That gluten ingestion may elicit gastrointestinal symptoms in non-CD patients has recently been shown in subjects affected with the D variant (diarrhea-predominant) of IBS, by Vazquez-Roque and coworkers. Subjects on a gluten containing diet (GCD) had more bowel movements per day, particularly those with HLA-DQ2 and/or DQ8 genotypes. The GCD was associated with higher small bowel permeability. Patients on the GCD had a small decrease in expression of zonula occludens 1 in small bowel mucosa, and significant decreases in expression of zonula occludens 1, claudin-1, and occludin in rectosigmoid mucosa; again the effects of the GCD on expression were significantly greater in HLA-DQ2/8–positive patients. On the other hand, the GCD *vs.* the GFD had no significant effects on gastrointestinal transit or histology. It was concluded that gluten alters bowel barrier functions in patients with IBS-D, particularly in HLA-DQ2/8–positive patients. These data provided mechanistic explanations for the observation that gluten withdrawal may improve patient symptoms in IBS [20].

How specific the effect of gluten withdrawal from the diet of patients with IBS is, still remains to be elucidated. Besides gluten, wheat, and wheat derivatives contain other constituents that could play a role in triggering symptoms in IBS patients, e.g., amylase-trypsin inhibitors (ATIs, see below) and fructans. In a second study, Biesiekirski *et al.* reported on 37 patients with IBS/self-reported NCGS investigated by a double-blind crossover trial. Patients were randomly assigned to a period of reduced low-fermentable, poorly-absorbed, short-chain carbohydrates (fermentable oligo-, di-, and mono-saccharides and polyols = FODMAPs) diet and then placed on either a gluten or whey proteins challenge. In all participants, gastrointestinal complaints consistently improved during reduced FODMAP intake, but significantly worsened to a similar degree when their diets included gluten or whey proteins [21]. FODMAPS list includes fructans, galactans, fructose, and polyols that are contained in several foodstuffs, including wheat, vegetables, and milk derivatives. These results raise the possibility that the positive effect of the GFD in patients with IBS is an unspecific consequence of reducing FODMAPs intake, given that wheat is one of the possible sources of FODMAPs. However, it should be stressed that FODMAPs cannot be entirely and exclusively responsible for the symptoms experienced by NCGS subjects, since these patients experience a resolution of symptoms while on a GFD despite continuing to ingest FODMAPs from other sources, like legumes (a much richer source of FODMPs than wheat). Nevertheless, based on the results reported by Biesiekirski *et al.* is also possible that there are IBS cases entirely due to FODMAPs that, therefore, cannot be classified as affected by NCGS [21].

6. Is Autism Part of the NCGS Spectrum?

Autism Spectrum Disorders (ASD) are chronic behavioral conditions, with onset before three years of age. ASD are one of the fastest growing developmental disabilities in the United States. They present with a wide range of stereotyped, repetitive behaviors, social and language impairment.

Function and outcome is affected not only by core deficits but also by associated behaviors such as hyperactivity, aggression, anxiety, and depression. Many studies have indicated that behavioral therapy and medication may be at least partially helpful in the management of children with ASD. Research on the effect of diet and nutrition on autism has been increasing in the past two decades, particularly on the symptoms of hyperactivity and attention. One of the most popular interventions for ASD is the gluten free casein free (GFCF) diet.

The possible effect of the GFCF in children with autism is not due to underlying CD, since an association between these two conditions has never been clearly confirmed by serological screening studies [22]. It has been hypothesized that some symptoms may be caused by opioid peptides formed from the incomplete breakdown of foods containing gluten and casein. Increased intestinal permeability, also referred to as the "leaky gut syndrome," has been suspected in ASD to be part of the chain of events that allows these peptides to cross the intestinal membrane, enter the bloodstream, and cross the blood-brain barrier, affecting the endogenous opiate system and neurotransmission within the nervous system. The resulting excess of opioids is thought to lead to behaviors noted in ASD, and the removal of these substances from the diet could determine a change in autistic behaviors [23]. The leaky gut/autism connection has fuelled a strong debate within the scientific community, far from being settled. A recent study has reported a high percentage of abnormal intestinal permeability test (as established by the lactulose/mannitol ratio) among patients with autism (36.7%) and their relatives (21.2%) compared with normal subjects (4.8%). Patients with autism on a reported GFCF diet had significantly lower intestinal permeability test values compared with those who were on an unrestricted diet and controls [24]. However, the degree of correlation between abnormal intestinal permeability to sugars (lactulose and mannitol) and proteins/peptides remains to be established. It should also be pointed out that, in a pilot study, Robertson *et al.* did not detect any changes in intestinal permeability in a small cohort of ASD children [25]. The finding of IgG class antibodies directed against food antigens is considered indirect evidence of increased intestinal permeability. Children with autism have significantly higher levels of IgG antibody (but not IgA) to gliadin compared with healthy controls, particularly in those with gastrointestinal symptoms [26]. Recent studies confirmed these findings and also reported an increase in antibodies directed to several other food allergens, including casein and whole milk [27].

Despite its popularity, the efficacy of the GFCF diet in improving autistic behavior remains not conclusively proven. A 2008 Cochrane review reported that only two small RCTs investigated the effect of GFCF diet in children with ASD ($n = 35$). There were only three significant treatment effects in favor of the diet intervention: overall autistic traits, mean difference (MD) = −5.60; social isolation, MD = −3.20 and overall ability to communicate and interact, MD = 1.70. In addition three outcomes were not different between the treatment and control group while differences for ten outcomes could not be analyzed because data were skewed. The review concluded that the evidence for efficacy of these diets is poor, and large scale, good quality randomized controlled trials are needed [28].

By using a two-stage, randomized, controlled study of GFCF diet of children with ASD, Whiteley and coworkers recently reported significant group improvements in core autistic and related behaviors after eight and 12 months on diet. The results showed a less dramatic change between children having been on diet for eight and children in diet for 24 months, possibly reflective of a plateau effect [29].

The above data suggest that removing gluten from the diet may positively affect the clinical outcome in some children diagnosed with ASD, indicating that autism may be part of the spectrum of NCGS, at least in some cases. However, a word of caution is necessary to stress the fact that only a small, selected sub-group of children affected by ASD may benefit from an elimination diet. Additional investigations are required in order to identify phenotypes based on best- and non-response to dietary modifications and assess any biological correlates including anthropometry before considering a dietary intervention.

7. Gluten-Related Disorders and Schizophrenia

An association between schizophrenia and CD was noted in reports spanning back to the 1960s [30]. In 1986 a double-blind gluten-free/gluten-load controlled trial of 24 patients conducted by Vlissides *et al.* showed changes in symptom profile of schizophrenics in response to exclusion of gluten from the diet [31]. On the other hand, a small blind study conducted by Potkin *et al.* showed no differences in the clinical status of eight schizophrenic patients on a 5-week gluten challenge in an in-patient setting, as measured by the Brief Psychiatric Rating Scale [32]. A subsequent study by Storms *et al.* tested 26 schizophrenic patients on a locked ward assigned to either a gluten-free or high gluten diet. No differences were found between the groups on their performance in a battery of psychological tests [33]. A recent study using blood samples from the Clinical Antipsychotic Trials of Intervention Effectiveness (CATIE) found that 5.5% of the subjects with schizophrenia had a high level of anti-tTG antibodies (compared to 1.1% in the healthy control sample) and 23.1% had AGA IgG positivity compared with 3.1% in controls. Interestingly enough, a large proportion of tTG positive subjects resulted EMA negative, questioning the possibility that their tTG positivity was related to CD. Indeed, only 2% of schizophrenic patients fulfilled the CD diagnostic criteria (both anti-tTG and EMA positive), questioning the role of CD in schizophrenia [34]. Additional studies revealed that most of the tTG positive subjects were tTG-6 positive, suggesting that these antibodies are more a biomarker of neuro-inflammation than CD [35]. This study indicated the existence of a specific immune response to gluten in some of these patients, probably related to NCGS. Other studies confirmed the high prevalence of antibodies to AGA among people with schizophrenia [36], however the exact mechanism underlying the observed improvement of symptoms in some patients with the GFD has remained elusive. Immunological mechanisms have been proposed, including the assertion that a subgroup of schizophrenics suffer from food intolerances that benefit from the adoption of a GFD. The beneficial effect of a GFD may also be achieved via circulating food-derived peptides (exorphins) exerting an influence on physiological processes in the brain (same mechanism as described in the autism paragraph). If it were true that a subset of schizophrenic patients did exhibit symptoms due to sensitivity to gluten, then not only would treatment for these individuals be easier and more efficient than neuroleptics but also their quality of life would improve.

In summary, the role of NCGS in conditions affecting the nervous system remains a highly debated and controversial topic that requires additional, well-designed studies to establish the real role of gluten as a triggering factor in these diseases.

8. Laboratory Evaluation

So far no specific biomarker of NCGS has been identified. Recently, Volta and colleagues reported on the pattern of CD serology found in 78 untreated patients affected with NCGS. Many patients displayed an elevated prevalence of high titer, "first-generation" IgG AGA directed against native gliadin (56.4%). The prevalence of IgG AGA detected in NCGS, although lower than that found in CD (81.2%), was much higher than other pathologic conditions such as connective tissue disorders (9%) and autoimmune liver diseases (21.5%) as well as in the general population and healthy blood donors (2%–8%). On the other hand, the prevalence of IgA AGA in NCGS patients was very low (7.7%). Noteworthy, the "best" CD markers, namely IgG deamidated gliadin peptide (DGP) antibodies, IgA tTGA, and IgA EMA, were always negative in NCGS patients, except for an isolated positivity at a very low titer for IgG DGP. The consistent negativity for IgG DGP, whose synthesis "*in vivo*" is an expression of the interaction between tissue transglutaminase and gliadin peptides, seems to exclude the involvement of adaptive immunity in NCGS pathogenesis. Interestingly enough, ELISA activities of IgA tTGA in NCGS patients were very low with 30% of them displaying values < 1 AU (none of them had IgA deficiency) [15].

The CD-predisposing HLA-DQ2 and DQ8 genotypes are found in 50% of NCGS patients, a prevalence that is lower than CD (95%) and only slightly higher than the general population (30%) [4].

In the work of Sapone and coworkers all subjects (11 patients with NCGS, 13 with CD, and seven controls), underwent upper duodenal endoscopy for small intestinal biopsy. Those with NCGS revealed normal to mildly inflamed mucosa (Marsh 0 to 1), while all CD patients showed partial or subtotal villous atrophy with crypt hyperplasia. As expected, CD patients had increased numbers of CD3+ IELs (>50/100 enterocytes) compared to controls, while NCGS patients had a number of CD3+ IELs intermediate between CD patients and controls in the context of relatively conserved villus architecture. The numbers of TCR-γδ IELs were only elevated in CD subjects (>3.4/100 enterocytes), while in NCGS patients the numbers of γδ IELs were similar to those in controls [2]. Recently, activation of circulating basophils [14] and increased infiltration of duodenal lamina propria with eosinophils [37] have been described.

9. Diagnosis

NCGS diagnosis is sometimes suspected by the patients themselves based on food withdrawal and introduction. Physicians may then concur if there has been the exclusion of other forms of gluten-induced disease (CD and WA) by appropriate serological and/or biopsy tests. Specific IgE might normalize if the patients are already on GFD and this might be a potential pitfall in diagnosis of WA The finding that symptoms disappear after gluten elimination adds weight to the diagnosis of NCGS, which is definitely proven by a double-blind (or open) oral gluten challenge performed after at least three weeks of GFD.

Based on a combination of clinical, biological, genetic and histological data, it is possible to differentiate the three gluten-related conditions (WA, CD, and NCGS), using recently published algorithms [4]. Since there is some degree of overlap between NCGS and other forms of wheat-exclusion responsive conditions (e.g., IBS responsive to low FODMAPs diet, non-IgE mediated

WA), periodical patient reassessment (e.g., every 6–12 months), including an accurate dietary interview, is strongly recommended.

10. Pathogenesis

The pathophysiology of NCGS is under scrutiny. In the study conducted by Sapone *et al.* [2], NCGS subjects showed a normal intestinal permeability and claudin-1 and ZO-1 expression compared with celiac patients, and a significantly higher expression of claudin-4. In the same NCGS patients, the up-regulation of claudin-4 was associated with an increased expression of toll-like receptor-2 and a significant reduction of T-regulatory cell marker FoxP3 relative to controls and CD patients. Additionally, an increase in IELs of the classes α and β, but no increase in adaptive immunity-related gut mucosal gene expression, including interleukin (IL)-6, IL-21, and interferon-γ (IFN-γ), was detected in NCGS. These changes suggested an important role of the intestinal innate immune system in NCGS, without any involvement of the adaptive immune response. In a study aimed at exploring and comparing the early mucosal immunological events in CD and NCGS, Brottveit *et al.* confirmed that CD patients mounted a concomitant innate and adaptive immune response to gluten challenge. NCGS patients only showed increased IFN-γ levels after gluten challenge and increased density of intraepithelial CD3(+) T cells at baseline [38]. These findings open the possibility of an adaptive component as well in the pathogenesis of NCGS.

The trigger/s of mucosal events leading to NCGS is not necessarily represented by the same array of gluten peptides responsible for CD development. Unlike the duodenal mucosa from patients with CD, upon incubation with gliadin, mucosa from patients with NCGS does not express markers of inflammation, and their basophils are not activated by gliadin [39]. *In vitro* studies suggest that wheat ATIs could play a major role as triggers of the innate immune response in intestinal monocytes, macrophages and dendritic cells eventually leading to NCGS. Wheat ATIs are a family of five or more homologous low-molecular-weight proteins highly resistant to intestinal proteolysis. They are known to be the major allergen responsible for baker's asthma. ATIs engage the TLR4-MD2-CD14 complex and lead to up-regulation of maturation markers and elicit release of pro-inflammatory cytokines in cells from celiac and non-celiac patients and in celiac patients' biopsies [40].

11. Current and Future Trends

The vast majority of celiac experts initially reacted with a great deal of skepticism to the concept of NCGS existence and the fact that it was a separate entity from CD. For those that witnessed the initial struggle of convincing health care professionals that CD was not confined within European boundaries this was a *déjà vu*. Indeed, we are now with NCGS where we probably were with CD forty years ago. In the 1980s we knew that CD existed, but we had little information on the mechanisms leading to the enteropathy, the genetic component of the disease, what kind of immune response was involved in the pathogenesis of the disease, its multifaceted clinical presentation, and its complication. We lacked robust screening tools to conduct well-design epidemiological studies and had little understanding on the most appropriate management of the disease and its complications. The confusion about NCGS stems from the few facts, and the many fantasies, currently available on this topic. The best testimonial of this concept is the comparison of the literature published on both conditions during the past

63 years. The publications on CD doubled every 20 years from approximately 2500 in the period of 1950–70 to ~9500 in the period 1991–2010, with already more than 2000 papers published between 2011 and 2013. Conversely, there were almost no scientific reports on NCGS before 1970 and only a handful number of papers have been published ever since, most of them after 2005. The increase interest in NCGS is testified by the decreased NCGS/CD publication ratio that dropped from 1:438 in the period 1950–70 to 1:10 in the period 2010–13 (Table 1).

Table 1. Trends in publication on celiac disease (CD) and non-celiac gluten sensitivity (NCGS) during the last decades.

Timeline	CD	NCGS	NCGS/CD ratio
1950–1970	2632	6	1:438
1971–1990	4915	118	1:43
1991–2010	9498	733	1:13
2011–2013	2014	188	1:10

Given the limited literature on the topic, it should not come as a surprise that there are still numerous questions about NCGS that should be addressed. Is NCGS permanent or transitory? Is the threshold of sensitivity the same for everybody, or change from subject to subject and in the same subject over time? How frequent is NCGS? The range reported in the literature is between 0.5% and 6%, based on poorly conducted studies and on definitions of the disease that varies widely from one report to another. Only recently, well-conducted studies based on double blind, placebo control design are providing evidence-based data on the prevalence of NCGS in specific clinical conditions, particularly IBS [13]. There is the strong need for more coordinated efforts to perform large multicenter studies for those conditions, including autism and schizophrenia, in which NCGS has been indicated as a possible cause in a subgroup of these patients. The lack of validated biomarkers for a diagnosis not based on exclusion criteria is judged to be of paramount importance by many experts in the field. Currently a large multicenter placebo-controlled study is underway to achieve this goal and, hopefully, will provide tools for a more correct diagnosis and for more rigorous studies to establish the prevalence of NCGS in specific conditions and in the general population. Recent studies raised the possibility that, beside gluten [13] and wheat ATIs [40], low-fermentable, poorly-absorbed, short-chain carbohydrates [21] can contribute to symptoms (at least those related to IBS) experienced by NCGS patients. These new findings need corroboration through additional studies involving larger numbers of subjects. If these studies will confirm these new findings, they will probably prompt a change in nomenclature from NCGS to wheat sensitivity to reflect the fact that, beside gluten, other components of wheat may be responsible for the symptoms reported by NCGS patients.

Acknowledgments

We wish to express our gratitude to Jacqueline Pante (Schär, Merano, Italy) and Andrea Comaschi (Weber Shandwick, Milan, Italy) for logistic support in the organization of the Munich Meeting.

References

1. Cooper, B.T.; Holmes, G.K.; Ferguson, R.; Thompson, R.A.; Allan, R.N.; Cooke, W.T. Gluten-sensitive diarrhea without evidence of celiac disease. *Gastroenterology* **1981**, *81*, 192–194.
2. Sapone, A.; Lammers, K.M.; Mazzarella, G.; Mikhailenko, I.; Cartenì, M.; Casolaro, V.; Fasano, A. Differential mucosal IL-17 expression in two gliadin-induced disorders: Gluten sensitivity and the autoimmune enteropathy celiac disease. *Int. Arch. Allergy Immunol.* **2010**, *152*, 75–80.
3. Sanders, D.S.; Aziz, I. Non celiac wheat sensitivity: Separating the wheat from the chaff. *Am. J. Gastroenterol.* **2012**, *107*, 1908–1912.
4. Sapone, A.; Bai, J.C.; Ciacci, C.; Dolinsek, J.; Green, P.H.; Hadjivassiliou, M.; Kaukinen, K.; Rostami, K.; Sanders, D.S.; Schumann, M.; *et al.* Spectrum of gluten-related disorders: Consensus on new nomenclature and classification. *BMC Med.* **2012**, *10*, 13.
5. Ludvigsson, J.F.; Leffler, D.A.; Bai, J.C.; Biagi, F.; Fasano, A.; Green, P.H.; Hadjivassiliou, M.; Kaukinen, K.; Kelly, C.P.; Leonard, J.N.; *et al.* The Oslo definitions for coeliac disease and related terms. *Gut* **2013**, *62*, 43–52.
6. Mäki, M. Lack of consensus regarding definitions of coeliac disease. *Nat. Rev. Gastroenterol. Hepatol.* **2012**, *9*, 305–306.
7. Koletzko, S.; Niggemann, B.; Arato, A.; Dias, J.A.; Heuschkel, R.; Husby, S.; Mearin, M.L.; Papadopoulou, A.; Ruemmele, F.M.; Staiano, A.; *et al.* European Society of Pediatric Gastroenterology, Hepatology, and Nutrition. Diagnostic approach and management of cow's-milk protein allergy in infants and children: ESPGHAN GI Committee practical guidelines. *J. Pediatr. Gastroenterol. Nutr.* **2012**, *55*, 221–229.
8. Tanpowpong, P.; Ingham, T.R.; Lampshire, P.K.; Kirchberg, F.F.; Epton, M.J.; Crane, J.; Camargo, C.A., Jr.; New Zealand Asthma and Allergy Cohort Study Group. Coeliac disease and gluten avoidance in New Zealand children. *Arch. Dis. Child.* **2012**, *97*, 12–16.
9. Tanpowpong, P.; Broder-Fingert, S.; Katz, A.J.; Camargo, C.A., Jr. Predictors of gluten avoidance and implementation of a gluten-free diet in children and adolescents without confirmed celiac disease. *J. Pediatr.* **2012**, *161*, 471–475.
10. Digiacomo, D.V.; Tennyson, C.A.; Green, P.H.; Demmer, R.T. Prevalence of gluten-free diet adherence among individuals without celiac disease in the USA: Results from the Continuous National Health and Nutrition Examination Survey 2009–2010. *Scand. J. Gastroenterol.* **2013**, *48*, 921–925.

11. Krosgaard, L.R.; Engsbro, A.L.; Bytzer, P. The epidemiology of irritable bowel syndrome in Denmark. A population-based survey in adults < 50 years of age. *Scand. J. Gastroenterol.* **2013**, *48*, 523–299.
12. Breckan, R.K.; Asfeldt, A.M.; Straume, B.; Florholmen, J.; Paulssen, E.J. Prevalence, comorbidity, and risk factors for functional bowel symptoms: A population-based survey in Northern Norway. *Scand. J. Gastroenterol.* **2012**, *47*, 1274–1282.
13. Biesiekierski, J.R.; Newnham, E.D.; Irving, P.M.; Barrett, J.S.; Haines, M.; Doecke, J.D.; Shepherd, S.J.; Muir, J.G.; Gibson, P.R. Gluten causes gastrointestinal symptoms in subjects without celiac disease: A double-blind randomized placebo-controlled trial. *Am. J. Gastroenterol.* **2011**, *106*, 508–514.
14. Carroccio, A.; Mansueto, P.; Iacono, G.; Soresi, M.; D'Alcamo, A.; Cavataio, F.; Brusca, I.; Florena, A.M.; Ambrosiano, G.; Seidita, A.; *et al.* Non-celiac wheat sensitivity diagnosed by double-blind placebo-controlled challenge: Exploring a new clinical entity. *Am. J. Gastroenterol.* **2012**, *107*, 1898–1906.
15. Volta, U.; Tovoli, F.; Cicola, R.; Parisi, C.; Fabbri, A.; Piscaglia, M.; Fiorini, E.; Caio, G. Serological tests in gluten sensitivity (non celiac gluten intolerance). *J. Clin. Gastroenterol.* **2012**, *46*, 680–685.
16. Mastrototaro, L.; Castellaneta, S.; Gentile, A.; Fontana, C.; Tandoi, E.; Dellatte, S.; Romagnoli, V.; Catassi, C.; Francavilla R. Gluten sensitivity in children: Clinical, serological, genetic and histological description of the first paediatric series. *Dig. Liver Dis.* **2012**, *44*, S254–S255.
17. Brottveit, M.; Vandvik, P.O.; Wojniusz, S.; Løvik, A.; Lundin, K.E.; Boye, B. Absence of somatization in non-coeliac gluten sensitivity. *Scand. J. Gastroenterol.* **2012**, *47*, 770–777.
18. Boettcher, E.; Crowe, S.E. Dietary proteins and functional gastrointestinal disorders. *Am. J. Gastroenterol.* **2013**, *108*, 728–736.
19. Sainsbury, A.; Sanders, D.S.; Ford, A.C. Prevalence of irritable bowel syndrome-type symptoms in patients with celiac disease: A meta-analysis. *Clin. Gastroenterol. Hepatol.* **2013**, *11*, 359–365.
20. Vazquez-Roque, M.I.; Camilleri, M.; Smirk, T.; Murray, J.A.; Marietta, E.; O'Neill, J.; Carlson, P.; Lamsam, J. A controlled trial of gluten-free diet in patients with irritable bowel syndrome-diarrhea: Effects on bowel frequency and intestinal function. *Gastroenterology* **2013**, *144*, 903–911.
21. Biesiekirski, J.R.; Peters, S.L.; Newnham, E.D.; Rosella, O.; Muir, J.G.; Gibson, P.R. No effects of gluten in patients with self-reported non-celiac gluten sensitivity following dietary reduction of low-fermentable, poorly absorbed, short-chain carbohydrates. *Gastroenterology* **2013**, *145*, 320–328.
22. Batista, I.C.; Gandolfi, L.; Nobrega, Y.K.; Almeida, R.C.; Almeida, L.M.; Campos Junior, D.; Pratesi, R. Autism spectrum disorder and celiac disease: No evidence for a link. *Arq. Neuropsiquiatr.* **2012**, *70*, 28–33.
23. Marcason, W. What is the current status of research concerning use of a gluten-free, casein-free diet for children diagnosed with autism? *J. Am. Diet. Assoc.* **2009**, *109*, 572.
24. De Magistris, L.; Familiari, V.; Pascotto, A.; Sapone, A.; Frolli, A.; Iardino, P.; Carteni, M.; de Rosa, M.; Francavilla, R.; Riegler, G.; *et al.* Alterations of the intestinal barrier in patients with autism spectrum disorders and in their first-degree relatives. *J. Pediatr. Gastroenterol. Nutr.* **2010**, *51*, 418–424.

25. Robertson, M.A.; Sigalet, D.L.; Holst, J.J.; Meddings, J.B.; Wood, J.; Sharkey, K.A. Intestinal permeability and glucagon-like peptide-2 in children with autism: A controlled pilot study. *J. Autism Dev. Disord.* **2008**, *38*, 1066–1071.
26. Lau, N.M.; Green, P.H.; Taylor, A.K.; Hellberg, D.; Ajamian, M.; Tan, C.Z.; Kosofsky, B.E.; Higgins, J.J.; Rajadhyaksha, A.M.; Alaedini, A. Markers of celiac disease and gluten sensitivity in children with autism. *PLoS One* **2013**, *8*, e66155.
27. De Magistris, L.; Picardi, A.; Siniscalco, D.; Riccio, M.P.; Sapone, A.; Cariello, R. Antibodies against food antigens in patients with autistic spectrum disorders. *BioMed. Res. Int.* **2013**, *2013*, 729349.
28. Millward, C.; Ferriter, M.; Calver, S.; Connell-Jones, G. Gluten- and casein-free diets for autistic spectrum disorder. *Cochrane Database Syst. Rev*. **2008**, *2*, CD003498.
29. Whiteley, P.; Haracopos, D.; Knivsberg, A.M.; Reichelt, K.L.; Parlar, S.; Jacobsen, J.; Seim, A.; Pedersen, L.; Schondel, M.; Shattock, P. The ScanBrit randomised, controlled, single-blind study of a gluten- and casein-free dietary intervention for children with autism spectrum disorders. *Nutr. Neurosci*. **2010**, *13*, 87–100.
30. Dohan, F.C. Cereals and schizophrenia data and hypothesis. *Acta Psychiatr. Scand.* **1966**, *42*, 125–152.
31. Vlissides, D.M.; Venulet, A.; Jenner, F.A. A double-blind glutenfree/gluten-load controlled trial in a secure ward population. *Br. J. Psychiatry* **1986**, *148*, 447–452.
32. Potkin, S.G.; Weinberger, D.; Kleinman, J.; Potkin, S.G.; Weinberger, D.; Kleinman, J.; Nasrallah, H.; Luchins, D.; Bigelow, L.; Linnoila, M.; *et al.* Wheat gluten challenge in schizophrenic patients. *Am. J. Psychiatry* **1981**, *138*, 1208–1211.
33. Storms, L.H.; Clopton, J.M.; Wright, C. Effects of gluten in schizophrenics. *Arch. Gen. Psychiatry* **1982**, *39*, 323–327.
34. Cascella, N.G.; Kryszak, D.; Bhatti, B.; Gregory, P.; Kelly, D.L.; Mc Evoy, J.P.; Fasano, A.; Eaton, W.W. Prevalence of celiac disease and gluten sensitivity in the United States clinical antipsychotic trials of intervention effectiveness study population. *Schizophr. Bull.* **2011**, *37*, 94–100.
35. Cascella, N.G.; Santora, D.; Gregory, P.; Kelly, D.L.; Fasano, A.; Eaton, W.W. Increased prevalence of transglutaminase 6 antibodies in sera from schizophrenia patients. *Schizophr. Bull.* **2013**, *39*, 867–871.
36. Dickerson, F.; Stallings, C.; Origoni, A.; Vaughan, C.; Khushalani, S.; Leister, F.; Yang, S.; Krivogorsky, B.; Alaedini, A.; Yolken, R. Markers of gluten sensitivity and celiac disease in recent-onset psychosis and multi-episode schizophrenia. *Biol. Psychiatry* **2010**, *68*, 100–104.
37. Holmes, G. Non coeliac gluten sensitivity. *Gastroenterol. Hepatol. Bed Bench* **2013**, *6*, 115–119.
38. Brottveit, M.; Beitnes, A.C.; Tollefsen, S.; Bratlie, J.E.; Jahnsen, F.L.; Johansen, F.E.; Sollid, L.M.; Lundin, K.E. Mucosal cytokine response after short-term gluten challenge in celiac disease and non-celiac gluten sensitivity. *Am. J. Gastroenterol*. **2013**, *108*, 842–850.
39. Bucci, C.; Zingone, F.; Russo, I.; Morra, I.; Tortora, R.; Pogna, N.; Scalia, G.; Iovino, P.; Ciacci, C. Gliadin does not induce mucosal inflammation or basophil activation in patients with non-celiac gluten sensitivity. *Clin. Gastroenterol. Hepatol*. **2013**, *11*, 1294–1299.

40. Junker, Y.; Zeissig, S.; Kim, S.J.; Barisani, D.; Wieser, H.; Leffler, D.A.; Zevallos, V.; Libermann, T.A.; Dillon, S.; Freitag, T.L.; *et al.* Wheat amylase trypsin inhibitors drive intestinal inflammation via activation of toll-like receptor 4. *J. Exp. Med.* **2012**, *209*, 2395–2408.

8

Vitamin and Mineral Deficiencies are Highly Prevalent in Newly Diagnosed Celiac Disease Patients

Nicolette J. Wierdsma [1,*], Marian A. E. van Bokhorst-de van der Schueren [1], Marijke Berkenpas [1], Chris J. J. Mulder [2] and Ad A. van Bodegraven [2]

[1] Department of Nutrition and Dietetics, VU University Medical Centre, P.O. Box 7057, Amsterdam 1007 MB, The Netherlands; E-Mails: m.vanbokhorst@vumc.nl (M.A.E.B.S.); m.berkenpas@vumc.nl (M.B.)

[2] Department of Gastroenterology, Celiac Centre Amsterdam, VU University Medical Centre, Amsterdam 1007 MB, The Netherlands; E-Mails: cjmulder@vumc.nl (C.J.J.M.); v.bodegraven@vumc.nl (A.A.B.)

* Author to whom correspondence should be addressed; E-Mail: N.Wierdsma@vumc.nl;

Abstract: Malabsorption, weight loss and vitamin/mineral-deficiencies characterize classical celiac disease (CD). This study aimed to assess the nutritional and vitamin/mineral status of current "early diagnosed" untreated adult CD-patients in the Netherlands. Newly diagnosed adult CD-patients were included (n = 80, 42.8 ± 15.1 years) and a comparable sample of 24 healthy Dutch subjects was added to compare vitamin concentrations. Nutritional status and serum concentrations of folic acid, vitamin A, B_6, B_{12}, and (25-hydroxy) D, zinc, haemoglobin (Hb) and ferritin were determined (before prescribing gluten free diet). Almost all CD-patients (87%) had at least one value below the lower limit of reference. Specifically, for vitamin A, 7.5% of patients showed deficient levels, for vitamin B_6 14.5%, folic acid 20%, and vitamin B_{12} 19%. Likewise, zinc deficiency was observed in 67% of the CD-patients, 46% had decreased iron storage, and 32% had anaemia. Overall, 17% were malnourished (>10% undesired weight loss), 22% of the women were underweight (Body Mass Index (BMI) < 18.5), and 29% of the patients were overweight (BMI > 25). Vitamin deficiencies were barely seen in healthy controls, with the exception of vitamin B_{12}. Vitamin/mineral deficiencies were counter-intuitively not associated with a (higher) grade of histological intestinal damage or (impaired) nutritional status. In conclusion, vitamin/mineral deficiencies are still common in newly "early diagnosed" CD-patients, even though the prevalence of obesity at initial diagnosis is rising. Extensive nutritional assessments seem warranted to guide nutritional advices and follow-up in CD treatment.

Keywords: vitamins; minerals; celiac disease; deficiency; adult; Body Mass Index

---

1. Introduction

Celiac disease (CD) is the most common food intolerance in the Western population, and currently represents a major health care issue. The prevalence of CD has been estimate to be 0.5%–1% in different parts of the world [1]. CD is an inflammatory, immune-mediated chronic disease of the mucosa of the proximal small intestine due to irreversible gluten intolerance in genetically susceptible individuals. Gluten refers to a set of amino acid sequences found in the prolamine fraction of wheat, barley and rye. The characteristic histopathological finding is a varying degree of villous atrophy and crypt hyperplasia, primarily in the duodenum and jejunum, with inflammatory changes leading to malabsorption. The first-line, and up-till-now only, treatment is a lifelong strict adherence to a gluten free diet (GFD). All other treatment modalities suppress the intestinal inflammatory response and do not treat the intolerance [2,3].

CD is a multi-system disorder which leads to striking differences in its clinical presentation. When present, gastrointestinal symptoms, including clinically evident malabsorption, may facilitate the diagnosis of CD. Over the last few decades, there appeared to be a changing clinical presentation of CD from the classical malabsorptive picture (diarrhoea, malabsorption and weight loss) towards one of a non-classical presentation with milder, non-specific symptoms such as tiredness, hematologic abnormalities, constipation and/or abdominal distension [4–6]. Nowadays, many patients present with no or only minor extra-intestinal symptoms. Indeed, microcytic or macrocytic anaemia, or folate deficiency may occasionally be the only clinical symptom to suggest CD. This leads to a great extent of underdiagnoses in several countries [7]. Currently, 20%–40% of newly diagnosed CD-patients are even classified as overweight (Body Mass Index (BMI) > 25 kg/m^2) instead of the anticipated underweight [8–12], although the prevalence of obesity seems lower than in the general population [13]. This makes the diagnosis of CD challenging. Greater clinical awareness—especially improved serological testing since the late 1990s, including that for anti-tissue transglutaminase (tTG) antibodies [14,15]—and the appearance of specialized centres has led to earlier recognition of CD-patients.

In the classically presenting CD-patients, malabsorption is frequently encountered [16], and micronutrient deficiencies may arise. Indeed, several studies demonstrate these deficiencies with varying results [17–21].

Our group recently demonstrated the specific functional insufficiency of the proximal small bowel in CD-patients by means of the citrulline generation test, in which the citrulline peak after glutamine administration and its conversion into citrulline in the enterocyte was delayed due to a decreased functional intestinal mass as a consequence of inflammatory changes [22].

Deficiencies of water-soluble vitamins, like B-vitamins, would be expected since they are absorbed in the proximal small bowel, which is the most prominent site affected in CD-patients. However, available data, in particular regarding vitamin B_2 and B_6 deficiencies, do not support this in untreated CD-patients [17,23]. Table 1 shows an overview of older and more recent literature on vitamin and mineral deficiencies in adult CD-patients.

Table 1. Literature overview on vitamin and mineral status in newly diagnosed adult celiac disease (CD)-patients.

Author, year	Patient Group	Outcome
	Till 2005	
Hallert,1981 [24]	CD (Folate)	Decreased serum folate concentration abnormality in adult CD. Predictive value of low folate for advice jejunal biopsy.
Stene-Larsen, 1988 [25]	CD ($n = 3$)	Vitamin B_{12} malabsorption by CD is emphasized as a pathogenic mechanism of megaloblastic anaemia.
Crofton, 1990 [20]	Untreated CD ($n = 8$) and healthy controls ($n = 5$) (Zinc)	Impaired turnover and loss of endogenous zinc in mild untreated CD. Zinc levels normal.
Kemppainen, 1995 [26]	Untreated CD ($n = 40$), CD in remission ($n = 52$) (Nutritional status)	Nutritional status quite good in both groups. 15%–38% deficiencies (HB, ferritin, iron or B_{12}) in untreated CD compared to 0%–20% in remission CD.
Kemppainen, 1998 [27]	Untreated CD ($n = 40$) (Nutritional status)	Anthropometric and biochemical nutritional status acceptable. Low ferritin and folate (enterocyte) levels, but normalised after 1 year GFD.
Alwitry, 2000 [23]	Celiac disease (Vitamin A)	Case report in vitamin A deficiency and eye deviation
Dahele, 2001 [18]	Untreated CD ($n = 39$) (Vitamin B12)	41% B12 deficient (<220 ng/L), 41% anaemic, and 31% folate deficient f the B_{12} deficient CD-patients.
Dickey, 2002 [28]	CD ($n = 159$) (Vitamin B12)	Low serum B_{12} is common in CD (12%) and is not due to autoimmune gastritis. 10% of B_{12} deficient group had atrophic gastritis. Advice to know B_{12} level before folate supplementation.
Hozyasz, 2003 [29]	Untreated CD Polish ($n = 18$), remission on GFD ($n = 12$) (Vitamin E)	All untreated CD-patients had reduced vitamin E levels. Vitamin A comparable to treated CD.
	2005–2013	
Harper, 2007 [30]	Untreated (3 mo after diagnosis) CD ($n = 405$) (Anaemia)	Iron deficiency in 31% of male and 19% of females, folate in 12%, B_{12} 5% and anaemia in 20% of CD-patients. Anaemia can not only be explained by nutritional deficiencies.
Dickey, 2008 [17]	Untreated CD ($n = 35$), persistent villous atrophy ($n = 34$, recovered ($n = 41$) (B-vitamins)	No compromised B_2 and B_6 in 3 groups. Homocysteine concentrations are inversely associated with serum and red cell folate and with B_{12}.

Table 1. *Cont.*

Henri-Bhargava, 2008 [19]	CD (Vitamin E, copper)	Neurological impairment due to vitamin E and copper deficiencies in CD.
Bergamaschi, 2008 [21]	Untreated CD (n = 150), after 1 year GFD (n = 53) (Anaemia)	34% anaemia at diagnosis. Iron, vitamin deficiencies and anaemia of chronic disease are common in CD. GFD treatment improves anaemia.
Lerner, 2012 [31]	CD (Spanish) (n = 22) and CD children (n = 120) (Spanish, Israeli), (Vitamin D)	Vitamin D levels correlate negatively with age. 55% of Adult CD-patients had vitamin D deficiency (25-hydroxy < 20 ng/mL) and should be supplemented.

It has been suggested that the current "early diagnosis" of CD might be associated with less vitamin and mineral deficiencies at the moment of diagnosis than the classical CD. Mineral and trace-element status of untreated CD-patients has not been widely studied. There is even a lack of recent reports in the literature (see Table 1) indicating which deficiencies should be checked in newly diagnosed celiacs in Western Europe. Therefore, we aimed to measure essential serum nutritional variables in order to assess the prevalence of vitamin and mineral deficiencies in untreated adult CD-patients from a tertiary referral Celiac Disease Centre, consuming a (gluten containing) standard Dutch (Western) diet before diagnosis. Secondly, we studied the nutritional status and differences in prevalence of vitamin and mineral deficiencies between patients with different grades of intestinal histological damage, nutritional status, and sex.

2. Materials and Methods

2.1. Patients

Eighty consecutively diagnosed adult patients (aged 18–75 years) with newly diagnosed CD were recruited from the Outpatient Clinic of the VU University Medical Centre, Amsterdam, the Netherlands, during the period 2005–2012. All patients consumed a normal (gluten-containing) Dutch-Western diet until inclusion. The mean daily gluten intake in the Netherlands is around 13 g [32]. Duodenal biopsy specimens were harvested to determine the grade of histological damage due to gluten sensitive enteropathy as classified by Marsh [33] and modified by Rostami [34,35]. Gastric (corpus) biopsies were routinely harvested to determine whether atrophic gastritis was present. CD associated antibodies, *i.e.*, anti-endomysial antibodies (EMA) and anti-tTG antibodies, were determined [36,37]. In addition, HLA-genotyping was performed, to analyse the presence of DQ_2 and DQ_8 (heterozygote or homozygote) as a prerequisite for a definitive diagnosis [38]. The diagnosis of CD was based on these histopathological, serological and genetic criteria.

Histopathological classification according to Marsh was used: intraepithelial lymphocytosis, crypt hyperplasia and villous atrophy Marsh IIIA, B and C (respectively, partial, subtotal and total villous atrophy) with or without elevated antibodies. Also, a group was added with low grade histopathological abnormalities Marsh I or Marsh II (lymphocytic enteritis with crypt hyperplasia) with gluten-dependent disorders, in case of elevated antibodies and the HLA-DQ_2 or HLA-DQ_8 genotype.

Blood samples were collected as part of routine clinical care. Patients were excluded if they had an established or suspected gastrointestinal abnormality other than CD, such as inflammatory bowel disease (IBD). A representative sample of 24 healthy Dutch subjects (comparable for sex, age and BMI) was added to compare concentrations of vitamin A, B_6, folic acid and B_{12} (see control subjects characteristics [39]). Both groups were studied in the same period, were living in a similar environment, and measurements were performed at the same clinical chemistry laboratory.

The study protocol was approved by the Medical Ethics Committee (2005, project code 05.153) of the VU University Medical Centre Amsterdam, The Netherlands.

2.2. Nutritional Status

Patient characteristics and demographic data (including age (year), body height (m), body weight (kg) and self-reported involuntary weight loss in the past 1 and 6 months) were collected, BMI was calculated and biochemical analyses were performed following diagnosis and before any dietary advice to initiate a GFD. Patients were subsequently classified as "malnourished" when they unintentionally lost more than 10% of their bodyweight in the past 6 months or more than 5% in the past month prior to diagnosis or as having "risk of malnutrition" when 5%–10% of the bodyweight was unintentionally lost in the 6 months before diagnosis. Moreover, patients were classified into 3 groups on the basis of baseline BMI; less than 18.5 kg/m^2 (underweight), 18.5–25.0 kg/m^2 (normal weight) and more than 25 kg/m^2 (overweight, or even "obese" in case of BMI above 30 kg/m^2) (according to the definition of the World Health Organisation (2000)).

2.3. Biochemical Analysis

Fasting venous blood samples were drawn and subsequently analysed at the endocrine and clinical chemistry laboratories of the VU University Medical Centre, Amsterdam. Samples for serum folic acid and serum vitamin B_{12} were analysed by competitive immunoassay (Luminescence, Abbott, IL, USA). Serum vitamin B_6 and vitamin A status were determined by high-performance liquid chromatography (HPLC). Vitamin (25-hydroxy) D was assessed with a competitive binding protein assay (Diasorin, Stillwater, MN, USA). Zinc status was assessed using Flame Atomic Absorption Spectroscopy (FAAS), serum haemoglobin by colorimetric methods (Cell Dyn Sapphire, Abbott, IL, USA) and ferritin values by electro-chemiluminescence immunoassay "ECLIA" (Roche, Mannheim, Germany) or "ACS CENTAUR" (Bayer, Mijdrecht, The Netherlands).

Vitamin B_6 and folic acid (both proximally absorbed) and vitamin B_{12} (distally absorbed) were considered to represent the water-soluble vitamin status. Vitamin A and vitamin (25-hydroxy) D were considered to represent the fat-soluble vitamin status, although sun exposure, even in The Netherlands, may have a strong influence on serum levels of vitamin D. Haemoglobin and ferritin levels below the reference ranges listed were used to establish a respective diagnosis of anaemia, iron-deficiency or iron-deficiency anaemia when both haemoglobin and ferritin were below reference ranges. Patients with a serum value below the lower limit of the reference value were considered "deficient". Reference values for the different parameters are displayed in Table 3.

2.4. Statistical Analysis

Data were tested for normal distribution and presented as means ± SD. The percentage of patients with values below the reference value and absolute number of deficient patients were additionally calculated for all assessed serum vitamin and mineral concentrations.

Data were analysed for the total group, and in stratified subgroups by sex, histological damage (Marsh classification) and BMI. To determine differences with regard to gender, a Student's *t*-test was applied in case of continuous data and Pearson's Chi-Square tests (χ^2) in the case of comparing proportions (% of deficient patients). Analysis of variance (ANOVA), with a Bonferroni correction when a statistical significant difference was achieved, was used to compare more than two groups. A Mann-Whitney U test (Wilcoxon) or in case of more than 2 variables, a Kruskal-Wallis test was applied for variables not found in a normal distribution. The level of statistical significance was determined a priori at $p < 0.05$. Statistical analyses were performed using SPSS (Statistical Package for Social Sciences Inc., Chicago, IL, USA—Windows version 20.0).

3. Results

3.1. Patient Characteristics and Nutritional Status

Patient characteristics are shown in Table 2; two-thirds of the population was female. Male patients were significantly older than female patients ($p = 0.006$). Approximately 46% (37/80) of the patients had partial villous atrophy (Marsh IIIA) and 42.5% showed subtotal (20/80) or total villous atrophy (14/80) (Marsh IIIB or IIIC, respectively). Histologically and serologically atrophic (corpus) gastritis was ruled out by a pathologist experienced in intestinal histology. Some of the CD patients reported to have used vitamin and mineral supplements before diagnosis of CD was made: 18 (22.5%) a multivitamin, folic acid or vitamin B-complex, 7 (8.8%) iron supplements and 14 (17.5%) a calcium supplement. The anthropometric data of 24 healthy controls were comparable to those of the patients included.

Patients had, on average, lost 2.4% (±6.3%) of their bodyweight during the 6 months prior to diagnosis. Approximately 17% was classified as malnourished (>10% weight loss) and 5% as being at risk of malnutrition (5%–10% previous weight loss). Six out of 80 patients (7.5%), and only females, were classified as underweight, whereas 29% (23/80) of patients were classified as overweight (female:male ratio =1:1). Of the overweight patients, 26% were even obese (6/80 of the total group, with female:male ratio = 1:1).

Table 2. Patient characteristics of untreated adult CD-patients by gender and compared to healthy controls.

		CD Patients			Healthy Controls *
N			80		24
Sex		All	Female (52)	Male (28)	F14/M11
Age (year)	mean ± SD (range)	42.8 ± 15.1 (18–75)	39.5 ± 14.3 ^	49.1 ± 14.9	43.0 ± 12.9
Height (m)	mean ± SD	1.73 ± 0.1	1.68 ± 0.09 ^	1.80 ± 0.08	1.76 ± 0.07 *[a]
Weight (kg)	mean ± SD	70.6 ± 15.3	66.0 ± 14.3 ^	79.1 ± 13.8	75.5 ± 11.6
BMI (kg/m^2)	mean ± SD	23.6 ± 4.0	23.2 ± 4.2	24.3 ± 3.6	24.1 ± 2.6
	<18.5	6 (7.5%)	6 (22.5%)	0	0
	18.5–25	51 (63.8%)	31 (59.6%)	20 (71.4%)	18 (72%)
	>25	23 (28.8%)	15 (28.8%)	8 (28.6%)	27 (28%)
Marsh classification *N* (%)	I/II #	9 (11.3%)	6 (11.5%)	3 (10.7%)	
	IIIA	37 (46%)	23 (44.2%)	14 (50.0%)	
	IIIB	20 (25%)	10 (19.2%)	10 (35.7%)	
	IIIC	14 (17.5%)	13 (25%)	1 (3.6%)	
Antibodies *N* (%)					
EMA	Negative	17 (21.3%)	11 (21.1%)	6 (22.0%)	
	doubtful	1 (1.3%)	1 (1.9%)	0	
	weak positive	5 (6.3%)	5 (9.6%)	0	
	positive	14 (17.5%)	10 (19.2%)	4 (14.3%)	
	strong positive	38 (47.5%)	23 (44.2%)	15 (53.6%)	
	n.d.	5 (6.3%)	2 (3.8%)	1 (3.6%)	
tTG	Negative	16 (20%)	9 (17.3%)	7 (25%)	
	doubtful	4 (5%)	3 (5.8%)	1 (3.6%)	
	weak positive	10 (12.5%)	9 (17.3%)	1 (3.6%)	
	positive	18 (22.5%)	12 (23.1%)	6 (21.4%)	
	strong positive	31 (38.8%)	19 (36.5%	12 (42.9%)	
	n.d.	1 (1.3%)	0	1 (3.6%)	
tTG (U/mL)	mean ± SD	171 ± 402	124 ± 378	274 ± 445	
	(range)	(3.2–2500)	(4–2500)	(3.2–1999)	
CD genotypes	$DQ_{2(hetero-/homozygote)}$	62 (77.5%)$_{(56/6)}$	42 (80.8%)$_{(37/5)}$	20 (71.4%)$_{(19/1)}$	
	$DQ_{8(hetero-/homozygote)}$	5 (6.3%)$_{(3/2)}$	3 (5.8%)$_{(2/1)}$	2 (7.1%)$_{(1/1)}$	
	DQ_2 and DQ_8	3 (3.8%)	2 (3.8%)	1 (3.6%)	
	DQ_2 nor DQ_8	3 (3.8%)	1 (1.9%)	2 (7.1%)	
	n.d.	7 (8.8%)	4 (7.7%)	3 (14.3%)	

BMI: Body Mass Index, EMA: anti-endomysial antibodies, tTG: anti-tissue transglutaminase, ^ Significantly different from men ($p < 0.05$) by Student's *t*-test, n.d. (not determined), # low grade histopathological abnormalities with HLA-DQ_2 and/or DQ_8 and elevated antibodies (EMA and/or tTG), * variables NS (not statistically significant from CD-patients ($p < 0.05$) by Mann-Whitney U test), *[a] statistical trend $p = 0.05$.

Table 3. Serum concentrations of nutritional biochemical parameters of untreated adult CD-patients (compared to healthy controls).

Serum Vitamin/Mineral [Reference Value]	Serum Concentration ^				Percentage deficient patients #			
	All	Male	Female	Healthy Controls	All	Male	Female	Healthy Controls
Vitamin A [1.2–3.0 nmol/L]	2.0 ± 0.7 0.1–4.0 (53)	2.2 ± 0.9 (17)	1.9 ± 0.6 (36)	2.5 ± 0.6 (1.4–4.0) $^{\%a}$ (25)	7.5% (4/53)	11.8% (2/17)	5.6% (2/36)	
Vitamin B_6 [13–80 nmol/L]	92.2 ± 142.7 6.0–593.0 (62)	56.1 ± 87.1 (20)	109.4 ± 160.8 (42)	70.1 ± 74.5 (21–384) (25)	14.5% (9/62)	25.0% (5/20)	9.5% (4/42)	
Folic acid [>5.6 nmol/L]	15.1 ± 15.0 2.1–90.1 (80)	10.4 ± 6.6 (28)	17.6 ± 17.6 ^{*a} (52)	20.4 ± 18.1 (4.4–91) $^{\%b}$ (25)	20.0% (16/80)	28.5% (8/28)	15.4% (8/52)	
Vitamin B_{12} [150–700 pmol/L)	231.2 ± 104.3 64.0–590.0 (80)	222.6 ± 75.6 (28)	235.7 ± 117.4 (52)	272.6 ± 112.5 (100–453) (25)	19.0% (15/80)	22.2% (6/27)	17.3% (9/52)	
Zinc [11–19 nmol/L]	10.3 ± 2.1 6.3–14.8 (40)	10.4 ± 2.2 (16)	10.2 ± 2.0 (24)		66.7% (26/40)	62.5% (10/16)	70.8% (17/24)	
Vitamin (25-hydroxy) D [30–150 nmol/L]	64.8 ± 26.8 29–120 (21)	64.5 ± 35.3 (8)	65.0 ± 21.6 (13)		4.8% (1/21)	12.5% (1/8)	0 (0/13)	
Haemoglobin [M 8.5–11/F 7.5–10 mmol/L]	8.0 ± 1.1 5.0–10.2 (71)	8.9 ± 0.8 (25)	7.5 ± 0.9 ^{*b} (46)		32.4% (23/71)	24.0% (6/25)	37.0% (17/46)	
Ferritin [20–250 µG/L]	48.1 ± 83.9 3.0–451.0 (39)	110.9 ± 147.2 (10)	26.4 ± 26.2 (29)		46.2% (18/39)	30.0% (3/10)	51.7% (15/29)	

^ Successively expressed as: mean ± SD, range, (*N*), * statistically significantly different from men (Student's *t*-test), ^{*a} $p = 0.04$, ^{*b} $p < 0.001$, # NS (not statistically significant ($p < 0.05$) by Pearson's Chi-Square tests (χ^2)), $^{\%}$ statistically significantly different from CD by Mann-Whitney U test, $^{\%a}$ $p = 0.006$, $^{\%b}$ $p = 0.030$, $^{\$}$ statistically significant by Pearson's Chi-Square tests ($^{\$a}$ $p = 0.049$, $^{\$b}$ $p = 0.066$.

3.2. Biochemical Analyses

Serum concentrations of vitamins and minerals of the untreated CD-patients are shown in Table 3. CD-patients were most frequently deficient for folic acid (20%, 16/80), followed by vitamin B_{12} (19%, 15/79), vitamin B_6 (14.5%, 9/62), vitamin A (7.5%, 4/53) and vitamin (25-hydroxy) D (4.5%, 1/21), respectively. Approximately 67% (26/39) of the patients had zinc deficiency, 32.4% (23/71) had anaemia, 46.2% (18/39) had insufficient iron storage evidenced by low ferritin and 25% (8/40) had iron-deficiency anaemia. CD-patients had lower values of vitamin A and folic acid than healthy controls. Overall, vitamin deficiencies were barely seen in healthy controls, with the exception of vitamin B_{12}. None of the healthy controls showed deficient levels (below the reference values) for vitamin A and vitamin B_6 and only one for folic acid.

Ten patients (12.5%) were not deficient for any of the assessed vitamins and minerals. These patients had similar base-line characteristics to the rest of the CD group. The remaining 70 patients (87.5%) were deficient in at least one of the nutritional parameters and 43 (53.8%) for two or more parameters.

Table 3 depicts the proportion of deficient patients, stratified by sex. As anticipated, serum haemoglobin concentrations were lower in women than in men ($p < 0.001$). While, on the other hand, serum folic acid concentrations were lower ($p = 0.040$) in men when compared to women. No statistically significant difference was found for any of the other nutritional parameters when comparing males and females. Notwithstanding, multivitamin use (including folic acid or vitamin B supplement) at their own volition or prescribed by the GP was more prevalent in women than men (30% *vs.* 13%). A statistical trend was seen for vitamin B_6, suggesting that men might be more often deficient than women ($p = 0.097$).

3.3. Association between Vitamin and Mineral Concentrations and Histological Damage (Marsh-Classification)

Table 4 depicts the mean serum vitamin and mineral values by Marsh strata. No statistically significant differences were found between the serum vitamin and mineral concentrations across the four Marsh strata, except for ferritin. Serum ferritin values decreased when the villous atrophy score increased ($p = 0.041$).

Table 4. Mean serum concentrations of vitamins and minerals (±SD) in untreated CD-patients by Marsh stratum.

Serum Vitamin/Mineral	Marsh Stratum			
	I/II # ($n = 9$)	IIIA ($n = 37$)	IIIB ($n = 20$)	IIIC ($n = 14$)
Vitamin A (nmol/L)	2.3 ± 0.4 (4/9)	2.0 ± 0.8 (28/37)	1.9 ± 0.44 (11/20)	1.9 ± 0.8 (10/14)
Vitamin B_6 (nmol/L)	129.8 ± 115.0 (7/9)	107.6 ± 170.7 (29/37)	55.7 ± 43.5 (15/20)	86.8 ± 163.9 (11/14)
Folic acid (nmol/L)	14.1 ± 8.5 (9/9)	14.7 ± 12.9 (37/37)	13.9 ± 15.5 (20/20)	18.4 ± 22.4 (14/14)

Table 4. *Cont.*

Vitamin B_{12} (pmol/L)	282.4 ± 151.7 (9/9)	225.2 ± 91.1 (37/37)	216.5 ± 80.2 (20/20)	234.7 ± 131.8 (14/14)
Vitamin (25-hydroxy) D (nmol/L)	89.3 ± 27.0 (3/9)	52.7 ± 16.4 (7/37)	63.0 ± 31.4 (6/20)	69.2 ± 29.2 (5/14)
Zinc (nmol/L)	11.0 ± 1.7 (5/9)	10.8 ± 2.3 (19/37)	9.8 ± 1.7 (11/20)	8.8 ± 1.7 (5/14)
Haemoglobin (mmol/L) *	8.5 ± 0.5 (7/9)	8.0 ± 1.2 (33/37)	8.0 ± 1.1 (18/20)	7.9 ± 1.0 (13/14)
Ferritin (μG/L) ^	123.8 ± 167.3 (6/9)	47.6 ± 66.3 (18/37)	18.8 ± 17.6 (10/20)	17.2 ± 22.0 (5/14)

Low grade histopathological abnormalities with HLA-DQ_2 and/or DQ_8 and elevated antibodies (EMA and/or tTG), * gender specific Females I/II 8.2 ± 0.29; IIIA 7.4 ± 0.95; IIIB 7.3 ± 0.84; IIIC 7.8 ± 0.97 and Male I/II 8.9 ± 0.78; IIIA 8.9 ± 0.96; IIIB 9.0 ± 0.67; IIIC 8.8 ± 0.72, ^ statistically significantly different (p = 0.041) by Kruskal-Wallis test.

3.4. Association between Vitamin and Mineral Concentrations and Nutritional Status

Table 5 depicts the mean serum concentrations of vitamins and minerals per BMI stratum. A trend was observed for underweight patients having a slightly higher serum folic acid concentration than patients with normal weight or overweight patients (p = 0.058). Besides, patients with >10% unintentional weight loss in the past 6 months had higher vitamin A and (a trend for) higher vitamin B_6 (p = 0.09) levels than patients without weight loss. Otherwise, no differences were observed between the different classes of nutritional status.

Table 5. Mean serum concentrations of vitamins and minerals (±SD) in untreated CD-patients by nutritional status (BMI stratum and unintentional weight loss).

Serum Vitamin/Mineral	**BMI Stratum (kg/m²) ^**			**Weight Loss (% in past 6 months)**	
	Under-Weight (<18.5) (n = 6)	**Normal Weight (18.5–25.0) (n = 51)**	**Over-Weight (>25) (n = 23)**	**Well-Nourished (0%–10%) (n = 64)**	**Mal-Nourished (>10%) (n = 13)**
Vitamin A (nmol/L)	1.7 ± 0.7 (5)	2.0 ± 0.7 (35)	2.0 ± 0.6 (13)	1.8 ± 0.6 (40)	2.6 ± 0.7 # (11)
Vitamin B_6 (nmol/L)	128.5 ± 207.8 (6)	99.3 ± 146.2 (39)	63.1 ± 109.0 (17)	68.1 ± 102.0 (48)	206 ± 240.8 (11)
Folic acid (nmol/L)	33.0 ± 29.9 (6)	14.5 ± 13.4 (51)	11.8 ± 10.0 (23)	13.4 ± 11.2 (64)	23.5 ± 27.1 (13)
Vitamin B_{12} (pmol/L)	216.3 ± 57.3 (6)	226.2 ± 114.5 (51)	246.0 ± 90.4 (23)	227.6 ± 104.0 (64)	250.8 ± 117.7 (13)
Vitamin (25-hydroxy) D (nmol/L)	52.0 (1)	63.4 ± 28.0 (11)	68.0 ± 27.9 (9)	67.1 ± 27.1 (17)	55.0 ± 26.5 (4)

Table 5. *Cont.*

Zinc (nmol/L)	8.8 ± 0.3 (2)	10.3 ± 2.1 (26)	10.6 ± 2.2 (12)	10.5 ± 2.1 (31)	9.8 ± 2.1 (7)
Haemoglobin (mmol/L)	7.6 ± 0.7 (6)	8.0 ± 1.1 (45)	8.2 ± 1.2 (20)	8.1 ± 1.1 (56)	7.8 ± 1.4 (12)
Ferritin (μG/L)	25.0 ± 2.1 (3)	34.9 ± 38.4 (26)	89.0 ± 151.9 (10)	48.5 ± 90.4 (33)	46.2 ± 38.3 (5)

^ NS (not statistically significant ($p < 0.05$) by Kruskal-Wallis test, # statistically significantly different from well-nourished patients (Student t-test), $p = 0.001$.

4. Discussion

The present study showed that the majority of an "early diagnosis" adult untreated CD patient group (with so-called non-classical presentation) in the Netherlands, had at least one, and often several, serum vitamin or mineral deficiencies at diagnosis. Almost 90% of CD-patients were found to be deficient in at least one or more of the assessed nutritional parameters, and half of patients were deficient for two or more nutritional serum variables. This was observed to be unrelated to severity of clinical presentation, nutritional status or (semi-quantified) histopathological damage (score).

In this study, no statistically significant difference in serum vitamin and mineral concentration was found between men and women, although (multi)vitamin use prior to diagnosis was more prevalent in women than men (30% *vs.* 13%). Information is lacking whether they took the vitamins at their own volition, or if they were prescribed by the general practitioner. In addition, the assessed serum deficiencies were independent of Marsh stratum (Table 4), nutritional status (Table 5) and age (data not shown). Folic acid deficiency was observed in 20% of the untreated CD-patients in this study. The prevalence of folate deficiency varies from 18% to 90% in varying older and newer reports of CD-patients [17,18,24,26]. In studies from Scotland and Finland, folate deficiency was reported in 42% [18] and 37% [27] of the untreated CD-patients, respectively. The difference in prevalence might at least partially be explained by technical aspects of measurement of "folate" (which is the natural form of folic acid) and "folic acid" since bioavailability of folic acid is twice that of folate [40]. Macrocytic anaemia in untreated CD-patients is usually caused by folate deficiency. In two large European studies, anaemia, mostly attributed to malabsorption, was reported to be present in 20%–34% of untreated CD-patients [20,30]. This corresponds with our results in which 25% of the CD-patients suffered from iron-deficiency anaemia.

The presence of vitamin B_6 deficiency has been reported in two studies, albeit in children with "acute celiac disease". A decreased pyridoxal phosphate was reported in serum samples and in duodenal mucosa, suggestive of vitamin B_6 deficiency [41,42] and indicative for decreased levels of vitamin B_6 in untreated CD children. We found water-soluble vitamin deficiencies (B_6, folic acid and B_{12}) in approximately one in seven (B_6) to one in five (folic acid and B_{12}) untreated CD-patients. This was despite the fact that more than 20% of the patients were using a prescribed or over-the-counter multivitamin/vitamin B-complex or a folic acid supplement before diagnosis.

Vitamin B_{12} deficiency was frequently observed in our CD-patient group (19%), in accordance with earlier studies, notably also in those without atrophic gastritis [17,18,26–28]. Intriguingly, this vitamin is typically absorbed in the terminal ileum. Apparently, the distal small bowel is functionally more affected than previously believed, based on patho-histological analysis of distal small bowel biopsy samples [43]. Vitamin B_{12} deficiency in untreated CD-patients has been confirmed in several previously conducted European studies [18,25–28], ranging from 12% up to 41%. It may be hypothesized that vitamin B_{12} deficiency is a result of a dysfunctional intrinsic factor [44]. Dickey reported that low vitamin B_{12} concentrations in CD were not due to auto-immune gastritis [28]. In this study, none of the patients had histologically or serologically demonstrated atrophic gastritis and, therefore, this was unlikely to be responsible for vitamin B_{12} deficiencies in CD.

In various small studies in Europeans, deficiencies of the fat soluble vitamins A [23,27], E [19,29] and D [45] in untreated CD-patients have been previously reported. The latter has been associated with osteomalacia. In clinical practice, many believe that the clinically relevant lower limit for vitamin D deficiency should be increased. As a consequence, the displayed (relatively low) deficiency percentages can therefore be an underestimation. The observed 7.5% of vitamin A deficient patients is less than the percentage reported in Finland (14%) for this vitamin [27]. From healthy subject studies, it is known that the vitamin A body storage is usually stable and sufficient for approximately one to two years [46]. This is confirmed by our healthy sample, in which none of the subjects showed a deficiency.

A majority of our untreated CD-patients had a zinc deficiency, which can probably be explained by increased endogenous losses of zinc, rather than abnormal zinc absorption [20]. Clinical relevance of zinc deficiency remains inconclusive and additional research is warranted. However, it is known that CD is associated with a wide array of skin lesions and manifestations, which may be partly ascribed to zinc deficiency [47–50], and cell mediated immunity and antioxidant buffer capacity may be compromised due to it as well [51].

Possible explanations for the high prevalence of nutritional deficiencies in untreated CD-patients might be an insufficient nutritional intake. This is supported by the presence of malnutrition in this cohort: 17% was malnourished based on the usual definition of >10% involuntary body weight loss prior to diagnosis and 7.5% had a BMI <18.5 kg/m^2. However, this seemed unlikely since patients did not report any changes (intentional or involuntary) in their habitual diet before diagnosis. Moreover, the observed presence of high serum folate levels, particularly in those classified as underweight, were contradictory as well. On the other hand, increased faecal losses of nutrients as a result of malabsorption might (partially) explain the high prevalence of deficiencies. However, since most patients did not report any clinical sign of malabsorptive diarrhoea, losses via the stools were thought to be of limited importance as well. Nevertheless, the observed findings in this study, sharing deficiencies in water and fat soluble vitamins, zinc and iron, indicate that maldigestion, malabsorption or a structurally moderately inadequate intake might have been present long before the clinical diagnosis of CD was established. It is known that the delay in diagnosing CD can be more than a decade [52]. One may hypothesize that this might be due to functional changes of the intestinal tract or due to changes in the intestinal microbiome [53]. In this study, even patients with mild CD (low grade pathohistological abnormalities) showed nutritional deficiencies and weight loss. A finding that was recently corroborated in a large Italian cohort showed that mild (histopathological) enteropathy did not necessarily mean mild intestinal dysfunction since, also in this group, alterations in bone marrow density and laboratory parameters were reported [54]. Remarkably, only female patients presented as underweight (approximately one in four females), while the female-male ratio was similar in the overweight and obese patients. A statistical trend for higher serum vitamin A and B concentrations was observed in patients classified as malnourished (low BMI or >10% unintentional weight loss prior to diagnosis). This may be explained by their more so-called classical CD presentation, which may trigger use of supplements due to a greater physicians' or patients' awareness when observing clinical signs of malnutrition.

Some considerations arise when interpreting the presented results: not all data were available in all subjects and some subgroups were relatively small, precluding detection of small effects or the drawing of firm conclusions in subgroups. Vitamin or mineral supplement use, whether at the patient's own initiative or prescribed by the GP, was based on self-reported information and can therefore be underestimated if patients forget to mention these "medicinal supplements". However, real numbers and frequencies of deficiencies or anaemia might be underestimated, since some patients were already taking these supplements before the initial diagnosis of CD, potentially leading to misclassification as "non-deficient" in this study. Besides, serum values of almost all vitamins or minerals do not fully represent total body stock or physiological function.

Based on our experience and supported by a recently published guideline on CD [3], we suggest monitoring body weight at diagnosis and nutritional serum parameters; at least vitamin B_6, folic acid, B_{12} and zinc and in any case (25-hydroxy) D of the fat soluble vitamins (due to its connection with presence of osteomalacia). Moreover, we suggest follow-up until serum values are at satisfying levels or upon indication (for instance, if bone density deviations, chronic diarrhoea, or skin lesions are present). Practically, a standard complete multivitamin supplement (100%–300% of RDA) should be considered for every newly diagnosed CD-patient. Continuation time has yet to be determined, since patients are at risk for vitamin deficiencies even after 10 years of a GFD [55]. Evidently, hypervitaminosis should be avoided, in particular regarding pyridoxine and iron [56,57]. It is demonstrated that bone-mineral density and nutritional status can improve after a GFD treatment [58] as well as that of general well-being, which can improve after vitamin B supplementation in CD-patients on a GFD [59].

5. Conclusions

In conclusion, deficiencies of vitamins or minerals are frequently observed in untreated adult Dutch CD-patients using a Western diet, although they are currently diagnosed earlier than in the previous century. This was observed even in obese patients. Almost 90% of the newly diagnosed CD-patients had one or more nutritional deficiencies. Malnutrition, expressed as an involuntary weight loss or being underweight, was found in 16% and 7.5% of patients, respectively, while overweight status (BMI > 25 kg/m^2) was present in almost 30% of the patients. Therefore, these results indicate that extensive nutritional assessment of body weight and serum nutritional parameters should be an integral part of celiac disease treatment to guide nutritional advices and follow-up in CD-treatment by means of an adequately composed individual-based, gluten free diet.

Acknowledgements

The authors thank the Department of Clinical Chemistry of the VU University Medical Centre in Amsterdam for their help with the analyses. And student Priyantha Malhoe for her assistance at the beginning of this manuscript.

Authorship Statement

NJW, AAvB and CJJM designed the protocol, NJW and MB conducted the research, NJW analyzed the data, NJW and AAvB wrote the paper, and all authors critically reviewed and approved the final version of the paper. NJW is primarily responsible for the contents of the paper and is acting as the submission's guarantor.

Financially Support

This study was funded in part by a grant received from the Dutch Society for Gastroenterology (Gastrostart). Gastrostart had no involvement in any of the study tasks.

References

1. Gujral, N.; Freeman, H.J.; Thomson, A.B. Celiac disease: Prevalence, diagnosis, pathogenesis and treatment. *World J. Gastroenterol.* **2012**, *18*, 6036–6059.
2. Green, P.; Cellier, C. Celiac disease. *N. Engl. J. Med.* **2007**, *357*, 1731–1743.
3. Bai, J.; Fried, M.; Corazza, G.; Schuppan, D.; Farthing, M.; Catassi, C.; Greco, L.; Cohen, H.; Ciacci, C.; Eliakim, R.; *et al.* World Gastroenterology Organisation global guidelines on celiac disease. *J. Clin. Gastroenterol.* **2013**, *47*, 121–126.
4. Tack, G.; Verbeek, W.H.; Schreurs, M.; Mulder, C.J.J. The spectrum of celiac disease: Epidemiology, clinical aspects and treatment. *Nat. Rev. Gastroenterol. Hepatol.* **2010**, *7*, 204–213.
5. Pare, P.; Douville, P.; Caron, D.; Lagace, R. Adult celiac sprue: Changes in the pattern of clinical recognition. *J. Clin Gastroenterol.* **1988**, *10*, 395–400.
6. Corazza, G.; Frisoni, M.; Treggiari, E.; Valentini, R.; Filipponi, C.; Volta, U.; Gasbarrini, G. Subclinical celiac sprue. Increasing occurence and clues to its diagnosis. *J. Clin. Gastroenterol.* **1993**, *16*, 16–21.
7. Gupta, R.; Reddy, D.; Makhari, G.; Sood, A.; Ramakrischna, B.; Yaccha, S.; Thapa, B.; Banerjee, R.; Anuradha, S.; Dutta, U.; *et al.* Indian task force for celiac disease: Current status. *World J. Gastroenterol.* **2009**, *15*, 6028–6033.
8. Cheng, J.; Brar, P.S.; Lee, A.R.; Green, P.H. Body mass index in celiac disease: Beneficial effect of a gluten-free diet. *J. Clin. Gastroenterol.* **2010**, *44*, 267–271.
9. Ukkola, A.; Maki, M.; Kurppa, K.; Collin, P.; Huhtala, H.; Kekkonen, L.; Kaukinen, K. Changes in body mass index on a gluten free diet in coeliac disease: A nationwide study. *Eur. J. Int. Med.* **2012**, *23*, 384–388.
10. Sinniah, R.; Roche, H.M. Letter: Rising incidence of obesity in the coeliac population—A malady or maladaptation? *Alliment. Pharmacol. Ther.* **2012**, *35*, 1483–1484.
11. Tucker, E.; Rostami, K.; Prabhakaran, S.; Al Dulaimi, D. Patients with coeliac disease are increasingly overweight or obese on presentation. *J. Gastrointest. Liver Dis.* **2012**, *21*, 11–15.

12. Tikkakoski, S.; Savilahti, E.; Kolho, K. Undiagnosed coeliac disease and nutritional deficiencies in adults screened in primary health care. *Scand. J. Gastroenterol.* **2007**, *42*, 60–65.
13. Kabbani, T.; Goldberg, A.; Kelly, C.; Pallav, K.; Tariq, S.; Peer, A.; Hansen, J.; Dennis, M.D.; Leffler, D. Body mass index and the risk of obesity in coeliac disease treated with gluten-free diet. *Alliment. Pharmacol. Ther.* **2012**, *35*, 723–729.
14. Evans, K.E.; Leeds, J.S.; Sanders, D.S. Be vigilant for patients with coeliac disease. *Practitioner* **2009**, *253*, 19–22.
15. Rostami, N.M.; Rostami, K.; Pourhoseingholi, M.A.; Nazemalhosseini, M.E.; Habibi, M.; Dabiri, H.; Zali, M.R. Atypical presentation is dominant and typical for coeliac disease. *J. Gastrointest. Liver Dis.* **2009**, *18*, 285–291.
16. McGough, N.; Cummings, J.H. Coeliac disease: A diverse clinical syndrome caused by intolerance of wheat, barley and rye. *Proc. Nutr. Soc.* **2005**, *64*, 434–450.
17. Dickey, W.; Ward, M.; Whittle, C.R.; Kelly, M.T.; Pentieva, K.; Horigan, G.; Patton, S.; McNulty, H. Homocysteine and related B-vitamin status in coeliac disease: Effects of gluten exclusion and histological recovery. *Scand. J. Gastroenterol.* **2008**, *43*, 682–688.
18. Dahele, A.; Ghosh, S. Vitamin B12 deficiency in untreated celiac disease. *Am. J. Gastroenterol.* **2001**, *96*, 745–750.
19. Henri-Bhargava, A.; Melmed, C.; Glikstein, R.; Schipper, H.M. Neurologic impairment due to vitamin E and copper deficiencies in celiac disease. *Neurology* **2008**, *71*, 860–861.
20. Crofton, R.W.; Aggett, P.J.; Gvozdanovic, S.; Gvozdanovic, D.; Mowat, N.A.; Brunt, P.W. Zinc metabolism in celiac disease. *Am. J. Clin. Nutr.* **1990**, *52*, 379–382.
21. Bergamaschi, G.; Markopoulos, K.; Albertini, R.; Di Sabatino, A.; Biagi, F.; Ciccocioppo, R.; Arbustini, E.; Corazza, G.R. Anemia of chronic disease and defective erythropoietin production in patients with celiac disease. *Haematologica* **2008**, *93*, 1785–1791.
22. Peters, J.H.; Wierdsma, N.J.; Teerlink, T.; van Leeuwen, P.A.; Mulder, C.J.; van Bodegraven, A.A. The citrulline generation test: Proposal for a new enterocyte function test. *Aliment. Pharmacol. Ther.* **2008**, *27*, 1300–1310.
23. Alwitry, A. Vitamin A deficiency in coeliac disease. *Br. J. Ophthalmol.* **2000**, *84*, 1079–1080.
24. Hallert, C.; Tobiasson, P.; Walan, A. Serum folate determinations in tracing adult coeliacs. *Scand. J. Gastroenterol.* **1981**, *16*, 263–267.
25. Stene-Larsen, G.; Mosvold, J.; Ly, B. Selective vitamin B12 malabsorption in adult coeliac disease. Report on three cases with associated autoimmune diseases. *Scand. J. Gastroenterol.* **1988**, *23*, 1105–1108.
26. Kemppainen, T.; Uusitupa, M.; Janatuinen, E.; Jarvinen, R.; Julkunen, R.; Pikkarainen, P. Intakes of nutrients and nutritional status in coeliac patients. *Scand. J. Gastroenterol.* **1995**, *30*, 575–579.
27. Kemppainen, T.A.; Kosma, V.M.; Janatuinen, E.K.; Julkunen, R.J.; Pikkarainen, P.H.; Uusitupa, M.I. Nutritional status of newly diagnosed celiac disease patients before and after the institution of a celiac disease diet—Association with the grade of mucosal villous atrophy. *Am. J. Clin. Nutr.* **1998**, *67*, 482–487.
28. Dickey, W. Low serum vitamin B12 is common in coeliac disease and is not due to autoimmune gastritis. *Eur. J. Gastroenterol. Hepatol.* **2002**, *14*, 425–427.

29. Hozyasz, K.K.; Chelchowska, M.; Laskowska-Klita, T. Vitamin E levels in patients with celiac disease. *Med. Wieku Rozwoj* **2003**, *7*, 593–604.
30. Harper, J.W.; Holleran, S.F.; Ramakrishnan, R.; Bhagat, G.; Green, P.H. Anemia in celiac disease is multifactorial in etiology. *Am. J. Hematol.* **2007**, *82*, 996–1000.
31. Lerner, A.; Shapira, Y.; Agmon-Levin, N.; Pacht, A.; Ben-Ami Shor, D.; Lopez, H.; Sanchez-Castanon, M.; Shoenfeld, Y. The clinical significance of 25OH-vitamin D status in celiac disease. *Clin. Rev. Allergy Immunol.* **2013**, *42*, 322–330.
32. Van Overbeek, F.M.; Uil-Dieterman, I.G.A.; Mol, I.W.; Kohler-Brands, L.; Heymans, H.S.A.; Mulder, C.J.J. The daily gluten intake in relatives of patients with coeliac disease compared with that of the general Dutch population. *Eur. J. Gastroenterol. Hepatol.* **1997**, *9*, 1097–1099.
33. Marsh, M.N. Gluten, major histocompatibility complex and the small intestine. A molecular and immunobiologic approach to the spectrum of gluten sensitivity (“celiac sprue”). *Gastroenterology* **1992**, *102*, 330–354.
34. Rostami, K. From microenteropathy to villous atrophy: What is treatable? *Dig. Liver Dis.* **2003**, *35*, 758–759.
35. Rostami, K.; Kerckhaert, J.; Tiemessen, R.; von Blomberg, B.M.; Meijer, J.W.; Mulder, C.J. Sensitivity of antiendomysium and antigliadin antibodies in untreated celiac disease: Disappointing in clinical practice. *Am. J. Gastroenterol.* **1999**, *94*, 888–894.
36. Hopper, A.D.; Hadjivassiliou, M.; Hurlstone, D.P.; Lobo, A.J.; McAlindon, M.E.; Egner, W.; Wild, G.; Sanders, D.S. What is the role of serologic testing in celiac disease? A prospective, biopsy-confirmed study with economic analysis. *Clin. Gastroenterol. Hepatol.* **2008**, *6*, 314–320.
37. Wahab, P.J.; Meijer, J.W.; Mulder, C.J. Histologic follow-up of people with celiac disease on a gluten-free diet: Slow and incomplete recovery. *Am. J. Clin. Pathol.* **2002**, *118*, 459–463.
38. Al-Toma, A.; Goerres, M.S.; Meijer, J.W.; Pena, A.S.; Crusius, J.B.; Mulder, C.J. Human leukocyte antigen-DQ2 homozygosity and the development of refractory celiac disease and enteropathy-associated T-cell lymphoma. *Clin. Gastroenterol. Hepatol.* **2006**, *4*, 315–319.
39. Wierdsma, N.J.; Peters, J.H.C.; van Bokhorst-de van der Schueren, M.A.E.; Mulder, C.J.J.; Metgod, I.; van Bodegraven, A.A. Bomb calorimetry, the gold standard for assessment of intestinal absorption capacity: Normative values in healthy ambulant adults. *J. Hum. Nutr. Diet.* **2013**, doi: 10.1111/jhn.12113.
40. Suitor, C.W.; Bailey, L.B. Food folate *vs*. synthetic folic acid: A comparison. *J. Am. Diet. Assoc.* **1999**, *99*, 285.
41. Reinken, L.; Zieglauer, H. Vitamin B-6 absorption in children with acute celiac disease and in control subjects. *J. Nutr.* **1978**, *108*, 1562–1565.
42. Reinken, L.; Zieglauer, H.; Berger, H. Vitamin B6 nutriture of children with acute celiac disease, celiac disease in remission, and of children with normal duodenal mucosa. *Am. J. Clin. Nutr.* **1976**, *29*, 750–753.
43. Hadithi, M.; Al-Toma, A.; Oudejans, J.J.; van Bodegraven, A.A.; Mulder, C.J.J.; Jacobs, M. The value of double-balloon enteroscopy in patients with refractory celiac disease. *Am. J. Gastroenterol.* **2007**, *102*, 987–996.

44. Fedosov, S.N.; Fedosova, N.U.; Krautler, B.; Nexo, E.; Petersen, T.E. Mechanisms of discrimination between cobalamins and their natural analogues during their binding to the specific B12-transporting proteins. *Biochemistry* **2007**, *46*, 6446–6458.
45. Deressa, E.; Wammer, A.C.; Falch, J.A.; Jahnsen, J. Bone metabolism in patients with newly diagnosed caeliac disease. *Tidsskr. Laegeforen.* **2006**, *126*, 1201–1204.
46. Tanumihardjo, S.A. Assessing vitamin A status: Past, present and future. *J. Nutr.* **2004**, *134*, 290S–293S.
47. Loche, F.; Bazex, J. Celiac disease associated with cuteanous sarcodosic granuloma. *Rev. Med. Interne* **1997**, *18*, 975–978.
48. Tasanen, K.; Raudasoja, R.; Kallioinen, M.; Ranki, A. Erythema elevatum diutinum in association with coeliac disease. *Br. J. Dermatol.* **1997**, *136*, 624–627.
49. Collin, P.; Reunala, T. Recognition and management of the cutaneous manifestations of celiac disease: A guide for dematologists. *Am. J. Clin. Dermatol.* **2003**, *4*, 13–20.
50. Addolorato, G.; Parente, A.; de Lorenzi, G.; D'angelo di Paola, M.E.; Abenavoli, L.; Leggio, G.; Capristo, E.; de Simone, C.; Rotoli, M.; Rapaccini, G.; *et al.* Rapid regression of psoriasis in a coeliac patient after gluten-free diet. A case report and review of the literature. *Digestion* **2003**, *68*, 9–12.
51. Prasad, A. Discovery of human zinc deficiency: Its impact on human health and disease. *Adv. Nutr.* **2013**, *4*, 176–190.
52. Nordstrom, F.; Lindholm, L.; Sandström, O.; Nordyke, K.; Ivarsson, A. Delay to celiac disease diagnosis and its implications for health-related quality of life. *BMC Gastroenterol.* **2011**, *11*, 118.
53. Blaser, M.J.; Falkow, S. What are the consequences of the disappearing human microbiota? *Nat. Rev. Microbiol.* **2009**, *7*, 887–894.
54. Zanini, B.; Caselani, F.; Magni, A.; Turini, D.; Ferraresi, A.; Lanzarotto, F.; Villanacci, V.; Carabellese, N.; Ricci, C.; Lanzini, A. Celiac disease with mild enteropathy is not mild disease. *Clin. Gastroenterol. Hepatol.* **2013**, *11*, 253–258.
55. Hallert, C.; Grant, C.; Grehn, S.; Granno, C.; Hulten, S.; Midhagen, G.; Strom, M.; Svensson, H.; Valdimarsson, T. Evidence of poor vitamin status in coeliac patients on a gluten-free diet for 10 years. *Aliment. Pharmacol. Ther.* **2002**, *16*, 1333–1339.
56. Snodgrass, S. Vitamin neurotoxicity. *Mol. Neurobiol.* **1992**, *6*, 41–73.
57. Gdynia, H.; Müller, T.; Sperfeld, A.; Kühnlein, P.; Otto, M.; Kassubek, J.; Ludolph, A.C. Severe sensorimotor neuropathy after intake of highest dosages of vitamin B6. *Neuromuscul. Disord.* **2008**, *18*, 156–158.
58. Sategna-Guidetti, C.; Grosso, S.B.; Grosso, S.; Mengozzi, G.; Aimo, G.; Zaccaria, T.; Di Stefano, M.; Isaia, G.C. The effects of 1-year gluten withdrawal on bone mass, bone metabolism and nutritional status in newly-diagnosed adult coeliac disease patients. *Aliment. Pharmacol. Ther.* **2000**, *14*, 35–43.

59. Hallert, C.; Svensson, M.; Tholstrup, J.; Hultberg, B. Clinical trial: B vitamins improve helath in patients with coeliac disease living on a gluten-free diet. *Alliment. Pharmacol. Ther.* **2009**, *29*, 811–816.

9

The Gluten-Free Diet: Testing Alternative Cereals Tolerated by Celiac Patients

Isabel Comino [1], María de Lourdes Moreno [1], Ana Real [1], Alfonso Rodríguez-Herrera [2], Francisco Barro [3] and Carolina Sousa [1,*]

1 Departamento de Microbiología y Parasitología, Facultad de Farmacia, Universidad de Sevilla, c/Profesor García González 2, 41012 Sevilla, Spain; E-Mails: icomino@us.es (I.C.); lmoreno@us.es (M.L.M.); arc@us.es (A.R.)
2 Instituto Hispalense de Pediatría, c/Guadalbullón 2, 41013 Sevilla, Spain; E-Mail: alfonsorodriguez@ihppediatria.com
3 Instituto de Agricultura Sostenible (C.S.I.C.), Alameda del Obispo s/n, 14004 Córdoba, Spain; E-Mail: fbarro@ias.csic.es

* Author to whom correspondence should be addressed; E-Mail: csoumar@us.es;

Abstract: A strict gluten-free diet (GFD) is the only currently available therapeutic treatment for patients with celiac disease, an autoimmune disorder of the small intestine associated with a permanent intolerance to gluten proteins. The complete elimination of gluten proteins contained in cereals from the diet is the key to celiac disease management. However, this generates numerous social and economic repercussions due to the ubiquity of gluten in foods. The research presented in this review focuses on the current status of alternative cereals and pseudocereals and their derivatives obtained by natural selection, breeding programs and transgenic or enzymatic technology, potential tolerated by celiac people. Finally, we describe several strategies for detoxification of dietary gluten. These included enzymatic cleavage of gliadin fragment by Prolyl endopeptidases (PEPs) from different organisms, degradation of toxic peptides by germinating cereal enzymes and transamidation of cereal flours. This information can be used to search for and develop cereals with the baking and nutritional qualities of toxic cereals, but which do not exacerbate this condition.

Keywords: celiac disease; gluten-free diet; cereals; pseudocereals; gluten detoxification

1. Introduction

Celiac disease is a food intolerant related syndrome that, despite being under-diagnosed, is one of the most frequent chronic gastrointestinal disorders. It develops in genetically predisposed individuals in whom unidentified environmental factors (infections, changes in microbial flora, *etc.*) can trigger intolerance to gluten contained in wheat, barley, rye and oats [1,2]. Gluten is a complex mixture of proteins called prolamins. This protein fraction has specific name: wheat prolamins are termed gliadins and glutenins, barley prolamins are hordeins, rye prolamins are secalin and those from oats are avenins. A common characteristic of these proteins is the presence of multiple proline and glutamine residues, making them resistant to gastrointestinal digestion and more exposed to deamination by tissue transglutaminase.

Several epitopes responsible for the toxicity of gluten have been identified based on their ability to stimulate proliferation of gluten-responsive T cells in celiac patient-derived small intestine biopsies. Considering only wheat, in the Immune Epitope Database (IEDB) [3] can be found 190 T-cell stimulatory epitopes related to celiac disease. Of these, 94 epitopes are located in α-gliadin genes, 74 in γ-gliadin genes, 12 in ω-gliadin genes, 8 in low molecular weight (LMW) glutenin genes, and 2 in high molecular weight (HMW) genes.

The most accepted model for explaining the immunopathogenesis of celiac disease is the two-signal model, characterized by a first innate immune response and a subsequent secondary adaptive response, which will promote a histological lesion characterized by a massive intraepithelial infiltration of lymphocytes, crypt hyperplasia and villous atrophy [2]. The ingestion of these proteins leads to the inflammation, atrophy, and hyperplasia of the small-intestinal crypts of the celiac patient. However, this disease not only affects the gut, but it is a systemic disease that may cause injury to the skin, liver, joints, brain, heart, and other organs.

Celiac disease goes in remission when the patients are put on a gluten-exclusion diet, and patients relapse when gluten is reintroduced into the diet [1,2]. Complying with a GFD is difficult and affects the patients' quality of life, but a strict diet is critical to reduce morbidity and mortality [4].

Gluten has many special characteristics that favor its use in various food products. Because a large amount of gluten is generated during the manufacture of starch, it has a relatively low price. This may turn out to be problematic for people on a GFD, since gluten proteins may be found in unexpected sources such as meat, fish or milk products. This is the reason why alternative approaches to the GFD are actively sought [5], which include the search for and development of new cereals or gluten with no or low immunogenic content. In this article, we will review the current status of alternative cereals and their derivatives obtained by natural selection, breeding programs and transgenic or enzimatic technology, which may be potential tolerated by patients with celiac disease.

2. Natural Varieties of Cereal and Pseudocereals Suitable for Patients with Celiac Disease

2.1. Wheat and Barley

Cultivated wheat is genetically very complex due to its origin from ancestral diploid species through a process of natural hybridization and subsequent polyploidization. The two wheat species of agricultural importance, the pasta wheat, and the bread wheat, are tetraploid (two genomes, AABB) and hexaploid (three genomes, AABBDD), respectively (Figure 1). The tetraploids originated in nature through spontaneous hybridization of two diploid species, each donor genomes A and B, between 0.5 and 2 million years ago. Bread wheat (AABBDD) originated in the fields, about 8000 years ago, through spontaneous hybridization between durum wheat (AABB) and *Aegilops tauschii*, the diploid donor of the D genome (Figure 1).

One species of wheat, *Triticum aestivum*, is predominantly used in the modern industrialized world, due to its increased protein production as well as its hardiness in colder climates. It has also been determined that the proteins that are the most immunogenic for celiac disease reside in the gliadin fraction of *T. aestivum*. However, there are almost 20 other species of wheat that are either not being cultivated by modern societies or are cultivated in select regions of the world [6]. With such a large number of wheat species available, a significant amount of research has been focused on the exploration of different species and cultivars of wheat as an alternative to a strict GFD for celiac patients [7].

Figure 1. Diagram showing the evolutionary relationships among species of wheat and related species of *Aegilops*. The dotted line separates the wild and domesticated species of wheat. Ancestral or unknown species are surrounded by a double dashed rectangle. Ploidy level and the number of chromosomes are indicated. Nomenclature according to van Slageren [8].

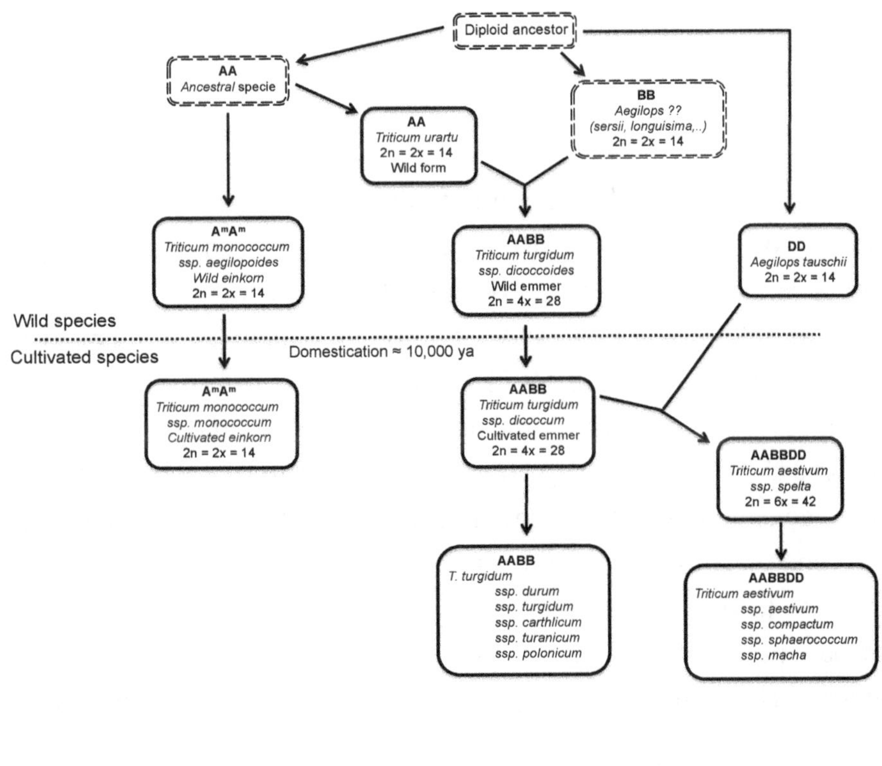

Attempts have been made to quantify the toxicity of a range of bread wheat and pasta wheat varieties and of species that contain only one of the three genomes of bread wheat [9,10]. Using specific T-cell clones and monoclonal antibodies, the results demonstrated that large quantitative differences exist in the presence of toxic gluten peptides, with some cultivars completely lacking particular harmful peptides [11]. Diploid wheat species are among the suitable candidates for their low capability to activate intestinal T cell responses in celiac patients [11,12]. Compared with tetraploid and hexaploid wheat, commonly used in the making of bread and pasta, the ancient diploid *Triticum monococcum* ssp. monococcum wheat showed a marked reduction, or even a lack, of toxicity *in vitro* cellular assays [13,14]. Gianfrani *et al.* [15] compared the immunological properties of 2 lines of diploid monococcum wheat, Monlis and ID331, with those of *T. aestivum.* They found that both lines activate celiac T cell response. However, ID331 was less effective to activate the innate immune pathways. The reduced ability of some diploid wheat lines to *in vitro* activate the innate immune response in celiac mucosa could render these cultivars less active in inducing celiac disease. However, more analyses are required to explore their potential use as new dietary opportunities for celiac patients.

Some approaches were performed to remove celiac toxic proteins in barley. Double-null hybrid plants, largely devoid of both B- and C-hordeins, were produced by conventional crossing [16]. Barley is a diploid and unlike the situation in bread wheat, the genetics of hordeins are relatively straightforward. There are four protein families of hordeins: B-, C-, D- and γ-hordeins, with the B- and C-hordeins together accounting for over 90% of barley hordeins. Isolation of hordein double-null barley lines from hybrids of Risø 56 and Risø 1508 has produced a line which does not accumulate B- or C-hordein and only has 3% of wild type hordein along with a 20-fold reduction in reactivity in T-cell assays [16,17]. In addition, studies carried out demonstrated that some malting lines (*Hordeum vulgare*) were less immunogenic compared with wild lines (*Hordeum chilense*) [18]. These findings could raise the prospect of breeding barley species with low levels of harmful gluten, and the attractive goal of developing non-toxic barley cultivars with a potential use in the manufacture of beverages as consumed worldwide as are the beers. However, nothing is known about the variability in celiac toxicity of other species or varieties of toxic cereals such as rye.

2.2. Oats

Cultivated oats are hexaploid cereals belonging to the genus *Avena* L., which is found worldwide in almost all agricultural environments [19]. Recently, oats have been receiving increasing interest as human food, mainly because the cereal could be suitable for consumptions by celiac patients. Several varieties of oats are available. It is a rich source of protein, contains a number of important minerals, lipids, β-glucan, a mixed-linkage polysaccharide, which forms an important part of oat dietary fiber, and also contains various other phytoconstituents like avenanthramides, an indole alkaloid-gramine, flavonoids, flavonolignans, triterpenoid saponins, sterols, and tocols. Traditionally oats have been in use since long and are considered as stimulant, antispasmodic, antitumor, diuretic, and neurotonic. Oat possesses different pharmacological activities like antioxidant, anti-inflammatory, antidiabetic, anticholesterolaemic, *etc.* [20].

The presence of oats in a GFD is still a subject of controversial. Oats differ from other cereals in their prolamin content. The percentage of proline and glutamine (amino acids abundant in toxic regions) in avenin is lower than in other toxic cereals. Some clinical researchers state that patients with celiac disease tolerate oats without signs of intestinal inflammation [21]. According to the Codex Alimentarius for food for special dietary use for persons intolerant to gluten, CODEX STAN118-1979 (revised 2008, [22]), oats can be tolerated by most but not all people who are intolerant to gluten. Moreover, according to the Commission Regulation (EC) No 41/2009 [23] concerning the composition and labeling of foodstuffs suitable for people intolerant to gluten, a major concern is the contamination of oats with wheat, rye or barley that can occur during grain harvesting, transport, storage and processing. Therefore, the risk of gluten contamination in products containing oats should be taken into consideration with regard to labeling of those products. In contrast, other studies confirmed the toxicity of oats in certain types of patients with celiac disease. Arentz-Hansen *et al.* [24] described the intestinal deterioration suffered by some patients with celiac disease following the consumption of oats while on a GFD. Avenin can trigger an immunological response in these patients similar to the response produced by the gluten of wheat, rye or barley. The monitoring of 19 adult patients with celiac disease who consumed 50 g/day of oats over 12 weeks showed that one of the subjects was sensitive to oats. Therefore, it is critical to clarify either qualitatively or quantitatively the potential immunotoxicity of oats to patients with celiac disease [21,24].

Comparison of the different studies are complicated by the different study designs, the different conditions used in the testing, the number of subjects included in each study and the reporting of the purity control of the oat material used in the clinical trials. Another relevant factor in different designs is the absence of information on the oat variety used. Silano *et al.* [25] investigated the immunogenic effect of avenins from four oat cultivars using peripheral lymphocytes from patients with CD. All the varieties of oats tested (Lampton, Astra, Ava, and Nave) by these investigators were immunogenic with differences in their capacity to induce a response. However, other study confirmed that *Avena genziana* and *Avena potenza* do not display *in vitro* activities related to CD pathogenesis [26].

The utility of the G12 antibody to identify potentially toxic oat varieties for celiac patients has been reported [27]. This finding allowed classification of oat varieties into three groups based in their degree of affinity for the G12 antibody: a highly recognized group, one of moderate recognition, and one with no reactivity [27]. These results were confirmed by MALDI-TOF, SDS-PAGE and western blot by showing that the number, relative intensity of the peaks and protein profile obtained for the nine oat varieties differ from one another. The potentially immunotoxicity of the different types of oats was determined by T cell proliferation and interferon γ release. The reactivity that T-cells isolated from celiac patients exhibited with three oat varieties (one from each of the classified groups) correlated directly with the moAb G12 reactivity. The diversity observed in the reactivity to the different oat cultivars suggests variations in the avenin composition, and therefore in the amount of immunotoxic epitopes similar to the 33-mer present in these varieties. This gives a rational explanation for why only some oats trigger an immunological response.

In comparison with wheat gliadins, the avenins have been little studied, and the number of full avenin genes present at the moment in the databases is limited and from few genotypes, so that the variability of avenin genes in oats is not well represented. It has recent been known that, like wheat, oat grains have both monomeric and polymeric avenins [28]. A direct correlation between the immunogenicity of the different varieties of oats and the presence of the specific peptides with a higher/lower potential immunotoxicity has been found, that could explain why certain varieties of oats are toxic for celiac patients and other not [28]. The incorporation of some varieties of oats in food products not only may improve the nutritional quality but also may provide a treatment for various illnesses and would be welcomed by patients with celiac disease.

2.3. Other Cereals and Pseudocereals

It is well-known that the high nutritional value of gluten containing cereals and the viscoelastic network generated by the gluten that enables an excellent aerated structure in food products. In contrast, cereal based gluten-free products can be rich in carbohydrates and fats, and they have deficiencies in macronutrients and micronutrients. In consequence, long time adherence to GFD could induce nutrients deficiencies. Different proteins have been proposed as alternative for both playing the polymer role and increasing the nutritional value of gluten-free products. The incorporation of other ingredients/nutrients like 3-omega lipids, specific proteins, *etc.* is an alternative to improve the nutritional composition of gluten-free products.

Figure 2. Taxonomic relation of known non-toxic cereals, minor cereals and pseudocereals in the context of celiac disease.

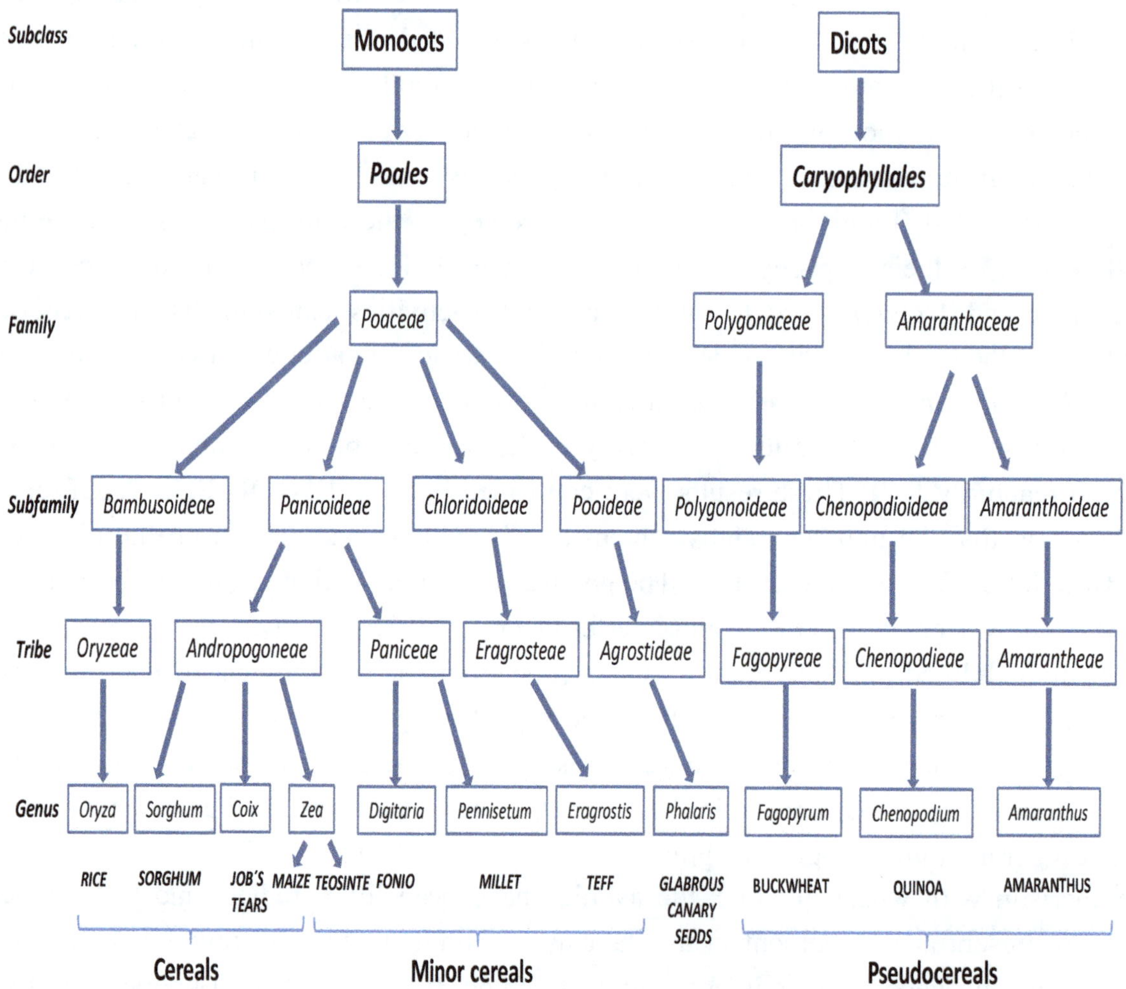

It is noteworthy that many grains (members of the grass family) that are closely related to wheat, rye and barley are considered toxic based on taxonomy. Furthermore, some studies focused on the protein homology in grains have supported molecular evidences [28,29]. However, member belonging to other tribes that appear to be related to corn, are considered safe (Figure 2) and can serve as substitutes and provide flours for cooking and baking for celiac and gluten-sensitive individuals. There are protein studies in support of this conclusion, although the studies are not sufficiently complete to provide more than guidance.

Non-gluten-containing sources frequently used in product formulation include cereals (rice, corn and sorghum), minor cereals (fonio, teff, millet, and job's tears) and pseudocereals (buckwheat, quinoa and amaranth). As the environmental conditions for growing these grains are variable, availability of regular supplies is not always assured.

2.3.1. Rice, Maize and Sorghum

Rice is the seed of the monocot plant of the genus *Oryza* and of the grass family Poaceae (formally Graminae), which includes twenty wild species and two cultivated ones, *Oryza sativa* (Asian rice) and *Oryza glaberrima* (African rice). Rice is one of the most important foods in the human diet and extended cereal crop. Rice is mainly consumed as white grain, but in the last decade, dozens of products containing rice as an ingredient have appeared on the food market [30]. There has been a notable increase in the use of rice flour in the formulation of gluten-free products for their hypoallergenic qualities or hypoallergenicity in spite of it is necessary to use a hydrocolloid, emulsifier, enzyme or protein to confer viscoelastic properties [30,31].

Maize (*Zea mays* subsp. *mays* L), also known as corn, is considered as a safe cereal for celiac patients. It is used as alternative to elaborate gluten-free foodstuffs. Some celiac patients considered refractory to the treatment with a GFD improved when a corn-free diet was prescribed [32]. However, some studies have showed the certain maize prolamins (zeins) contain amino acid sequences that resemble the wheat gluten immunodominant peptides and their integrity after gastrointestinal proteolysis is unknown [33]. Darewickz *et al.* [34] detected amino acid sequences with a high degree of identity to the celiac-toxic peptides in maize prolamins (zeins). This could be because the zeins, like other storage proteins, have its origin in the alpha-amylase inhibitors [35].

Sorghum (genus of numerous species of grasses) is a drought-and heat-tolerant cereal grain that grows in semiarid conditions. Whereas sorghum traditionally has been used primarily as animal feed in western countries, nearly 40% of the world sorghum production is used for human food in Africa and India. Immunological studies and *in vitro* and *in vivo* challenges of sorghum food products have supported that sorghum might provide a good basis for gluten-free foods [36]. In a recent study, Pontieri *et al.* [37] by using *in silico* approaches and biochemical/immunochemical experiments have demonstrated that sorghum can be definitively considered safe for consumption by people with celiac disease for the absence of toxic gliadin-like peptides.

2.3.2. Minor Cereals

Minor cereals, so called because they are less common and are only grown in a few small regions of the world, included fonio, teff, millet, teosinte and Job's tears [38].

Fonio (*Digitaria exilis*) is a typically cereal in Sudan or Ethiopia where it is considered to be the tastiest of all cereals [38]. Fonio can survive in poor soil conditions such as sandy and acidic soils and its composition is similar to that of other millets: limited in lysine, but rich in methionine [39].

Teff (*Eragrostis tef*) is the smallest of all grains in the world and it is classified on the basis of seed color, ranging from milky white to almost black. Teff is a cereal traditionally grown in Ethiopia and used to make *injera* or flat bread.

Millet refers to a number of different species of the *Pennisetum* genus, all of which are small-grained, annual cereal grasses. The most important type for food consumption is pearl millet that is similar in texture to rice flour [38].

Job's tears (*Coix lacryma-jobi*), also known as Chinese Pearl Barley, is a type of millet wild tropical Asian grass related to maize. Job's tears is naturally gluten-free, but similar to other grains it may be contaminated during processing by comingling with gluten grains such as wheat. It is used as a source of food and drinks.

2.3.3. Pseudocereals

Pseudocereals are non-grasses plants which grains are used in the same way that true cereals. Pseudocereals seeds can be ground into flour and then to produce derived products like bread and pasta. Recently, the use of pseudocereals producing small grain-like seeds like amaranthus and quinoa (Amaranthaceae family), belonging to dicotyledons (Magnoliopsida class), have been considered for the preparation of gluten-free food products because the lack toxic seed proteins and have high nutritional value [40]. However, the believed lack of toxicity for most of these pseudocereals was based on their taxonomical classification rather than a direct evaluation of their inmunostimulator activity.

Several studies affirmed that amaranth and quinoa have high quality protein in terms of digestibility, efficiency ratio and nutrition balance, almost equivalent to that of milk protein casein [41,42]. Additionally, these pseudocereals are also rich in polyunsaturated fatty acids (high linolenic:linoleic acid ratio) and bioactive compounds such as γ- and β-tocopherol, polyphenols and flavonoids.

The genus *Amaranthus* L. contains more than 60 species; *A. caudatus*, *A. cruentus* and *A. hypochondriacus* are those most used for human nutrition. Amaranth proteins consist mainly of albumins and globulins, where prolamins, the toxic proteins for celiac patients, are very scarce. The essential amino acids content is high in amaranth seeds and the amino acid composition is better balanced than in most cereals. It is a good source of riboflavin, vitamin E, calcium, magnesium and irons, among minerals [40]. Studies focused on investigate from the molecular point of view the protein patterns from different amaranth cultivars to verify their suitability for the diet of subjects suffering from celiac disease, suggested that amaranth may be safely included in a GFD. However, controlled clinical studies are necessary to confirm the results and support the inclusion in the celiac's diet [40].

Quinoa (*Chenopodium quinoa*) is an Andean grain that has been consumed for thousands of years in South America and was a staple of the Incas. There are hundreds of varieties of quinoa, ranging in color from white to red and purple to black [38]. Quinoa has a high biological value (83%) because of its high concentration of proteins (<23%), providing all of the essential amino acids [43–45]. Quinoa has important applications in the food and pharmaceutical industries. Due to its excellent nutritional value and a potential for production in various climates, quinoa has been classified as one of the humanity's most promising crops [46]. Several studies to examine the suitability of quinoa for patients with celiac disease have been carried out in last years and concluded that quinoa could be a safe addition to a GFD. However, 2 cultivars had celiac-toxic epitopes that could activate the adaptive and innate immune responses in some patients with celiac disease [45]. A complete *in vivo* characterization of quinoa protein reactivity is needed to recommend their consumption by patients with celiac disease [45,47,48].

Buckwheat (*Fagopyrum* spp.) is botanically classified as a fruit and it is thought to have originated in China. It can be consumed as grains or as flour. The toasted grains are known as Kasha. Buckwheat is a highly nutritious pseudocereal known as a dietary source of protein with favorable amino acid composition and vitamins [49], starch, and dietary fiber [50], essential minerals (Steadman and others 2001), and trace elements [51]. Two species of buckwheat are cultivated for food consumption, *Fagopyrum esculentum* or common buckwheat and *Fagopyrum tartaricum* or tartary buckwheat [52]. Common buckwheat is primarily consumed in Asian countries. However, consumption in western countries including the United States is increasing due to it is the substitute for wheat flour for gluten-sensitive patients and as a health food because of its nutrient content [53,54]. It has been reported cases of buckwheat allergy in Japan, Korea and Europe [55].

2.3.4. Other Cereals

An alternative grain that may potentially be considered for celiac patients is glabrous canary seed (*Phalaris canarienses* L.) that belongs to the Poaceae (Gramineae) family. In a recent study carried out by Boye *et al.* [30] confirmed that glabrous canary seeds were a good alternative gluten-free cereal and reported three techniques able to be used to support gluten-free labeling of products that contain it.

3. Modified Harmless Cereal Varieties

3.1. Gluten Detoxification by Biotechnological Methods

The use of genetic engineering to down-regulate gene expression by RNA interference (RNAi) technology [56] is now routine in many crops, including wheat, and is therefore an attractive opportunity for reducing the immunotoxic components of gluten and, hence the incidence of gluten-related allergies and intolerance in wheat. Several groups have taken advantage of the possibilities that the RNAi technology offers for the silencing of multigene families, and they have addressed the down-regulation of more than one group of gliadins and/or glutenins.

This technology was applied to down-regulated the expression of α-gliadins [57], γ-gliadins [58,59], ω-gliadins [60], all gliadins [61], and gliadins and LMW-GS [62] in bread wheat. These examples show the usefulness of RNAi to silence specific genes corresponding to gluten proteins, which are the known sources of immunogenic epitopes. However, only transgenic lines deficient in γ-gliadins [58] and in all three gliadin fractions [61] have been tested by monoclonal antibodies and T-cell assays for these transgenic lines to be used in foodstuff tolerated by many patients with celiac disease or other gluten-related pathologies.

Results reported by Gil-Humanes *et al.* [58] and Piston *et al.* [59] used two hpRNA construct to silence the γ-gliadins in two genotypes of the bread wheat cv "Bobwhite". They reported 18 transgenic lines with reduction of the γ-gliadin fraction, from 65 to 97% depending of the transgenic line [59]. The reduction of γ-gliadins was also accompanied by an increase in other storage proteins, in particular, the ω- and α-gliadins, and the HMW-GS and LMW-GS. However, the total gliadin content did not show significant differences in the transgenic lines relative to the wild types. Later, two hpRNA constructs designed using a chimeric sequence encompassing highly conserved genes among α-, ω-, and γ-gliadins were reported [61]. They showed that the chimeric fragment was able to effectively down-regulate the expression of genes from all three gliadin groups. The gliadin composition of the transgenic lines, determined by RP-HPLC, showed a significant reduction of the gliadin content in all of the transgenic lines, ranging from 70% to 88%. Overall, the gluten proteins were decreased up to 56% while the non-gluten proteins albumins and globulins were increased in some transgenic lines [63], as consequence, the total nitrogen content of the grain was not significantly affected.

These lines hold good potential to be used in foodstuff tolerated by many patients with celiac disease or other gluten-related pathologies. The competitive ELISA system based on monoclonal antibody [64] is a good assay for quantifying the amount of gluten in foods [65]. For transgenic lines with γ-gliadins silenced [58,61], gliadin content (ppm) did not decrease significantly but increased for some lines as consequence of the compensatory effects with other gliadins, specifically α- and ω-gliadins. However, when gluten proteins from transgenic lines, deficient in all three groups of gliadins, were tested by the monoclonal antibody, there was a significant reduction of the gliadin content in all of the transgenic lines, with the average reduction of 92% and a range between 90% and 98% [61]. Total gluten proteins were extracted for T-cell assays, treated with recombinant human TG2, and tested in serial dilution for stimulation of DQ2- and DQ8-restricted T-cell clones of celiac patients [61]. The transgenic lines deficient only in γ-gliadins retained high amounts of α- and ω-gliadins, and the DQ2-γ-VII–specific T-cell clone gave strong response to the total gluten extract from those lines [61]. In contrast, a pronounced reduction in proliferative responses was seen in some transgenic lines deficient in all three gliadin fractions. There was about a 2-log reduction in the expression of the DQ2-α-II epitope in these transgenic lines. The responses of the T-cell clones specific for the other epitopes (DQ2-γ-VII, DQ8-α-I, and DQ8-γ-I) were at or below detection level for the highest concentration of gluten protein tested. They concluded that transgenic lines containing around 30% of ω-gliadin, 10% of α-gliadin, and only 1% of γ-gliadin compared with their wild-type control, were particularly inefficient to stimulate the celiac disease lesion-derived T cells [61].

One important question is how quality is affected by the silencing of gliadins, or other gluten proteins. The rheological and gluten properties, and baking quality of wheat lines with the α-gliadins down-regulated were reported [66]. They showed that the deficiency of α-gliadins did not substantially affect the baking performance of wheat flour, although breads made using flour from lines with α-gliadins silenced had lower volumes (−11%) compared to that of wild type breads. The mixing properties of 18 transgenic lines with the γ-gliadins down-regulated were determined by using the mixograph and sodium dodecyl sulfate sedimentation (SDSS) test [59]. They concluded that the reduction of γ-gliadins seems not to have a direct effect on the mixing and bread-making properties of wheat dough, but the compensatory effect on the synthesis of the other prolamins can provide stronger doughs with improved overmixing resistance. Although gliadins are not the main component affecting the bread-making quality of wheat, it is unknown the effect that the silencing of all three groups of gliadins [61], or gliadins and LMW-GS [62] will have on wheat quality. Preliminary results reported [61] based on SDSS test, showed that most of transgenic lines with ω-, γ- and α-gliadins down regulated had SDSS volumes comparable with those of wild types, and five lines had SDSS volume values significantly lower than wild types. However, SDSS volumes of these five lines were still comparable with those of the medium-quality bread wheat. The addition of non-toxic oat flour [67], or other flours from gluten-free cereals or pseudocereals, such as sorghum, buckwheat and quinoa [37,68], might compensate the lack of gliadins, enhancing the quality of the new wheat varieties.

3.2. Gluten Detoxification by Enzymatic Methods

Food proteins are usually degraded into small peptides and amino acids by gastric, pancreatic and brushborder enzymes. However, gluten proteins are highly resistant to complete proteolytic digestion due to their high proline and glutamine content. Since the pioneering experiments carried out by Frazer *et al.* [69], who determined that celiac-toxic proteins could be partially hydrolyzed by gastrointestinal enzymes without loss toxicity, several strategies have been considered for detoxification of dietary gluten. Some of these strategies have been based on treatment with special peptidases that hydrolyze toxic protein and peptides to nontoxic fragments.

The beginning for the enzymatic strategies was the findings that the toxicity was abolished by complete acidic hydrolysis [70]. However, researches about gluten detoxification were not developed until 21st century. The approaches included enzymatic cleavage of gliadin fragment by PEP from different organisms, degradation of toxic peptides by germinating cereal enzymes and transamidation of cereal flours [5].

3.2.1. Prolyl Endopeptidases

Shan *et al.* [71] were the first in propose that PEPs could catalyze breakdown of gluten peptides and thereby diminish its toxic effects. This hypothesis was based on that the abundance and location of proline residues is a crucial factor for the gastrointestinal resistance, and the unique ability of these enzymes to hydrolyze the peptide bond on the carboxyl side of a proline residue. Since then, further studies have shown that the fermentation of wheat, rye and barley flours with selected peptidases cause a significant decrease of gluten toxicity. The PEPs are widely distributed in bacteria, fungi, animals and plants, but it is known that lactic acid bacteria (lactobacilli) have a very complex peptidase system [72]. Lactobacilli species isolated from sourdoughs have been screened with respect to gluten degradation, finding that a pool of peptidases is needed to degraded α-gliadin fragments [73]. Studies based on use lactobacillus as microbial inoculum during fermentation of flour mixture has shown a potential ability to hydrolyze wheat prolamins by *in vitro* and *in vivo* assays [74]. Despite that, the gluten concentration remains high, therefore studies based on more complex formulas were developed. Recently, the combination of lactobacilli and fungal peptidases has been selected to eliminate the toxicity of wheat flour during long-time fermentation. Thus, food processing by selected proteases opens new perspectives toward an efficient approach to eliminate gluten toxicity.

3.2.2. Germinating Cereals

The role of the proline- and glutamine-rich storage proteins of cereals is to supply the embryo with nitrogen and amino acids during the first period of seedling development. Therefore, it is likely that endogenous cereal proteases synthesized during germination would be capable of extensively hydrolyzing these proteins [75]. Given evidences about this capacity, the use of proteases from germinating wheat seeds was proposed to create safe cereal products for celiac patients [76,77]. The analysis of protein content by RP-HPLC during kernels germination of wheat, rye and barley demonstrated a remarkable degradation of prolamins. In further experiments, protease extracts from these germinated cereals cleave peptides rapidly into non-toxic fragments with less than nine amino acids [75]. Comparative studies of proteases efficacy from different cereals by *in vitro* models have revealed that barley enzymes were superior in diminish the toxicity of gliadin and secalin, but there were only minor differences between the three enzyme mixtures (oats, wheat and barley) [78]. On the other hand, it should be pointed out that germinating cereal proteases have distinct advantages in comparison to bacterial and fungal peptidases. These enzymes derive from a naturally safe food source being excellent alternatives to recombinant proteases, which might not be accepted by many celiac patients. Indeed, the production of germinated cereals, just like the extraction of highly active proteases, is simple and well-established technological process [75]. Altogether, these enzymes from germinating cereals might be utilized in food processing to develop high quality food safe for celiac patients.

3.2.3. Transamidation

The enzyme transglutaminase (TG) catalyzes two classes of reactions, transamidation and deamidation. The first one transforms the primary γ-carboxamide group to a secondary one, and in the second reaction, the glutaminyl residue is converted to a glutamyl residue [79]. Tissue transglutaminase 2 (tTG) has been describe as one of the key factor in the immunopathogenesis of celiac disease because of gluten peptides increase their immunogenicity due to the deamidation [80]. Considering that only the transamidation might be use for gluten detoxification, several studies have been focused to know the ratio between these two reactions [81,82]. It seems that the ratio can vary considerably depending on different factors like the presence of primary amines, the peptide sequence as well as enzyme concentration. In general terms, it has been found highest rate of deamidation in tTG, however, the few studies carry out with TGs from other origins have shown a considerably lower deamidation *versus* transamidation activity in microbial TG (mTG) [83,84]. Based on that, Gianfrani *et al.* [85] treated wheat flour with mTG and lysine methyl ester to abolish gluten activity, detecting the decrease of the activity mediated by T-cell. Thus, they suggested a food-grade enzyme and an appropriate amine donor to block the T cell-mediated gliadin activity [85]. Recently, Mazzarella *et al.* [86] has shown in a randomized single blinded trial that transamidated gluten reduced the number of clinical relapses in challenged patients with no changes of baseline values for serological/mucosal celiac markers and an unaltered kidney function. Other application has been use the mTG from *S. mobaraensis* to detoxify cereal-based beverages since the beer treatment with mTG will lead to crosslinking of residual gluten peptide. If that aggregate exceeds a certain MW, they lose their solubility and can be removed from the beer resulting in beverages with gluten content below 20 mg/kg [87]. Therefore, although mTG is not able to degrade gluten, it could be used to immunodetoxify gluten.

4. Conclusions

Currently the only treatment for celiac disease is a lifelong GFD. However, adherence to the GFD is not easy, due to the ubiquitous nature of gluten, cross-contamination of foods and social constraints. While many patients are content with their GFD, others would welcome alternative treatments and/or food products that would allow more flexibility.

Here, we review the status of potential alternative cereals and pseudocereals and their derivatives under consideration for celiac disease. Diploid wheat species appear to be among the suitable candidates for their low capability to activate intestinal T cell responses in celiac patients. Compared with tetraploid and hexaploid wheats commonly used in the making of bread and pasta, the ancient diploid *Triticum monococcum* ssp. monococcum wheat showed a marked reduction of toxicity *in vitro* assays. Moreover, the use of genetic engineering to down-regulate gene expression by RNAi technology represents an attractive opportunity for reducing the immunotoxic components of wheat. Simultaneous silencing of the full complement of gliadins results effective for the reduction of T-cell epitopes in celiac disease.

Several studies have been demonstrated that oat immunogenicity for patients with celiac disease varies according to the cultivars. The incorporation of some varieties of oats in food products not only may improve the nutritional quality, but may provide a treatment for various illnesses and would be welcomed by patients with celiac disease.

Non-gluten-containing sources frequently used in product formulation include cereals (rice, corn and sorghum), minor cereals (fonio, teff, millet, and job's tears) and pseudocereals (buckwheat, quinoa and amaranth). However, new studies seem to show that certain cereals and pseudocereals such as corn and quinoa, traditionally considered safe for celiac patients, could activate the immune response in some celiac patients.

More recently, studies have been showed several strategies for detoxification of dietary gluten based on treatment with special peptidases that hydrolyze toxic protein and peptides to nontoxic fragments. These included enzymatic cleavage of gliadin fragment by PEPs from different organisms, degradation of toxic peptides by germinating cereal enzymes and transamidation of cereal flours. Food processing by selected proteases opens new perspectives toward an efficient approach to eliminate gluten toxicity, which could allow the development of foods with reduced or absent levels of gluten.

Acknowledgments

This work was supported by the Spanish Ministry of Economy and Competitiveness (AGL2010-19643-C02-02 and TRA2009_0047), the European Regional Development Fund (FEDER) and Junta de Andalucía (Project P09AGR-4783).

References

1. Sollid, L.M. Coeliac disease: Dissecting a complex inflammatory disorder. *Nat. Rev. Immunol.* **2002**, *2*, 647–655.
2. Bernardo, D.; Peña, A.S. Developing strategies to improve the quality of life of patients with gluten intolerance in patients with and without coeliac disease. *Eur. J. Intern. Med.* **2012**, *23*, 6–8.
3. Immune Epitope Database and Analysis Resourse. Available online: http://www.iedb.org/ (accessed on 14 October 2013).
4. Corrao, G.; Corazza, G.R.; Bagnardi, V.; Brusco, G.; Ciacci, C.; Cottone, M.; Sategna Guidetti, C.; Usai, P.; Cesari, P.; Pelli, M.A.; *et al.* Mortality in patients with coeliac disease and their relatives: A cohort study. *Lancet* **2001**, *358*, 356–361.
5. Rashtak, S.; Murray, J.A. Review article: Coeliac disease, new approaches to therapy. *Aliment. Pharmacol. Ther.* **2012**, *35*, 768–781.
6. Feldman, M.; Levy, A.A. Genome evolution in allopolyploid wheat—A revolutionary reprogramming followed by gradual changes. *J. Genet. Genomics* **2009**, *36*, 511–518.
7. Marietta, E.V.; Murray, J.A. Testing the safety of alternative wheat species and cultivars for consumption by celiac patients. *Am. J. Clin. Nutr.* **2012**, *96*, 1247–1248.
8. Van Slageren, M.W. *Wild wheats: A Monograph of Aegilops L. and Amblyopyrum (Jaub. & Spach) Eig (Poaceae)*; Wageningen Agriculture University: Wageningen, The Netherlands, 1994.
9. Auricchio, S.; de Ritis, G.; de Vincenzi, M.; Occorsio, P.; Silano, V. Effects of gliadin-derived peptides from bread and durum wheats on small intestine cultures from rat fetus and coeliac children. *Pediatr. Res.* **1982**, *16*, 1004–1010.
10. Van Herpen, T.W.; Goryunova, S.V.; van der Schoot, J.; Mitreva, M.; Salentijn, E.; Vorst, O.; Schenk, M.F.; van Veelen, P.A.; Koning, F.; van Soest, L.J.; *et al.* Alpha-Gliadin genes from the A, B, and D genomes of wheat contain different sets of celiac disease epitopes. *BMC Genomics* **2006**, *10*, 7–11.
11. Spaenij-Dekking, L.; Kooy-Winkelaar, Y.; van Veelen, P.; Drijfhout, J.W.; Jonker, H.; van Soest, L.; Smulders, M.J.; Bosch, D.; Gilissen, L.J.; Koning, F. Natural variation in toxicity of wheat: Potential for selection of nontoxic varieties for celiac disease patients. *Gastroenterology* **2005**, *129*, 797–806.
12. Molberg, O.; Uhlen, A.K.; Jensen, T.; Flaete, N.S.; Fleckenstein, B.; Arentz-Hansen, H.; Raki, M.; Lundin, K.E.; Sollid, L.M. Mapping of gluten T-cell epitopes in the bread wheat ancestors: Implications for celiac disease. *Gastroenterology* **2005**, *128*, 393–401.
13. Pizzuti, D.; Buda, A.; D'Odorico, A.; D'Incà, R.; Chiarelli, S.; Curioni, A.; Martines, D. Lack of intestinal mucosal toxicity of *Triticum monococcum* in coeliac disease patients. *Scand. J. Gastroenterol.* **2006**, *41*, 1305–1311.
14. Vincentini, O.; Maialetti, F.; Gazza, L.; Silano, M.; Dessi, M.; de Vincenzi, M.; Pogna, N.E. Environmental factors of coeliac disease: Cytotoxicity of hulled wheat species *Triticum monococcum*, *T. turgidum* ssp. *dicoccum* and *T. aestivum* ssp. *spelta*. *J. Gastroenterol. Hepatol.* **2007**, *22*, 1816–1822.

15. Gianfrani, C.; Maglio, M.; Rotondi Aufiero, V.; Camarca, A.; Vocca, I.; Iaquinto, G.; Giardullo, N.; Pogna, N.; Troncone, R.; Auricchio, S.; *et al.* Immunogenicity of monococcum wheat in celiac patients. *Am. J. Clin. Nutr.* **2012**, *96*, 1339–1345.
16. Tanner, G.J.; Howitt, C.A.; Forrester, R.I.; Campbell, P.M.; Tye-Din, J.A.; Anderson, R.P. Dissecting the T-cell response to hordeins in coeliac disease can develop barley with reduced immunotoxicity. *Aliment. Pharmacol. Ther.* **2010**, *32*, 1184–1191.
17. Tanner, G.J.; Blundell, M.J.; Colgrave, M.L.; Howitt, C.A. Quantification of hordeins by ELISA: The correct standard makes a magnitude of difference. *PLoS One* **2013**, *8*, e56456.
18. Comino, I.; Real, A.; Gil-Humanes, J.; Pistón, F.; de Lorenzo, L.; Moreno, M.L.; López-Casado, M.Á.; Lorite, P.; Cebolla, A.; Torres, M.I.; *et al.* Significant differences in coeliac immunotoxicity of barley varieties. *Mol. Nutr. Food. Res.* **2012**, *56*, 1697–1707.
19. Suttie, J.M.; Reynolds, S.G. Fodder oats: A world overview, 2004. Food and Agriculture Organization of the United Nations (FAO). Available online: http://www.fao.org/docrep/008/y5765e/y57 65e00.htm (accessed on 16 October 2012).
20. Eppendorfer, W.H. Nutritive value of oat and rye grain protein as influenced by nitrogen and amino acid composition. *J. Sci. Food Agric.* **2006**, *28*, 152–156.
21. Pulido, O.; Gillespie, Z.; Zarkadas, M.; Dubois, S.; Vavasour, E.; Rashid, M.; Switzer, C.; Godefroy, S.B. Introduction of oats in the diet of individuals with coeliac disease: A systematic review. *Adv. Food Nutr. Res.* **2009**, *57*, 235–285.
22. Codex Alimentarius International Food Standars. Available online: http://www.codexalimentarius.net/web/more_info.jsp?id_sta=291 (accessed on 28 August 2013).
23. COMMISSION REGULATION (EC) No 41/2009 of 20 January 2009 Concerning the Composition and Labelling of Foodstuffs Suitable for People Intolerant to Gluten. Available online: http://eur-lex.europa.eu/LexUriServ/LexUriServ.do?uri=OJ:L:2009:016:0003:0005:EN:PDF (accessed on 21 January 2009).
24. Arentz-Hansen, H.; Fleckenstein, B.; Molberg, Ø.; Scott, H.; Koning, F.; Jung, G.; Roepstorff, P.; Lundin, K.E.; Sollid, L.M. The molecular basis for oat intolerance in patients with coeliac disease. *PLoS Med.* **2004**, *1*, 84–92.
25. Silano, M.; di Benedetto, R.; Maialetti, F.; de Vincenzi, A.; Calcaterra, R.; Cornell, H.J.; de Vincenzi, M. Avenins from different cultivars of oats elicit response by coeliac peripheral lymphocytes. *Scand. J. Gastroenterol.* **2007**, *42*, 1302–1305.
26. Maglio, M.; Mazzarella, G.; Barone, M.V.; Gianfrani, C.; Pogna, N.; Gazza, L.; Stefanile, R.; Camarca, A.; Colicchio, B.; Nanayakkara, M.; *et al.* Immunogenicity of two oat varieties, in relation to their safety for celiac patients. *Scand. J. Gastroenterol.* **2011**, *46*, 1194–1205.
27. Comino, I.; Real, A.; de Lorenzo, L.; Cornell, H.; López-Casado, M.Á.; Barro, F.; Lorite, P.; Torres, M.I.; Cebolla, A.; Sousa, C. Diversity in oat potential immunogenicity: Basis for the selection of oat varieties with no toxicity in celiac disease. *Gut* **2011**, *60*, 915–922.
28. Real, A.; Comino, I.; de Lorenzo, L.; Merchán, F.; Gil-Humanes, J.; Giménez, M.J.; López-Casado, M.Á.; Torres, M.I.; Cebolla, Á.; Sousa, C.; *et al.* Molecular and immunological characterization of gluten proteins isolated from oat cultivars that differ in toxicity for celiac disease. *PLoS One* **2012**, *7*, e48365.

29. Tye-Din, J.A.; Stewart, J.A.; Dromey, J.A.; Beissbarth, T.; van Heel, D.A.; Tatham, A.; Henderson, K.; Mannering, S.I.; Gianfrani, C.; Jewell, D.P.; *et al.* Comprehensive, quantitative mapping of T cell epitopes in gluten in celiac disease. *Sci. Transl. Med.* **2010**, *2*, 41ra51.
30. Rosell, C.M.; Marco, C. Rice. In *Gluten Free Cereal Products and Beverages*; Arendt, E.K., dal Bello, F., Eds.; Elsevier Science: London, UK, 2008; pp. 81–100.
31. Boye, J.I.; Achouri, A.; Raymond, N.; Cleroux, C.; Weber, D.; Koerner, T.B.; Hucl, P.; Patterson, C.A. Analysis of Glabrous canary seeds by ELISA, Mass spectrometry, and western blotting for the absence of cross-reactivity with major plant food allergens. *J. Agric. Food Chem.* **2013**, *61*, 6102–6112.
32. Accomando, S.; Albino, C.; Montaperto, D.; Amato, G.M.; Corsello, G. Multiple food intolerance or refractory celiac sprue? *Dig. Liver Dis.* **2006**, *38*, 784–785.
33. Cabrera-Chávez, F.; Iamett, S.; Miriani, M.; Calderón de la Barca, A.M.; Mamone, G.; Bonomi, F. Maize prolamins resistant to peptic-tryptic digestion maintain immune-recognition by IgA from some celiac disease patients. *Plant Foods. Hum. Nutr.* **2012**, *67*, 24–30.
34. Darewicz, M.; Dziuba, J.; Minkiewicz, P. Computational characterization and identification of peptides for in silico detection of potentially celiac-toxic proteins. *Food Sci. Technol. Int.* **2007**, *13*, 125–133.
35. Shewry, P.R.; Napier, J.A.; Tatham, A.S. Seed storage proteins: Structures and biosynthesis. *Plant Cell* **1995**, *7*, 945.
36. Ciacci, C.; Maiuri, L.; Caporaso, N.; Bucci, C.; del Giudice, L.; Rita Massardo, D.; Pontieri, P.; di Fonzo, N.; Bean, S.R.; Ioerger, B.; *et al.* Celiac disease: *In vitro* and *in vivo* safety and palatability of wheat-free sorghum food products. *Clin. Nutr.* **2007**, *26*, 799–805.
37. Pontieri, P.; Mamone, G.; de Caro, S.; Tuinstra, M.R.; Roemer, E.; Okot, J.; de Vita, P.; Ficco, D.B.; Alifano, P.; Pignone, D.; *et al.* Sorghum, a healthy and gluten-free food for celiac patients as demonstrated by genome, biochemical, and immunochemical analyses. *J. Agric. Food. Chem.* **2013**, *61*, 2565–2571.
38. Saturni, L.; Ferretti, G.; Bacchetti, T. The gluten-free diet: Safety and nutritional quality. *Nutrients* **2010**, *2*, 16–34.
39. Arendt, E.K.; Dal Bello, F. *Gluten-Free Cereal, Products and Beverages (Food Science and Technology)*; Academic press: London, UK, 2011.
40. Ballabio, C.; Uberti, F.; di Lorenzo, C.; Brandolini, A.; Penas, E.; Restani, P. Biochemical and immunochemical characterization of different varieties of amaranth (*Amaranthus* L. ssp.) as a safe ingredient for gluten-free products. *J. Agric. Food. Chem.* **2011**, *59*, 12969–12974.
41. Ranhotra, G.S.; Gelroth, J.A.; Glaser, B.K.; Lorenz, K.J.; Johnson, D.L. Composition and protein nutritional quality of quinoa. *Cereal. Chem.* **1993**, *70*, 303–305.
42. Repo-Carrasco, R.; Esponiza, C.; Jacobsen, S.-E. Nutritional value and use of the Andean crops: Quinoa (*Chenopodium quinoa*) and kañiwa (*Chenopodium pallidicaule*). *Food Rev. Int.* **2003**, *19*, 179–189.
43. Abugoch, J.L.E. Quinoa (*Chenopodium quinoa* Wild.): Composition, Chemistry, Nutritional, and Functional Properties. In *Advances in Food and Nutrition Research*; Taylor, S.L., Ed.; Academic Press: Lincoln, NE, USA, 2009; Volume 58, pp. 1–31.

44. Gonzalez, J.A.; Konishi, Y.; Bruno, M.; Valoy, M.; Prado, F.E. Interrelationships among seed yield, total protein and amino acid composition of ten quinoa (*Chenopodium quinoa*) cultivars from two different agroecological regions. *J. Sci. Food Agric.* **2012**, *92*, 1222–1229.
45. Zevallos, V.F.; Ellis, H.J.; Suligoj, T.; Herencia, L.I.; Ciclitira, P.J. Variable activation of immune response by quinoa (*Chenopodium quinoa* Wild.) prolamins in celiac disease. *Am. J. Clin. Nutr.* **2012**, *96*, 337–344.
46. Mäkinen, O.E.; Zannini, E.; Arendt, E.K. Germination of oat and quinoa and evaluation of the malts as gluten free baking ingredients. *Plant Foods Hum. Nutr.* **2013**, *68*, 90–95.
47. De Vincenzi, M.; Silano, M.; Luchetti, R.; Carratu, B.; Boniglia, C.; Pogna, N.E. Agglutinating activity of alcohol-soluble proteins from quinoa seed flour in celiac disease. *Plant Foods Hum. Nutr.* **1999**, *54*, 93–100.
48. Berti, C.; Ballabio, C.; Restani, P.; Porrini, M.; Bonomi, F.; Iametti, S. Immunochemical and molecular properties of proteins in *Chenopodium quinoa*. *Cereal Chem.* **2004**, *81*, 275–277.
49. Bonafaccia, G.; Marocchini, M.; Kreft, I. Composition and technological properties of the flour and bran from common and tartary buckwheat. *Food Chem.* **2003**, *80*, 9–15.
50. Skrabanja, V.; Kreft, I.; Golob, T.; Modic, M.; Ikeda, S.; Ikeda, K.; Kreft, S.; Bonafaccia, G.; Knapp, M.; Kosmelj, K. Nutrient content in buckwheat milling fractions. *Cereal Chem.* **2004**, *81*, 172–176.
51. Bonafaccia, G.; Gambelli, L.; Fabjan, N.; Kreft, I. Trace elements in flour and bran from common and Tartary buckwheat. *Food Chem.* **2003**, *83*, 1–5.
52. Ikeda, K. Buckwheat: Composition, chemistry and processing. *Adv. Food Nutr. Res.* **2002**, *44*, 395–434.
53. Stember, R.H. Buckwheat allergy. *Allergy Asthma Proc.* **2006**, *27*, 393–395.
54. Wieslander, G. Review on buckwheat allergy. *Allergy* **1996**, *51*, 661–665.
55. Panda, R.; Taylor, S.L.; Goodman, R.E. Development of a Sandwich Enzyme-Linked Immunosorbent Assay (ELISA) for detection of buckwheat residues in food. *J. Food Sci.* **2010**, *75*, 110–117.
56. Watanabe, Y. Overview of Plant RNAi. In *Methods in Molecular Biology*; Kodama, H., Komamine, A., Eds.; Humana Press: Totowa, NJ, USA, 2011; Volume 744, pp. 1–11.
57. Becker, D.; Wieser, H.; Koehler, P.; Folck, A.; Mühling, K.H.; Zörb, C. Protein composition and techno-functional properties of transgenic wheat with reduced α-gliadin content obtained by RNA interference. *J. Appl. Bot. Food Qual.* **2012**, *85*, 23.
58. Gil-Humanes, J.; Pistón, F.; Hernando, A.; Álvarez, J.B.; Shewry, P.R.; Barro, F. Silencing of γ-gliadins by RNA interference (RNAi) in bread wheat. *J. Cereal Sci.* **2008**, *48*, 565–568.
59. Pistón, F.; Gil-Humanes, J.; Rodríguez-Quijano, M.; Barro, F. Down-Regulating γ-gliadins in bread wheat leads to non-specific increases in other gluten proteins and has no major effect on dough gluten strength. *PLoS One* **2011**, *6*, e24754.
60. Altenbach, S.B.; Allen, P.V. Transformation of the US bread wheat "Butte 86" and silencing of omega-5 gliadin genes. *GM Crops* **2011**, *2*, 66–73.
61. Gil-Humanes, J.; Pistón, F.; Tollefsen, S.; Sollid, L.M.; Barro, F. Effective shutdown in the expression of celiac disease-related wheat gliadin T-cell epitopes by RNA interference. *Proc. Natl. Acad. Sci. USA* **2010**, *107*, 17023–17028.

62. Wen, S.; Wen, N.; Pang, J.; Langen, G.; Brew-Appiah, R.A.T.; Mejias, J.H.; Osorio, C.; Yang, M.; Gemini, R.; Moehs, C.P.; *et al.* Structural genes of wheat and barley 5-methylcytosine DNA glycosylases and their potential applications for human health. *Proc. Natl. Acad. Sci. USA* **2012**, *109*, 20543–20548.
63. Gil-Humanes, J.; Pistón, F.; Shewry, P.R.; Tosi, P.; Barro, F. Suppression of gliadins results in altered protein body morphology in wheat. *J. Exp. Bot.* **2011**, *62*, 4203–4213.
64. Valdés, I.; García, E.; Llorente, M.; Méndez, E. Innovative approach to low-level gluten determination in foods using a novel sandwich enzyme-linked immunosorbent assay protocol. *Eur. J. Gastroenterol. Hepatol.* **2003**, *15*, 465–747.
65. Codex Alimentarius International Food Standars. Available online: http://www.codexalimentarius.org (accessed on 28 August 2013).
66. Wieser, H.; Koehler, P.; Folck, A.; Becker, D. Characterization of Wheat with Strongly Reduced α-Gliadin Content. In *Gluten Proteins*; Lookhart, L.G., Ng, W.P.K., Eds.; AACC International: St Paul, MN, USA, 2006; pp. 13–16.
67. Van den Broeck, H.C.; Gilissen, L.J.W.J.; Smulders, M.J.M.; van der Meer, I.M.; Hamer, R.J. Dough quality of bread wheat lacking alpha-gliadins with celiac disease epitopes and addition of celiac-safe avenins to improve dough quality. *J. Cereal Sci.* **2011**, *53*, 206–216.
68. Alvarez-Jubete, L.; Auty, M.; Arendt, E.K.; Gallagher, E. Baking properties and microstructure of pseudocereal flours in gluten-free bread formulations. *Eur. Food Res. Technol.* **2010**, *230*, 437–445.
69. Frazer, A.C.; Fletcher, R.F.; Ross, C.A.C.; Shaw, B.; Sammons, H.G.; Schneider, R. Gluten-Induce enteropathy the effect of partially digested gluten. *Lancet* **1959**, *2*, 252–255.
70. Van de Kamer, J.H.; Weijers, H.A. Celiac disease. V. Some experiments on the cause of the harmful effect of wheat gliadin. *Acta Pediatr. Scand.* **1955**, *44*, 465–469.
71. Shan, L.; Molberg, Ø.; Parrot, I.; Hausch, F.; Gray, G.M.; Sollid, L.M.; Khosla, C. Structural basis for gluten intolerance in celiac sprue. *Science* **2002**, *297*, 2275–2279.
72. Di Cagno, R.; de Angelis, M.; Lavermicocca, P.; de Vincenzi, M.; Giovanini, C.; Faccia, M.; Gobbetti, M. Proteolysis by sourdough lactic acid bacteria: Effects on wheat flour protein fractions and gliadin peptides involved in human cereal intolerance. *Appl. Environ. Microbiol.* **2002**, *68*, 623–633.
73. Gerez, C.L.; Font de Valdez, G.; Rollan, G.C. Functionality of lactic acid bacteria peptidase activities in the hydrolysis of gliadin-like fragments. *Appl. Microbiol.* **2008**, *47*, 427–432.
74. Di Cagno, R.; de Angelis, M.; Auricchio, S.; Greco, L.; Clarke, C.; de Vincenzi, M.; Giovanini, C.; D'Archivio, M.; Landolfo, F.; Parrilli, G.; *et al.* Sourdough bread made from wheat and nontoxic flours and started with selected lactobacilli is tolerated in celiac sprue patients. *Appl. Environ. Microbiol.* **2004**, *70*, 1088–1096.
75. Hartmann, G.; Koehler, P.; Wieser, H. Rapid degradation of gliadin peptides toxic for celiac disease patients by proteases from germinating cereals. *J. Cereal Sci.* **2006**, *44*, 368–371.
76. Kiyosaki, T.; Matsumoto, I.; Asakura, T.; Funaki, J.; Kuroda, M.; Misaka, T.; Arai, S.; Abe, K. Gliadain, a gibberellin-inducible cysteine proteinase occurring in germinating seeds of wheat, *Triticum aestivum* L., specifically digests gliadin and is regulated by intrinsic cystatins. *FEBS J.* **2007**, *274*, 1908–1917.

77. Michalcova, E.; Potoka, E.; Chmelova, D.; Ondrejovic, M. Study of wheat protein degradation during germination. *J. Microbiol. Biotechnol.* **2012**, *1*, 1439–1447.
78. Stenman, S.M.; Lindfors, K.; Venäläinen, J.I.; Hautala, A.; Mänistö, P.T.; Garcia-Horsman, J.A.; Kaukorvita-Norja, A.; Auriola, S.; Mauriala, T.; Mäki, M.; *et al.* Degradation of celiac disease-inducing rye secalin by germinating cereal enzymes: Diminishing toxic effects in intestinal epithelial cells. *Clin. Exp. Immunol.* **2010**, *161*, 242–249.
79. Wieser, H.; Koehler, P. Detoxification of gluten by means of enzymatic treatment. *J. AOAC Int.* **2012**, *95*, 356–363.
80. Van de Wal, Y.; Kooy, Y.; van Veelen, P.A.; Pena, S.; Mearin, L.; Papadopoulus, G.; Koning, F. Selective deamidation by tissue transglutaminase strongly enhances gliadin-specific T cell reactivity. *J. Immunol.* **1998**, *15*, 1585–1588.
81. Skovbjerg, H.; Koch, C.; Anthonsen, D.; Sjoestroem, H. Deamidation and cross-linking of gliadin peptides by transglutaminases and the relation to celiac disease. *Biochim. Biophys. Acta* **2004**, *1690*, 220–230.
82. Stamnaes, J.; Fleckenstein, B.; Sollid, L.M. The propensity for deamidation and transamidation of peptides by transglutaminase 2 is dependent on substrate affinity and reaction conditions. *Biochim. Biophys. Acta* **2008**, *1784*, 1804–1811.
83. Ohtsuka, T.; Umezawa, Y.; Nio, N.; Kubota, K. Comparison of deamidation activity of transglutaminases. *J. Cereal Sci.* **2001**, *66*, 25–29.
84. Nonaka, M.; Sawa, A.; Matsuura, Y.; Motoki, M.; Nio, N. Deamidation of several food proteins using free and immobilized Ca^{2+}-independent microbial transglutaminase. *Biosci. Biotechnol. Biochem.* **1996**, *60*, 532–533.
85. Gianfrani, C.; Siciliano, R.A.; Facchiano, A.M.; Camarca, A.; Mazzeo, M.F.; Costantini, S.; Salvati, V.M.; Maurano, F.; Mazzarella, G.; Iaquinto, G.; *et al.* Transamidation of wheat flour inhibits the response to gliadin of intestinal T cells in celiac disease. *Gastroenterology* **2007**, *133*, 780–789.
86. Mazzarella, G.; Salvati, V.M.; Laquinto, G.; Stefanile, R.; Capobianco, F.; Luongo, D.; Bergamo, P.; Maurano, F.; Giardullo, N.; Malamisura, B.; *et al.* Reintroduction of gluten following flour transamidation in adult celiac patients: A randomized, controlled clinical study. *Clin. Dev. Immunol.* **2012**, *2012*, 329150.
87. Pasternack, R.; Marx, S.; Jordan, D. Prolamin-Reduced Beverages and Methods for the Preparation Thereof. Int. Pat. WO 2006051093 A1, 18 May 2006.

10

The Gluten-Free Diet: Safety and Nutritional Quality

Letizia Saturni [1,*], Gianna Ferretti [1,2] and Tiziana Bacchetti [1,2]

[1] Centro Interdipartimentale di Educazione Sanitaria e Promozione alla Salute, Ancona, 60035 Italy; E-Mails: g.ferretti@univpm.it (G.F.); t.bacchetti@univpm.it (T.B.)

[2] Dipartimento di Biochimica, Biologia e Genetica - Università Politecnica delle Marche - Ancona, 60035, Italy

* Author to whom correspondence should be addressed; E-Mail: lsaturni@univpm.it;

Abstract: The prevalence of Celiac Disease (CD), an autoimmune enteropathy, characterized by chronic inflammation of the intestinal mucosa, atrophy of intestinal villi and several clinical manifestations has increased in recent years. Subjects affected by CD cannot tolerate gluten protein, a mixture of storage proteins contained in several cereals (wheat, rye, barley and derivatives). Gluten free-diet remains the cornerstone treatment for celiac patients. Therefore the absence of gluten in natural and processed foods represents a key aspect of food safety of the gluten-free diet. A promising area is the use of minor or pseudo-cereals such as amaranth, buckwheat, quinoa, sorghum and teff. The paper is focused on the new definition of gluten-free products in food label, the nutritional properties of the gluten-free cereals and their use to prevent nutritional deficiencies of celiac subjects.

Keywords: celiac disease; gliadin; gluten-free diet; hordein; minor cereals; pseudo-cereals; secalin; avenin

1. Celiac Disease

Celiac disease (CD) is a chronic systemic autoimmune disorder caused by a permanent intolerance to gluten proteins in genetically susceptible individuals [1,2]. Currently CD is thought to resemble a multisystem immunological disorder rather than a disease restricted to the gastrointestinal tract [1,2]. The first accurate clinical description of CD evidenced broad flat villi and a dense chronic lymphoepithelial inflammatory cell infiltrate in the small intestinal mucosa of patients [3]. Later the progression of the abnormalities of the intestinal mucosal in response to gluten has been described in CD patients [4]. The clinical symptoms of CD differ greatly and depend on age of the patient, duration and the extent of extra-intestinal manifestations [5-7]. CD was thought to be a rare disease, with a prevalence of about 0.02%, however using serology and biopsy, recent studies carried out in Europe, India, South America, Australasia and USA indicate that the prevalence may be between 0.33 and 1.06% in children and between 0.18–1.2% in adults [8-11]. The highest prevalence (5.66%) in childhood has been observed in Sahrawi [12]. In other African countries, CD is rarely diagnosed, this reflects in a much lower prevalence. Population studies also indicate that a large proportion of celiac people remain undiagnosed; this is due to many clinicians being unfamiliar with the condition.

2. Pathogenesis and Molecular Mechanism

As summarized in the Figure 1, environmental, genetic and immunologic factors are involved in the pathogenesis of celiac disease [13]. Interactions between gluten peptides and intestinal epithelium [14], autoantigen (the ubiquitous enzyme tissue transglutaminase (tTG) [15] are involved and some molecular mechanisms have been hypothesized.

Figure 1. Factors involved the pathogenesis of celiac disease.

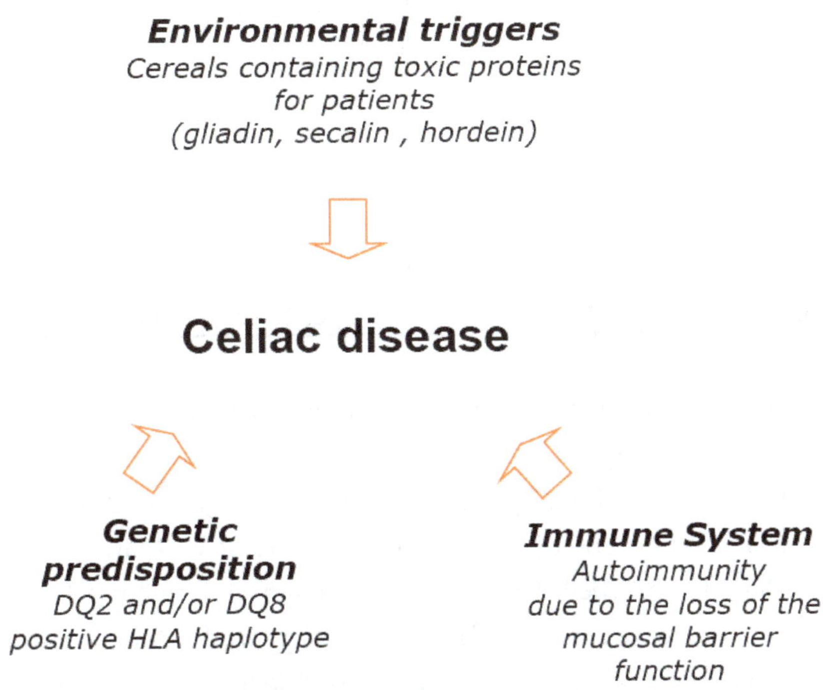

Gluten is a general term used to describe a mixture of wheat storage proteins (prolamins and glutenins). However other cereals have proteins that exert a toxic effect for CD patients; toxic prolamins include gliadin in wheat, secalin in rye and hordein in barley. Prolamins are characterized by a particular amino acid composition with domains with a high content of proline and glutamine. It has been demonstrated that these protein domains are resistant to degradation by gastric, pancreatic and proteases in the human intestinal brush border membrane. This results in an accumulation of relatively large peptide fragments (such as a recently described 33mer sequence) [13-16]. The study of the molecular mechanisms about the toxic effect of protein fragments has demonstrated that these peptides both *in vivo* and *in vitro* induce mucosal damage [14,16] and/or behave as "immunogenic" (*i.e.* are able to specifically stimulate HLA-DQ2 or HLA-DQ8) [17]. In fact, peptides such as the 33mer sequence, are able to stimulate intestinal immunitary cells and T cells. It has been hypothesized that one of the first events in CD pathogenesis might be a direct effect of certain wheat peptides, distinct from those recognized by T cells, on the intestinal epithelium of patients.

3. Gluten Free Diet

3.1. Nutritional State of Celiac Subjects

Previous studies have demonstrated that 20-38% of celiac patients [18-21] have some nutritional deficiencies such as calorie/protein [22], dietary fibre [23-25], minerals [26-35] and vitamins [27,32,36-39] (Table1).

Table 1. Common nutrient deficiencies in celiac subjects at diagnosis and after Gluten Free Diet (GFD).

At diagnosis	*Long term GFD*
Calorie/Protein	Fibre
Fibre	
Iron	
Calcium	
Magnesium	
Vitamin D	
Zinc	
Folate, Niacin, Vitamin B12, Riboflavin	Folate, Niacin, Vitamin B12

Malabsorption of iron, folate, and calcium is common, as these nutrients are absorbed in the proximal small bowel. In particular, it has been reported that the frequency of iron-deficiency in celiac disease varies from 12% to 69% [36,37]. The incidence of vitamin B-12 deficiency in untreated patients ranges from 8% to 41% [36,38], though there is a relative sparing of villous atrophy in the ileum where vitamin B-12 is absorbed. Calcium, phosphorus, and vitamin D deficiencies may occur due to malabsorption or a decreased intake of milk and dairy products in an effort to avoid lactose, in fact secondary lactose intolerance resulting from decreased lactase production by the damaged villi is also common [40]. The severity of the aforementioned nutritional deficiencies is modulated by different factors: the length of time that people has lived with the active, but undiagnosed disease, the extent of damage to the gut intestinal tract and the degree of malabsorption.

Previous studies have demonstrated that most of these nutritional deficiencies disappear after following strictly a gluten free diet [22,26,32]. Other authors have shown that gluten free diet does not guarantee adequate nutritional intake [24,25] and some nutritional deficiencies have been described after treatment with a long-term GFD for about 8-12 years (Table 1) [25,32]. The analysis of diet of 47 adults in USA showed that the recommended amount of calcium, iron and fibers was consumed only by 32, 44 and 46% of women included in the study [25]. The inadequate fiber intake is likely to be related to the composition of many GF foods made with starches and /or refined flours with low content in fiber [23-25]. In fact during refining, the outer layer of grain containing most of the fibre is removed, leaving only the starchy inner layer.

Previous studies have investigated the nutritional composition of processed gluten–free products and it has been demonstrated that they have high levels of lipids, sugars and salt. Subjects with celiac disease tend to compensate for the restrictions of a gluten-free diet by eating foods containing high levels of fat, sugar and calories, therefore celiac patients may show an excessive consumption of total fats and saturated fats [41]. Mariani *et al.* [41] reported that diet of CD adolescent patients was hyperproteic and hyperlipidic and contained low amounts of carbohydrates, iron, calcium, and fiber. Polito *et al.* [42] and Rea *et al.* [43] observed an excess in energy, animal protein, and lipid intake, which was partially responsible for the high percentage of overweight patients. As far as concerns fat composition of gluten-free products, it has been evidenced that they contain *trans* fatty acids [44] that may provoke metabolic imbalance when in association with a inadequate intake of essential fatty acids [45]. All these components have a negative effect on health and this should be seriously taken in account because the limited choice of food products in the diet of celiac induces a high consume of packaged gluten-free products, such as snacks and biscuits [44]. A high intake of dietary lipids is a major factor influencing the development of diseases such as coronary heart disease and obesity [46]. Therefore, it has been suggested that paradoxically, a strict gluten-free diet may be a nutritional risk factor for CD patients, because it leads these subjects to incorrect alimentary choices [41].

3.2. Safety and Nutritional Aspects of Gluten Free-Diet

It has to be stressed that there are many aspects related to the food safety such as contamination by biological (micro-organisms such as bacteria, viruses, parasites, moulds), by physical factors or chemical substances (acrylamide, PCBs and dioxins, persistent organic pollutants). The contamination of foods may occur also through environmental toxins (heavy metals, PCBs, and dioxins), or through the intentional use of various chemicals, such as pesticides, animal drugs, and other agrichemicals. All these factors may pose significant health risks to consumers, including celiac subjects. In the present study, the term "safety" was referred mainly to the naturally gluten-free foods or foods specially processed to reduce gluten content. Since the discovery that wheat was a key environmental factor that triggered celiac disease in susceptible individuals, the relationship between the disease and the ingestion of wheat gluten proteins has became an essential part of the definition of "Gluten Free Diet". GFD means that CD subjects have to exclude all foods and medications containing gluten.

As summarized in Table 2, cereals containing gluten (wheat, rye, barley) and hybrids such as Khorosan wheat (Kamut®), spelt (sometimes called *Farro*) and triticale (a combination of wheat and rye) are not allowed. Other products such as semolina (durum wheat), einkorn, bulgur and wheat derivatives (wheat germ, wheat bran, whole wheat and cracked wheat) have also to be avoided. Additionally all foods derived from gluten-containing cereals including pasta, breads and crackers are not allowed. Malt is also toxic for CD subjects because it is a partial hydrolysate of barley prolamins [47]. Therefore barley malt, malt syrup, malt extract, malt flavorings cannot be inserted in CD diet. Beer usually contains appreciable quantities of hordein (barley gluten prolamin) [47], however some low gluten beer has been presented in the market.

For several years oat have been excluded from the CD diet because it was thought that avenin (the storage protein found in oats) was also toxic to CD patients. Moreover the use of oats in GFD is still debated in relation to a possible cross-contamination with gluten-containing grains, as demonstrated in some commercial products in the United States. However some studies have demonstrated gluten contamination either in naturally gluten free products (soybean, rice, millet, corn, buckwheat) or in industrially-purified gluten free flours [49]. As far as concern oat, recent studies have revealed that when consumed in moderation, oat free from cross-contamination with gluten-containing grains, is well-tolerated by most children and adults with CD even in long-term use [48,50-53]. The literature also suggests that pure oats can be beneficial to those individuals with CD who tolerate it, and its palatability may help to increase compliance with a gluten-free diet [54] and improve the nutritional value [55-57].

Table 2. Vegetable and animal foods allowed or not allowed in gluten-free diet.

ALLOWED	NOT ALLOWED
Vegetable foods	
Cereals	**Cereals**
Corn	Wheats (Spelt ,semolina, durum)
Rice	Rye
Sorghum	Barley
Oat *	Triticale
Minor cereals	Kamut®
Fonio	Malt
Teff	
Millet	
Teosinte	
Job's tears	
Pseudo-cereals	
Buckwheat	
Quinoa	
Amaranth	
Vegetables	
Fruits	
Pulses	
Nuts	
Other plant foods	
Tapioca	
Soybean	
Potato	
Root crops	
Vegetable oils	

Table 2. *Cont.*

Animal foods
Milk and derivatives
Plain meat
Fish
Egg
Butter

* oat, oat bran and oat syrup could be allowed in the GFD only if they are recommended by patient's healthcare team

As mentioned, several cereals containing gluten have to be avoided, however a lot of other vegetable and animal foods such as fish, poultry and meats, as well as fruits and vegetables, are permitted in their natural state. Rice, corn and potatoes have been widely used as substitute of gluten-containing grains. A number of nutrient dense grains, seeds, pulses offer increased variety, improved palatability and high nutritional quality for the GFD (Table 2) [54,59,61]. Minor cereals - so called because they are less common and are only grown in a few small regions of the world- such as fonio, teff, millet, teosinte and Job's tears, and pseudo-cereals producing small grain-like seeds (buckwheat, Tartarian buckwheat, quinoa and amaranth grain) are allowed (Table 3). Minor cereals and pseudo-cereals may be sold whole, milled into flour, flakes or grits, puffed and /or incorporated into pasta, cereals, crackers and other gluten-free specialty products. In the last years, the range of processed gluten-free products is increased: breads, biscuits, and pasta produced by gluten-free ingredients and food additives have been proposed on the market. Therefore, celiac patients need to pay attention to food labels, looking for words such as wheat starch, wheat bran, graham flour, kamut® and hydrolyzed wheat protein.

Table 3. Characteristics of some plant (pseudo-cereals and minor cereals) gluten-free alternative.

Teff	*Teff* is a grass native to Ethiopia, that belongs to the Poaceae family. It is also grown in India, Australia and Northwestern USA. Teff is the smallest of all grains in the world (about 100-150 teff grains equal the size if 1 wheat kernel) and its grains range from milky white to almost black. Teff has a unique nutty, mild molasses-like flavour and is sold as whole grain and as flour. In Ethiopia flour is fermented 1-3 days to make "Injera", a sour-dough-type flat bread .
Fonio	*Fonio* is a typically cereal in Sudan or Ethiopia where it is considered to be the tastiest of all cereals
Millet	The term *millet* refers to various grasses that grown in semi-arid regions of the world. There are a lot of species, but only pearl and finger millets are used for food consumption. Millet is closely related to corn and belongs to Gramineae family. Milled seeds are very small and can be yellow, white, gray or red. It is similar in texture to rice flour.

Table 3. *Cont.*

Amaranth	*Amaranth* is a broad-leafed plant which produces florets containing thousands of tiny grain-like, tan-colored seeds. Although it is used as grain, it is not an actual grain but a member of the Amaranthaceaea family. Amaranth seeds have been used as a staple by many ancient civilizations around the word. It has a robust nutty flavour.
Buckwheat	*Buckwheat* is thought to have originated in China. The larger producers of buckwheat today are China, Japan, Russia and North America, although it is also grown in Europe, India, Australia. Buckwheat is botanically classified as a fruit, not a cereal grain and is of the Polygonaceae family, which is closely related to rhubarb. It is triangular in shape and has a black shell. The outer shell is removed and the kernel inside is known as a great.
Quinoa	*Quinoa* has been consumed for thousands of years in South America and was a staple of the Incas. It is not actually a grain but the seeds of a broad-leafed plant from the Chenopodiaceae family which is a close relative of the weed, lamb's quarters. There are hundreds of varieties of quinoa, ranging in colour from white to red and purple to black.

3.3. Food Labelling and Legislative Aspects

The absence of gluten in natural and processed foods represents a key aspect of food safety of the gluten free diet. The term "gluten free" was introduced in food labels several years ago. The current Codex Standard for GF foods was adopted by the Codex Alimentarius Commission of the World Health Organization (WHO) and by the Food and Agricultural Organization (FAO) in 1976 and amended in 1983 (Codex Alimentarius Commission, 1983). The definition came under review in the 1990s.

It has to be stressed that gluten contamination in processed GF products cannot be totally avoided. There is no agreement about the amount of dietary gluten that CD subjects may introduce without damaging the mucosa of the small intestine. Some authors consider safe a threshold for which gluten contamination should be set: less than 30 mg of gluten per day [62]; between 10 and 100 mg intake daily [63]; higher than 50 mg per day [64].

In USA, Food and Drug Administration (Codex Standard, 2007) is proposing to define the term gluten-free to mean that a food bearing this claim does not contain: an ingredient that is not allowed (wheat, rye, barley or their crossbred hybrids); an ingredient that is derived from a prohibited grain and that has not been processed to remove gluten; an ingredient that is derived from a prohibited grain that has been processed to remove gluten, if the use of that ingredient results in the presence of 20 ppm or more gluten in the food and, at last, 20 ppm or more gluten.

Recently, European countries have accepted the definition of GF designed by Codex Alimentarius (the gluten free certification organization, 2007) [65]. The term 'gluten-free' will refer only to foods containing less than 20 ppm of gluten (Table 4). In addition, the claim 'very low gluten' will be used for foods such as bread, produced using cereals that have been specially processed to remove most of the gluten and containing gluten less than 30 mg daily. Manufacturers can use the new labeling system immediately; however, they have time to adapt to the new rules until 1 January 2012.

We may expect that new type of labeling will help CD subjects to make safer and more informed food choices.

Table 4. New Codex Alimentarious Standards for Gluten-Free foods.

- Gluten-free foods are dietary foods
a) consisting of or made only from one or more ingredients which do not contain wheat (*i.e.*, all Triticum species, such as durum wheat, spelt and kamut®), rye, barley, oats[1] or their crossbred varieties, and the gluten level does not exceed 20 mg/kg in total, based on the food as sold or distributed to the consumer,
and/or
b) consisting of one or more ingredients from wheat (*i.e.*, all Triticum species, such as durum wheat, spelt, and kamut®), rye, barley, oats[1] or their crossbred varieties, which have been specially processed to remove gluten, and the gluten level does not exceed 20 mg/kg in total, based on the food as sold or distributed to the consumer.
- Foods specially processed to reduce gluten content to a level above 20 up to 100 mg/kg
These foods consist of one or more ingredients from wheat (*i.e.*, all Triticum species, such as durum wheat, spelt, and kamut®), rye, barley, oats[1] or their crossbred varieties, which have been specially processed to reduce the gluten content to a level above 20 up to 100 mg/kg in total, based on the food as sold or distributed to the consumer.
[1] Oats can be tolerated by most but not all people who are intolerant to gluten. Therefore, the allowance of oats that are not contaminated with wheat, rye or barley in foods covered by this standard may be determined at the national level.

3.4. General Dietary Advices for Celiac Subjects

Even if studies related to nutritional state of CD are limited for duration and study design, all demonstrated that nutritional therapy is an essential part of a management of CD.

Different countries show different lifestyles and nutritional habits; therefore is not easy to suggest dietary recommendations that could be applied to celiac people of different ethnic groups. Here we describe some dietary advices and the nutritional properties of some foods that can be included in the gluten-free diet to prevent malnutrition.

Carbohydrate. Complex and simple carbohydrates intake should represent about 55% of total calories. As aforementioned, even if the grain sources of carbohydrate are limited in the GFD, legumes and a wide variety of grains and seeds are permitted (Table 2). In the last years, the nutrient composition of minor cereals and pseudo-cereals has been characterized and it has been demonstrated that they represent a good source of carbohydrate (Table 5), dietary fibre, minerals, vitamins and phenols [66-72].

Table 5. Chemical composition (% dry mass) of Amaranth, Quinoa, Oat and Buckwheat compared to Wheat.

Component	Amaranth	Quinoa	Buckwheat	Oat	Wheat
Starch	67.3	69.0	67.2	**nd**	61.0
Protein	15.2	13.3	10.9	**13**	11.7
Fat	8.0	7.5	2.7	**7.5**	2.0
Minerals	3.2	2.6	1.59	**3.1**	1.8

Dietary fibre. Dietary fibre is a complex mixture of plant materials and molecules that are resistant to breakdown (digestion). Some fibre components exert physiological roles and are metabolized by gut bacteria. Several studies have demonstrated that high-fibre diets prevent many human diseases, colon cancer, coronary heart disease and diabetes [73]. An adequate intake (20-35g/d) of fibre has to be recommended in CD subjects. As aforementioned, some studies have reported that GFD is associated with a lower intake of dietary fibre [23,24]. As summarized in Table 6, the fibre content in minor cereals and pseudo-cereals range from 7 to 10 g/100 g [68]. These levels are higher with respect to other plant foods fruits, nuts, pulses and cereals such as corn and rice. Therefore, their use in GDF can help to increase fibre intake in CD patients.

Table 6. Fibre content in different plant foods.

	Fibre (g/100g)
Cereals	
Oat	10.3
Wheat	9.5
Barley	9.2
Teff	8.0
Corn	7.3
Spelt	6.8
Rice	2.8
Pseudo-cereals	
Buckwheat	10.0
Quinoa	7.0
Amaranth	6.7
Fruit and vegetable	0.5-5.0
Nuts	4.0-12.0
Pulses	5.0-18.0

Protein. Dietary protein intake should represent about 15% of total calories. In GDF the main dietary source of protein are animal foods such as meat, milk and dairy products, eggs and fish. Plant foods which are useful sources of protein include legumes, nuts, seeds and gluten free cereals. In the last years, the protein content of pseudo-cereals and minor cereals has been investigated and it has been demonstrated that is higher with respect to wheat (Table 5), moreover the quality of the protein is much better [74,75]. In particular lysine, the limiting amino acid in cereals can be found in high amounts. The high content of arginine and histidine, both essential for infants and children, makes Amaranth and Quinoa interesting for the nutrition of CD children. Moreover pseudo-cereals and minor cereals contain amino acids like methionine and cysteine which are essential to human health. Protein quality not only depends on the amino acid composition, but also on the bioavailability or digestibility. Protein digestibility, available lysine, net protein utilisation (NPU) or protein efficiency ratio (PER) are widely used as indicators for the nutritional quality of proteins. In this respect, the values for pseudo-cereal proteins are definitively higher when compared to cereals and are close to those of casein [74,75].

Lipids. Total fat intake should represent about 25-30% or less of total calories. The intake of unsaturated fat (monounsaturated and polyunsaturated) should be preferred. Monounsaturated and polyunsaturated fatty acids should provide more than 15% and 10% of total calories, respectively (50% and 25% of total fat) (Table 4). In fact, monounsaturated fats and omega-3 fatty acids intake has been associated with reduced cardiovascular disease risk [76]. They are found in foods such as vegetable oils, nuts, seeds and higher fat fish including salmon, trout and herring. On the contrary saturated fatty acids, manly found in animal foods (meat, poultry, whole milk dairy products) and in tropical oils, should be limited (8-10% of total calories). Also *trans* fatty acids play a negative effect on development of atherosclerosis [45], therefore their intake should be limited at less than 1% of total calories (about 5g/die). As previously described the levels of saturated and *trans* fatty acids in processed gluten free products are higher with respect to conventional foods [44]. Therefore, it is important that celiac subjects pay attention to the food label and to hydrogenated fats content.

Although the lipid content of pseudo-cereals is higher compared to other plant foods (Table 5), they are characterised by a higher content of unsaturated fatty acids in particularly of linolenic acid [71,77], an omega-3 fatty acid essential for all mammals. A consumption of α-linolenic acid (2 to 3 g per day) has been considered important for the primary and secondary prevention of coronary heart disease [78]. Amaranth contains a high amount of squalene, a highly unsaturated open chain triterpen, which is usually only found in liver of deep see fish and other maritime species [71,77].

Micronutrients. To avoid micronutrient deficiencies in celiac subjects, the amount of fruits and vegetables should be increased. An intake of at least five portions of fruit or vegetable a day has been recommended to help to reduce the risk of some diseases (cancer, heart disease). Fruit and vegetables are low in energy and rich in vitamins and minerals. Moreover, they contain phytochemicals and antioxidant compounds that exert a protective effect against diseases associated with oxidative damage [79,80].

Mineral salts. These are essential nutrients. They include major minerals (calcium, phosphorus, sodium, potassium, chloride and magnesium) and trace elements (iron, zinc, selenium). In addition to animal products, also vegetable foods contain a significant amount of minerals. The total content of minerals in amaranth, quinoa and oats is about twice as high as in other cereals (Table 4) [77,81,82]. In teff, iron and calcium contents (11-33 mg and 100-150 mg, respectively) are higher than those of wheat, barley, or sorghum and rice. In Ethiopia, an absence of anaemia seems to correlate with the levels of teff consumption and is presumed to be due to the grain's high content of iron. The content of minerals in buckwheat seeds is lower than in wheat. However, except for calcium, buckwheat is a richer source of nutritionally important minerals than many cereals such as rice, sorghum, millet and maize [77,81]. Minerals are located in the germ; therefore, we may expect that they are not completely lost during the refining process.

Vitamins. An adequate intake of vitamins is particularly important for celiac patients to prevent vitamin deficiencies. Folic acid is present in green leafy vegetable, liver and cereals. High concentration of folic acid has been found in gluten free cereals such as quinoa (78.1 μg/100 g) and amaranth (102 μg/100g) with respect to wheat (40 μg/100 g). Both amaranth, quinoa and oats are also good sources of riboflavin, vitamin C and vitamin E [72,82,83]. The vitamins B2 and B6 are also present in buckwheat seeds [83]. Finally, it should be noted that a growing number of gluten-free specialty products are now being fortified with vitamins and minerals.

Table 7. Phenolic acid content in different plant foods and derivatives.

Sample	Phenolic acid (mg/100g)
Whole Grains:	
Foxtail millet	390.7
Pearl millet	147.8
Rye	136.2
Wheat	134.2
Barley	45.0–134.6
Sorghum	38.5–74.6
Finger millet	61.2
Maize	60.1
Oat	47.2
Rice	19.7–37.6
Brans	
Wheat	452.7
Rye	419.0
Oat	65.1
Fruit and beverages	
Coffee	97
Blueberry	85
Green and black teas	30–36
Dark plum	28

Phytochemicals. All plant-derived foods contain phytochemicals such as polyphenols which affect their organoleptic and nutritional properties. Awareness of their importance in human nutrition has been aroused because of their potential beneficial effects on human health (in fact they are able to reduce risk of cardiovascular disease, ischemic stroke, type II diabetes, metabolic syndrome and gastrointestinal cancers [73]. Moreover they have been reported to have antiviral, anti-allergic, antiplatelet, anti-inflammatory, antitumor and antioxidant activities [79,80]. As previously reported, the main food sources of these compounds are fruits, vegetables, wine, teas [79,80]. However, more recently it has been reported that cereals and pseudo-cereals could represent a good source of polyphenols. The levels of total phenolic acids in some cereals and gluten-free products are summarized in table 7 [85-87]. Flavonoids are polyphenolic compounds (flavonols, flavones, flavanones, isoflavones, catechins, anthocyanidins and chalcones) occurring in fruits, vegetables and beverages (tea, coffee, beer, wine and fruit drinks). They contribute to the colour of several fruits and vegetables. Flavonoids have been reported also in the pericarp of pigmented varieties of barley, maize, rice, rye and wheat [83]. The levels of antocyanins in different fruits and pigmented cereal grains are summarized in Table 8 [88,89]. Other flavonoids mainly found in fruits and vegetables are also reported in cereals. For example the flavone apigenin, a typical compound found in parsley and celery, is also reported in millet, oats and sorghum. Flavonones, have been quantified in sorghum and oats [85-87].

Table 8. Anthocyanin content of different fruits and pigmented cereal grains (mg/100 g).

Sample	**Anthocyanin (mg/100g)**
Blue barley	0.4
Pink maize	9.3
Red maize	56
Blue maize	22.5
Purple maize	96.5
Black rice	22.8–32.7
Black sorghum	94.4
Corn shaman blue	32.7
Blue wheat	10.6–21
White wheat	0.7
Purple wheat	1.3–13.9
Blackberry cultivars	131 to 256

Several phytochemicals behave as antioxidants *in vitro*. Recently the total antioxidant capacity of gluten free cereals has been studied. The results have shown that buckwheat and quinoa possess the highest antioxidant potential among the studied cereals and pseudo-cereals [85-87,90].

4. Conclusions

The prevalence of celiac disease is increased in the last years. Previous studies have demonstrated that gluten free diet products are poor sources of minerals (such as iron), vitamins (such as folate, thiamine niacin and riboflavin) and fibre [23,24], therefore the nutritional content of gluten-free foods is an increasing area of concern. A promising area is the use of minor or pseudo-cereals such as amaranth, buckwheat, quinoa, sorghum and teff. Minor cereals and pseudo-cereals may be used to prepare several gluten-free specialty products. The technological and nutritional properties of these alternative cereals as wheat replacements have been investigated and it has been suggested that their use could improve intakes of protein, iron, calcium and fibre of celiac patients [54]

In a systematic review of literature on oat inclusion in the gluten-free diet, Størstud *et al.* [55] noted that the inclusion of oats would increase the variety and nutrient content of the gluten-free diet. Other authors have confirmed that oats exert a positive effect on GDF [56]. Recently, Lee *et al.* [54] demonstrated that the adding of three servings of gluten-free alternative grains, including oats and quinoa, positively impacts the nutrient profile (fibre, thiamine, riboflavin, niacin, folate and iron) of the grain portion of the gluten-free diet. Minor cereals and pseudo-cereals are important sources of proteins and carbohydrates, especially fibre, and would permit a wider choice of foods for celiac individuals when selecting foods.

As far as concerns food price, Stevens *et al.* [92] have reported previously that commercially available products labelled gluten-free were significantly more expensive than comparable products. Lee *et al.* [54] have suggested that the alternative grains such as oats and quinoa could represent less expensive alternative with respect to standard gluten-free diet choices, quinoa and oats could increase dietary compliance also by reducing the economic burden of the diet. However further studies are necessary to better investigate whether the use of pseudo-cereals and minor cereals can contribute to reduce nutritional deficiencies of treated CD subjects and decrease prices of gluten free foods.

References

1. Green, P.H.; Rostami, K; Marsh, M.N. Diagnosis of coeliac disease. *Best Pract. Res. Clin. Gastroenterol.* **2005**, *19*, 389-400.
2. Murray, J.A.; Van Dyke, C.; Plevak, M.F.; Dierkhising, R.A.; Zinsmeister, A.R.; Melton, L Trends in the identification and clinical features of celiac disease in a North American community, 1950-2001. *Clin. Gastroenterol. Hepatol.* **2003**, *1*, 9-27
3. Paulley, J.W. Observation on the aetiology of idiopathic steatorrhoea; jejunal and lymph-node biopsies. *Br. Med. J.* **1954**, *2*, 1318-21.
4. Marsh, M.N. Gluten, major histocompatibility complex, and the small intestine. A molecular and immunobiologic approach to the spectrum of gluten sensitivity ('celiac sprue').*Gastroenterology* **1992**, *102*, 330-54.
5. Fasano, A. Clinical presentation of celiac disease in the pediatric population. *Gastroenterology* **2005**, *128*, S68-73.
6. Chand, N.; Mihas, A.A. Celiac disease: current concepts in diagnosis and treatment. *J. Clin. Gastroenterol.* **2006**, *40*, 3-14.
7. Green, P.H.; Jabri, B. Coeliac disease. *Lancet* **2003**, *362*, 383-391.
8. Barker, J.M.; Liu, E. Celiac disease: pathophysiology, clinical manifestations, and associated autoimmune conditions. *Adv. Pediatr.* **2008**, *55*, 349-365.
9. Fasano, A.; Berti, I.; Gerarduzzi, T. ;Not, T.; Colletti, R.B.; Drago, S.; Elitsur, Y.; Green, P.H.; Guandalini, S.; Hill, I.D.; Pietzak, M.; Ventura, A.; Thorpe, M.; Kryszak, D.; Fornaroli, F.;

Wasserman, S.S.; Murray, J.A.; Horvath, K. Prevalence of celiac disease in at-risk and not-at-risk groups in the United States: A large multicenter study. *Arch. Intern. Med.* **2003**, *163*, 286-292.

10. Dube, C.; Rostom, A.; Sy, R.; Cranney, A.; Saloojee, N.; Garritty, C.; Sampson, M.; Zhang, L.; Yazdi, F.; Mamaladze, V.; Pan, I.; Macneil, J.; Mack, D.; Patel, D.; Moher, D. The prevalence of celiac disease in average-risk and at-risk Western European populations: A systematic review. *Gastroenterology* **2005**, *128*, S57-S67.
11. Sood, A.; Midha, V.; Sood, N.; Malhotra, V. Adult celiac disease in Northern India. *Indian J. Gastroenterol.* **2003**, *22*, 124-126.
12. Catassi,C.; Rätsch, I.M.; Gandolfi, L.; Pratesi, R.; Fabiani, E.; El Asmar, R.; Frijia, M.; Bearzi, I.; Vizzoni, L. Why is coeliac disease endemic in the people of the Sahara? *Lancet* **1999**, *354*, 647-8.
13. Shan, L.; Molberg, O.; Parrot. I.; Hausch, F.; Feliz, F.; Gray, G.M.; Sollid, L.M.;Khosla, C. Structural basis for gluten intolerance in celiac sprue. *Science* **2002**, *297*, 2275-2279.
14. van de Wal, Y.; Kooy, Y.M.; van Veelen, P.; Vader, W.; August, S.A.; Drijfhout, J.W.; Pena, S.A.; Koning, F. Glutenin is involved in the gluten driven mucosal T cell response. *Eur. J. Immunol.* **1999**, *10*, 3133-3139.
15. Dieterich, W.; Ehnis, T.; Bauer, M.; Donner, P.;Volta, U.; Riecken, E.O.; Schuppan, D. Identification of tissue transglutaminase as the autoantigen of celiac disease. *Nat. Med.* **1997**, *3*, 797-801.
16. Dewar, D.H.; Amato, M.; Ellis, H.J.; Pollack, E.L.; Gonzalez-Cinca, N.; Wieser, H.; Ciclitira, P.J. The toxicity of high molecular weight glutenin subunits of wheat to patients with coeliac disease. *Eur. J. Gastroenterol. Hepatol.* **2006**, *18*, 483-491.
17. Ciccocioppo, R.; Di Sabatino, A.; Corazza, G.R. The immune recognition of gluten in coeliac disease. *Clin. Exp. Immunol.* **2005**, *140*, 408-16.
18. Kemppainen, T.; Uusitupa, M.; Janatuinen, E.; Järvinen, R.; Julkunen, R.; Pikkarainen, P. Intakes of nutrients and nutritional status in coeliac patients. *Scand. J. Gastroenterol.* **1995**, *30*, 575-579
19. Kinsey, L.; Burden, S.T.; Bannerman, E. A dietary survey to determine if patients with celiac disease are meeting current healthy eating quidelines and how their diet compares to that of British general population. *Eur. J. Clin. Nutr.* **2008**, *62*, 1333-1342
20. Bode S, Gudmand-Hoyer E. Symptoms and haemotological features in consecutive adult coeliac patients. *Scand. J. Gastroenterol.* **1996**, *31*, 54-60
21. Kemppainen T. *Oat meal as a component of a gluten-free diet, nutrient intakes, nutritional status and osteopenia in coeliac patients*; Kuopio University publications D, Medical Sciences: Kuopio, Finland, 1997; p. 188.
22. Bardella, M.T.; Fredella, C.; Prampolini, L.; Molteni, N.; Giunta, A.M.; Bianchi, P.A. Body composition and dietary intakes in adult celiac disease patients consuming a strict gluten-free diet. *Am. J. Clin. Nutr.* **2000**, *72*, 937-9.
23. Thompson, T. Folate, iron, and dietary fiber contents of the gluten free diet. *J. Am. Dietetic Assoc.* **2000**, *100*, 1389-1396.
24. Thompson, T. Thiamin, riboflavin, and niacin contents of the gluten-free diet: Is there cause for concern? *J. Am. Dietetic Assoc.* **1999**, *99*, 858-862.

25. Thompson, T.; Dennis, M.; Higgins, L.A.; Lee, A.R.; Sharrett, M.K.Gluten-free diet survey: are Americans with coeliac disease consuming recommended amounts of fibre, iron, calcium and grain foods? *J. Hum. Nutr. Diet.* **2005**, *18*, 163-9.
26. Annibale, B.; Severi, C.; Chistolini, A.; Antonelli, G.; Lahner, E. *et al.*. Efficacy of gluten-free diet alone on recovery from iron deficiency anemia in adult celiac patients. *Am. J. Gastroenterol.* **2001**, *96*, 132-7.
27. Barton, S.H.; Kelly, D.G.; Murray J.A.. Nutritional deficiencies in celiac disease, *Gastroenterol. Clin. North Am.* **2007**, *36*, 93-108
28. See, J.; Murray, J.A. Gluten-free diet: The medical and nutrition management of celiac disease, *Nutr. Clin. Pract.* **2006**, *21*, 1-15.
29. Halfdanarson, T.R.; Litzow, M.R.; Murray, J.A. Hematological manifestations of celiac disease, *Blood* **2006**, *109*, 412-421.
30. Jameson, S. Coeliac disease, insulin-like growth factor, bonemineral density, and zinc. *Scand. J. Gastroenterol.* **2000**, *35*, 894-896.
31. Mautalen, D.; Gonzalez, R.; Mazure, H.; Vazquez, M.P.; Lorenzetti, E.; Maurino, S.; Niveloni, S.; Pedreira, Smecuol E.; Boerr, L.A.; Bai, J.C. Effect of treatment on bone mass, mineral metabolism, and body composition in untreated celiac disease patients. *Am. J. Gastroenterol.* **1997**, *92*, 313-318.
32. Hallert, C.; Grant, C.; Grehn, S.; Grännö, C.; Hultén, S.; Midhagen, G.; Ström, M.; Svensson, H.; Valdimarsson, T. Evidence of poor vitamin status in coeliac patients on a gluten-free diet for 10 years. *Aliment Pharmacol. Ther.* **2002**, *16*, 1333-9.
33. Farrell, R.J.; Kelly, C.P. Celiac sprue. *N. Engl. J. Med.* **2002**, *346*, 180-188.
34. Scott, E.M.; Gaywood, I.; Scott, B.B. Guidelines for osteoporosis in celiac disease and inflammatory bowel disease: British Society of Gastroenterology. *Gut* **2000**, *46*, 1-8.
35. Rude, R.K.; Olerich, M. Magnesium deficiency: possible role in osteoporosis associated with gluten-sensitive enteropathy. *Osteoporos Int.* **1996**, *6*, 453-61.
36. Halfdanarson, T.R.; Litzow, M.R.; Murray J.A. Hematological manifestations of celiac disease. *Blood* **2006**, *109*, 412-421.
37. Tikkakoski, S.; Savilahti, E.; Kolho, K.L. Undiagnosed celiac disease and nutritional deficiencies in adults screened in primary health care. *Scand. J. Gastroenterol.* **2007**, *42*, 60-65.
38. Dahele, B.; Ghosh, S. Vitamin B12 deficiency in untreated celiac disease. *Am. J. Gastroenterol.* **2001**, *96*, 745-750.
39. Bode, M.; Gudmand-Hoyer E. Symptoms and haematologic features in consecutive adult celiac patients. *Scand. J. Gastroenterol.* **1996**, *31*, 54-60.
40. Ojetti, V.; Nucera, G.; Migneco, A.; Gabrielli, M.; Lauritano, C.; Danese, S.; Zocco, M.A.; Nista, E.C.;Cammarota, G.; De Lorenzo, A.; Gasbarrini, G.; Gasbarrini, A. High prevalence of celiac disease in patients with lactose intolerance. *Digestion* **2005**, *71*, 106-110.
41. Mariani, P.; Viti, M.G.; Montuori, M.; La Vecchia, A.; Cipolletta, E.; Calvani, L.; Bonamico, M. The gluten-free diet: a nutritional risk factor for adolescents with celiac disease? *J. Pediatr. Gastroenterol. Nutr.* **1998**, *27*, 519-23.
42. Polito, C.; Olivieri, A.C.; Marchese, L.; Desiderio, G.; Pullano, F.; Rea, F. Weight overgrowth of coeliac children on gluten-free diet. *Nutr. Res.* **1992**, *12*, 353-8.

43. Rea, F.; Polito, C Marotta; A.; Di Toro, A.; Iovene, A.; Collini, R.; Rea, L.; Sessa, G. Restoration of body composition in celiac children after one year of gluten-free diet. *J. Pediatr. Gastroenterol. Nutr.* **1996**, *23*, 408-12.
44. Caponio, F.; Summo, C.; Clodoveo, M.L.; Pasqualone, A. Evaluation of the nutritional quality of the lipid fraction of gluten-free biscuits. *Euro. Food Res. Technol.* **2008**, *223*, 135-139.
45. Judd, J.T.; Clevidence, B.A.; Muesing, R.A.; Wittes, J.; Sunkin, M.E.; Podczasy, J.J. Dietary trans fatty acids: effects on plasma lipids and lipoproteins of healthy men and women. *Am. J. Clin. Nutr.* **1994**, *59*, 861-8.
46. Lissner, L.; Heitmann, B.L. Dietary fat and obesity: evidence from epidemiology. *EJCN* **1995**, *49*, 79-90.
47. Ellis, H.J.; Doyle, A.P; Day, P.; Wieser, H.; Ciclitira, P.J. Demonstration of the presence of coeliac-activating gliadin-like epitopes in malted barley. *Int. Arch. Allergy Immunol.* **1994**, *104*, 308-10.
48. Thompson, T. Oats and the gluten-free diet. *J. Am. Diet. Assoc.* **2003**, *103*, 376-9.
49. Lohiniemi, S., Collin, P., Mäki, M., Eds.; *Changing features of celiac disease*; The Finnish Coeliac Society: Tampere, Finland, 1988.
50. Haboubi, N.Y., Taylor, S.; Jones, S. Coeliac disease and oats: a systematic review. *Postgrad. Med. J.* **2006**, *82*, 672-678.
51. Størsrud, S.; Olsson, M.; Arvidsson, R.; Lenner, L.; Nilsson, Å.; Nilsson, O.; Kilander, A. Adult celiac patients do tolerate large amounts of oats. *Eur. J. Clin. Nutr.* **2003**, *57*, 163-169.
52. Janatuinen, E.K.; Kemppainen, T.A.; Julkunen, R.J.K.; Kosma, V-M.; Mäki, M.; Heikkinen, M.; Uusitupa, M.I.J. No harm from five year ingestion of oats in coeliac disease. *Gut* **2002**, *50*, 332-335
53. Kemppainen, T.; Janatuinen, E.; Holm, K.; Kosma, V.M.; Heikkinen, M.; Mäki, M.; Laurila, K.; Uusitupa, M.; Julkunen, R. No observed local immunological response at cell level after five years of oats in adults coeliac disease. *Scand. J. Gastroenterol.* **2007**, *42*, 54-59
54. Lee, A.R.; Ng, D.L.; Dave, E.; Ciaccio, E.J.; Green, P.H. The effect of substituting alternative grains in the diet on the nutritional profile of the gluten-free diet. *J. Hum. Nutr. Diet.* **2009**, *22*, 359-63.
55. Størsrud, S.; Hulthen, L.R.; Lenner, R. Beneficial effects of oats in the gluten-free diet of adults with special reference to nutrient status, symptoms and subjective experiences. *Brit. J. Nutr.* **2003**, *90*, 101-107.
56. Kemppainen, T.; Heikkinen, M.T.; Ristikankare, M.K.; Kosma, V-M.; Julkunen, R.J. Nutrient intakes during diets including unkilned and large amounts of oats in celiac disease. *Eur. J. Clin. Nutr.* **2009**, *10*, 113
57. Lee, A.R.; Ng, D.L.; Dave, E.; Ciaccio, E.J.; Gree, P.H.R. The effect of substituting alternative grains in the diet on the nutritional profile of the gluten-free diet. *J. Hum. Nutr. Diet.* **2009**, *22*, 359-363
58. Thompson, T. Gluten contamination of commercial oat products in the United States. *N. Engl. J. Med.* **2004**, *351*, 2021-2.
59. Gambus, H.; Gambus, F.; Sabat, R. The research on quality improvement of gluten-free bread by amaranthus flour addition. *Zywnosc* **2002**, *9*, 9-112.

60. Schoenlechner, R., Berghofer, E. Investigation of the processing aspects of the pseudocereals amaranth and quinoa. In *Proceedings of the International Association of Cereal Chemists Conference* Montreal, Canada, October **2002**; pp. 73-79.
61. Gallagher, E.; Gormley, T.R.; Arendt, E.K. Recent advances in the formulation of gluten-free cereal-based products. *Food Sci. Technol.* **2004**, *15*, 143-52.
62. Collin, P.; Thorell, L.; Kaukinen, K.; Mäki, M. The safe threshold for gluten contamination in gluten-free products. Can trace amounts be accepted in the treatment of coeliac disease? *Aliment. Pharmacol. Ther.* **2004**, *19*, 1277-83.
63. Hischenhuber, C.; Crevel, R.; Jarry, B.; Mäki, M.; Moneret-Vautrin, D.A.; Romano, A.; Troncone, R.; Ward, R. Review article: safe amounts of gluten for patients with wheat allergy or coeliac disease. *Aliment. Pharmacol. Ther.* **2006**, *23*, 559-75.
64. Catassi, C.; Fabiani. E.; Iacono, G.; D'Agate, C.; Francavilla, R.; *et al.*. A prospective, double-blind, placebo-controlled trial to establish a safe gluten threshold for patients with celiac disease. *Am. J. Clin. Nutr.* **2007**, *85*, 160-6.
65. Codex Alimentarius Commission. *Draft revised codex standard for foods for special dietary use for persons intolerant to gluten Joint FAO/WHO Food Standards Programme*; WHO: Geneva, Switzerland, 2007.
66. Krauss, M.R.; Eckel, R.H.; Howard, B.; Appel, J.L.; Daniels, S.R.; Deckelbaum, R.J.; Erdman, J.W.; Kris-Etherton, P.; Goldberg, I.R. AHA Scientific Statement: AHA Dietary Guidelines Revision 2000: A Statement for Healthcare Professionals From the Nutrition Committee of the American Heart Association. *J. Nutr.* **2001**, *131*, 132-146.
67. Gabrovská, D.; Fiedlerová, V.; Holasová, M.; Masková, E.; Smrcinov, H.; Rysová, J.; Winterová, R.; Michalová, A.; Hutar, M. The nutritional evaluation of underutilized cereals and buckwheat. *Food Nutr. Bull.* **2002**, *23*, 246-9.
68. Ötles, S.; Cagindi, Ö. Cereal based functional foods and nutraceuticals. *Acta Sci. Pol. Technol. Aliment* **2006**, *5*, 107-112.
69. Gutzma´n-Maldonado, S.H.; Paredes-Lopez, O. Functional products of plants indigenous to Latin America: amaranth, quinoa, common beans, and botanicals. In *Functional Foods. Biochemical & Processing Aspects*; Mazza, G, Ed.; Technomic Publishing Press: Lancaster, UK, 1999; pp. 293-328.
70. Kim, S.L.; Kim, S.K.; Park, C.O. Introduction and nutritional evaluation of buckwheat sprouts as a new vegetable. *Food Res. Int.* **2004**, *37*, 319-327.
71. Yánez, E.; Zacarías, I.; Granger, D.; Vásquez, M.; Estévez, A.M. Chemical and nutritional characterization of amaranthus (Amaranthus cruentus)] *Arch. Latinoam. Nutr.* **1994**, *44*, 57-62.
72. Coulter, L.; Lorenz, K. Quinoa –composition, nutritional value, food applications. *Lebensm WissTechnol.* **1990**, *23*, 203-207.
73. Anderson, J.W.; Baird, P.; Davis, R.H.; Ferreri, Jr., S.; Knudtson, M.; Koraym, A.; Waters, V.; Williams, C.L. Health benefits of dietary fiber. *Nutr. Rev.* **2009**, *67*, 188-205.
74. Gorinstein, S.; Pawelzik, E.; Delgado-Licon, E.; Haruenkit, R.; Weisz M.; Trakhtenberg, S. Characterization of pseudocereal and cereal proteins by protein and amino acid analyses. *J. Sci. Food Agr.* **2002**, *82*, 886-891

75. Abdel-Aal, E.S.M.; Hucl, P. Amino acid composition and in vitro protein digestibility of selected ancient wheats and their end products. *J. Food Comp. Anal.* **2002**, *15*, 737-747.
76. Temple, N.J. Dietary fats and coronary heart disease. *Biomed. Pharmacother.* **1996**, *50*, 261-8.
77. Adeyeye, A.; Ajewole, K. Chemical composition and fatty acid profiles of cereals in Nigeria. *Food Chem.* **1992**, *44*, 41-44.
78. Mozaffarian, D. "Does α-linolenic acid intake reduce the risk of coronary heart disease? A review of the evidence". *Altern. Ther. Health Med.* **2005**, *11*, 24-30.
79. Yao, L.H.; Jiang, Y.M.; Shi, J.; Tomás-Barberán, F.A.; Datta, N.; Singanusong, R.; Chen, S.S. Flavonoids in food and their health benefits. *Plant Foods Hum. Nutr.* **2004**, *59*, 113-22.
80. Stevenson, D.E.; Hurst, R.D.Polyphenolic phytochemicals--just antioxidants or much more? *Cell Mol. Life Sci.* **2007**, *64*, 2900-16.
81. Dyner, L.; Drago, S.R.; Piñeiro, A.; Sánchez, H.; González, R.; Villaamil, E.; Valencia, M.E. Composition and potential contribution of iron, calcium and zinc of bread and pasta made with wheat and amaranth flours. *Arch. Latinoam Nutr.* **2007**, *57*, 69-77.
82. Sadiq Butt, M.; Tahir-Nadeem, M.; Khan, M.K.; Shabir, R.; Butt, M.S. Oat: unique among the cereals. *Eur. J. Nutr.* **2008**, *47*, 68-79.
83. Fabjan, N.; Rode, J.; Košir, I.J.; Wang, Z.; Zhang, Z.; Kreft, I. Tartary buckwheat (Fagopyrum tataricum Gaertn.) as a source of dietary rutin and quercetin. *J. Agric. Food Chem.* **2003**, *51*, 6452-6455.
84. Jones, J.M. Grain-based foods and health. *Cereals Foods World* **2006**, *51*, 108.
85. Zielin´ski, H.; Kozlowska, H. Antioxidant activity and total phenolics in selected cereal grains and their different morphological fractions. *J. Agric. Food Chem.* **2000**, *48*, 2008-2016.
86. Paśkoa, P.; Bartońa, H.; Zagrodzkia, P.; Gorinstein, S.; Fołta, M.; Zachwieja, Z. Anthocyanins, total polyphenols and antioxidant activity in amaranth and quinoa seeds and sprouts during their growth. *Food Chem.* **2009**, *115*, 994-998.
87. Gorinstein, S.; Vargas, O.J.M.; Jaramillo, N.O.; Salas, I.A.; Ayala, A.L.M.; Arancibia-Avila, P.; Toledo, F.; Katrich E.; Trakhtenberg, S. The total polyphenols and the antioxidant potentials of some selected cereals and pseudocereals. *Eur. Food Res. Technol.* **2007**, *225*, 321-328.
88. Abdel-Aal, el-S.M.; Young, J.C.; Rabalski, I. Anthocyanin composition in black, blue, pink, purple, and red cereal grains. *J. Agric. Food Chem.* **2006**, *54*, 4696-704.
89. Siebenhandl, S.; Grausgruber, H.; Pellegrini, N.; Del Rio, D.; Fogliano, V.; Pernice, R.; Berghofer, E. Phytochemical profile of main antioxidants in different fractions of purple and blue wheat, and black barley. *J. Agric. Food Chem.* **2007**, *55*, 8541-7.
90. Zduńczyk, Z.; Flis, M.; Zieliński, H.; Wróblewska, M.; Antoszkiewicz, Z.; Juśkiewicz, J. In vitro antioxidant activities of barley, husked oat, naked oat, triticale, and buckwheat wastes and their influence on the growth and biomarkers of antioxidant status in rats. *J. Agric. Food Chem.* **2006**, *54*, 4168-75.

91. Peraaho, M.; Kaukinen, K.; Mustalahti, K.; Vuolteenaho, N.; Maki, M.; Laippala, P.; Collin, P. Effect of an oats containing gluten-free diet on symptoms and quality of life in celiac disease, a randomized study. *Scand. J. Gastroenterol.* **2004,** *39*, 27-31.

92. Stevens, L.; Rashid, M. Gluten-free and regular foods: a cost comparison. *Can. J. Diet. Pract. Res.* **2008**, *69*, 147-50.

11

Lectin Staining Shows No Evidence of Involvement of Glycocalyx/Mucous Layer Carbohydrate Structures in Development of Celiac Disease

Henrik Toft-Hansen [1,2,*], Christian Nielsen [2], Matteo Biagini [3], Steffen Husby [1] and Søren T. Lillevang [2]

[1] Hans Christian Andersen Children's Hospital, Odense University Hospital, Sdr. Boulevard 29, Odense 5000, Denmark; E-Mail: steffen.husby@rsyd.dk

[2] Department of Clinical Immunology, Odense University Hospital, Sdr. Boulevard 29, Odense 5000, Denmark; E-Mails: christian.nielsen@rsyd.dk (C.N.); soren.lillevang@rsyd.dk (S.T.L.)

[3] Department of Pathology, Odense University Hospital, J.B. Winsløws Vej 15, 2., Odense 5000, Denmark; E-Mail: matteo.biagini@rsyd.dk

* Author to whom correspondence should be addressed; E-Mail: htoft-hansen@health.sdu.dk;

Abstract: The presence of unique carbohydrate structures in the glycocalyx/mucous layer of the intestine may be involved in a susceptibility to celiac disease (CD) by serving as attachment sites for bacteria. This host-microbiota interaction may influence the development of CD and possibly other diseases with autoimmune components. We examined duodenal biopsies from a total of 30 children, of which 10 had both celiac disease (CD) and type 1 diabetes (T1D); 10 had CD alone; and 10 were suspected of having gastrointestinal disease, but had normal duodenal histology (non-CD controls). Patients with both CD and T1D were examined before and after remission following a gluten-free diet. We performed lectin histochemistry using peanut agglutinin (PNA) and Ulex europaeus agglutinin (UEA) staining for Gal-β(1,3)-GalNAc and Fucα1-2Gal-R, respectively, of the glycocalyx/mucous layer. The staining was scored based on dissemination of stained structures on a scale from 0 to 3. Evaluation of the scores revealed no difference between biopsies obtained before and after remission in the group of children with both CD and T1D. A comparison of this pre-remission group with the children who had CD alone or the non-CD controls also showed no significant differences. Based on our material, we found no indication that the presence of Gal-β(1,3)-GalNAc or Fucα1-2Gal-R is involved in the susceptibility to CD, or that the disease process affects the expression of these carbohydrates.

Keywords: pediatric celiac disease; type 1 diabetes; duodenal biopsies; glycosylation; lectin staining

---

1. Introduction

The role of the adaptive immune system in celiac disease (CD) has been studied in detail over the past few decades, and its association with HLA-DQ2 and DQ8 is well established [1]. Association with other genomic regions has been demonstrated, but the individual impact of each region is small, and, in combination, these regions can only explain about 5% of the total genetic disease susceptibility [2]. Recently, there has been a surge of interest in the possible role of the microbiota in the etiology of CD and a wide range of other diseases, particularly with autoimmune components [3,4].

The glycocalyx/mucous layer covers the gastrointestinal tract, and acts as a semi-permeable barrier between the lumen and the epithelium. Bacteria in the host microbiota may use carbohydrate structures in the glycocalyx/mucous layer as attachment sites [5]. Inherited differences in expression of certain carbohydrates could lead to a predisposition to colonization with particular strains of bacteria, which may influence the susceptibility to CD. Alternatively, the presence of certain bacteria independent of inherited factors could cause an environmental predisposition to CD by altering the expression of carbohydrates. Also, the disease process involving inflammation of the gut mucosa could affect the expression of carbohydrates [6].

Bacteria that are decreased or enriched in the gut of CD patients compared to healthy controls could be important in maintaining gut homeostasis in the healthy individuals or in compromising the epithelial function in CD [7]. It has been shown that rod-shaped bacteria were frequently found in the mucosa of pediatric CD patients with active disease, as well as in another group of pediatric CD patients in remission on a gluten-free diet (GFD), though not in controls with no known food intolerances [8]. Since the rod-shaped bacteria were also present in the children in remission, this indicates that CD patients could be genetically predisposed to colonization with these particular bacteria, perhaps due to the expression of particular carbohydrates.

The prevalence of CD in patients with Type 1 Diabetes (T1D) is estimated to be around 8% compared to around 1% in the general population [9]. CD and T1D share genetic risk factors with a strong association to HLA-DQ2 or DQ8 for both diseases [10]. According to Danish guidelines, all children diagnosed with T1D are screened by serology for the presence of CD-associated antibodies. In contrast to children with CD alone, biopsies are also taken after the implementation of a gluten-free diet in children with both diseases. By studying biopsies obtained from the same children with CD and T1D before and after remission, as well as children with CD alone or no CD at all, we aimed to investigate whether or not the expression of unique carbohydrate structures appeared to be genetically determined or affected by the inflammatory status of the tissue.

2. Materials and Methods

2.1. Study Design

We obtained duodenal biopsies from a total of 30 children. Among this group, 10 had both celiac disease (CD) and type 1 diabetes (T1D) (aged 5–11 years, mean = 8.6); 10 had CD but not T1D (aged 1–14 years, mean = 5.9); and 10 were non-CD controls, verified to have normal duodenal histology (aged 2–17, mean = 7.9), but who could have other gastrointestinal diseases, chiefly gastroesophageal reflux disease. The group with both CD and T1D were examined both before and after remission (2–4 years after first biopsy) following introduction of gluten-free diet (GFD). Biopsies were scored according to the Modified Marsh classification [11] (Table 1).

Table 1. Biopsy Marsh scores for individual patients. Group A consists of patients with both celiac disease (CD) and type 1 diabetes, so each patient has two scores: untreated and after remission (GFD). Group B patients have CD only, and Group C patients do not have CD (normal biopsies), but may have other diseases.

Group A Patient ID	CD + T1D Untreated	CD + T1D GFD	Group B Patient ID	CD	Group C Patient ID	Non-CD
A1	3A	0	B1	2	C1	0
A2	3C	0	B2	3B	C2	0
A3	2	0	B3	3C	C3	0
A4	2	0	B4	3B	C4	0
A5	3B	0	B5	3B	C5	0
A6	3C	0	B6	3C	C6	0
A7	3C	0	B7	3C	C7	0
A8	3A	0	B8	3C	C8	0
A9	3B	0	B9	3C	C9	0
A10	3C	0	B10	3C	C10	0

2.2. Lectin Histochemistry

We performed lectin histochemistry using peanut agglutinin (PNA) and Ulex europaeus agglutinin (UEA) staining carbohydrates in glycolipids or glycoproteins of the glycocalyx/mucous layer. PNA specifically binds the galactose sequence Gal-β(1,3)-GalNAc, and UEA specifically binds the fucose sequence Fucα1-2Gal-R [12]. Briefly, duodenal biopsies were embedded and snap-frozen in liquid nitrogen immediately after gastroscopy. Cryosections were fixed, followed by blocking of endogen biotin with an Avidin Biotin kit (DAKO, Glostrup, Denmark) and then incubated with biotinylated lectin, rinsed, and followed by incubation with horse radish peroxidase (HRP)-conjugated streptavidin (DAKO). Bound lectins were visualized using the HRP substrate carbazol.

The staining was scored based on dissemination of stained structures in the epithelial cell layer on a scale from 0 to 3, where 0 represents no staining of the epithelial cell layer, 1 represents staining in the cytoplasm of epithelial cells, 2 represents staining of cytoplasm and glycocalyx, and 3 represents staining of cytoplasm and glycocalyx, in addition to villus goblet cells. The observed staining pattern was hierarchical as described. Staining of crypt goblet cells was not considered in the analysis. Intensity of staining was not included in the score.

2.3. Ethics

The study was approved by the Regional Committee for Biomedial Research (VF-20050134) and by the Danish Data Protection Agency (DOK 2709660991).

2.4. Statistical Methods

Statistical analysis was performed with non-parametrical tests using the GraphPad Prism software [13]. A statistical significance limit of $p < 0.05$ was chosen.

3. Results

PNA staining patterns are illustrated in Figure 1 with examples of staining in samples from a CD patient (Figure 1a), a CD + T1D patient untreated and treated with a GFD (Figure 1b,c, respectively), and finally a non-CD patient (Figure 1d). Some degree of PNA staining was evident in all samples in all groups (Table 2) with a score of 1 as the lowest (Figure 1a), where only cytoplasmic was observed. Figure 1b,c show PNA staining of biopsies obtained from the same patient (A7) with both CD and T1D before and after treatment with GFD. In the case of patient A7, the score went up from 2 in the untreated state to 3 after treatment, but this was not a consistent trend for this group of patients as a whole. A score of 2 (Figure 1b) includes staining of the brush border as well as cytoplasm, and a score of 3 (Figure 1c,d) indicates additional staining in some, but not necessarily all villus goblet cells. The PNA staining in goblet cells appeared localized to spots inside the cells.

Figure 1. Peanut agglutinin (PNA) staining. (**a**) Patient B3 (CD, untreated), score 1; (**b**) Patient A7 (CD+T1D, untreated), score 2; (**c**) Patient A7 (CD + T1D, on GFD), score 3; (**d**) Patient C2 (non-CD), score 3. Thin arrows mark staining of cytoplasm of epithelial cells. Thick arrows mark staining of glycocalyx. Arrowheads mark staining in goblet cells.

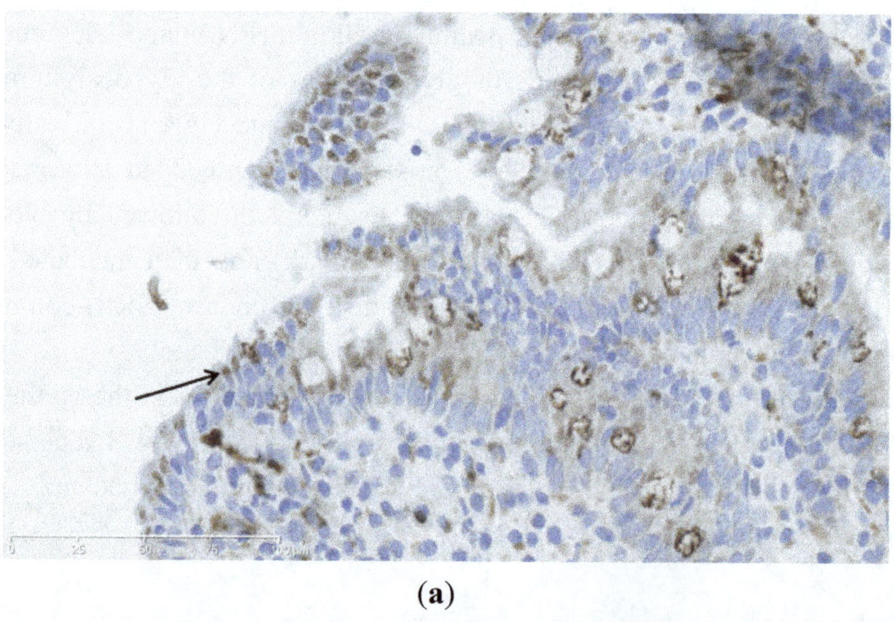

(**a**)

Figure 1. *Cont.*

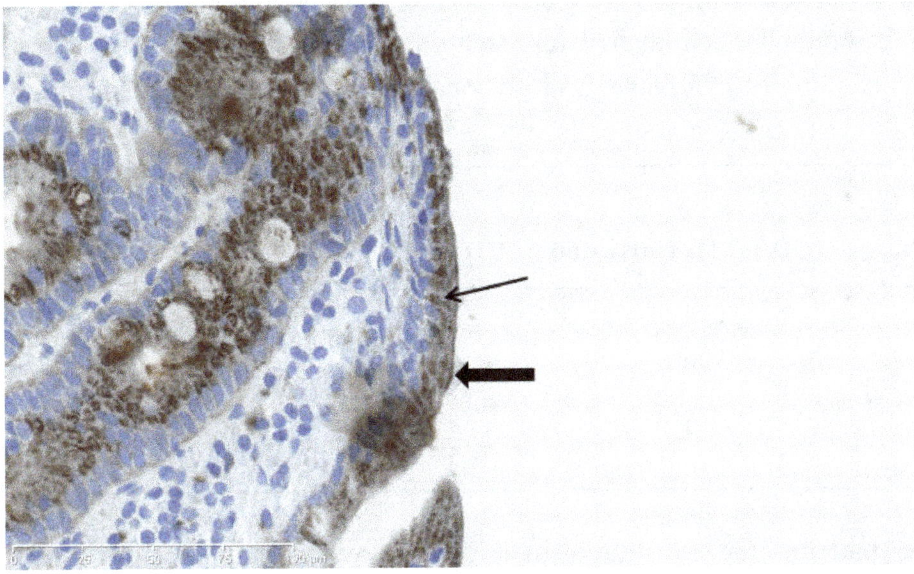

(b)

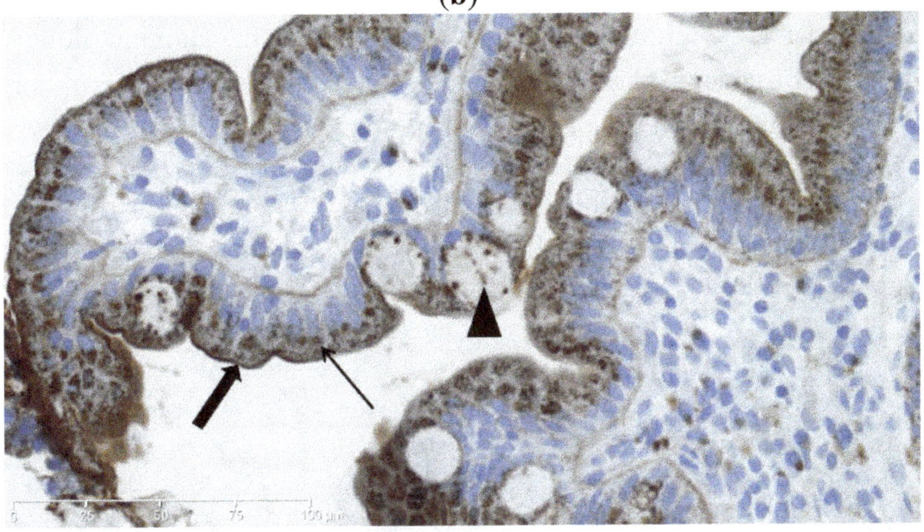

(c)

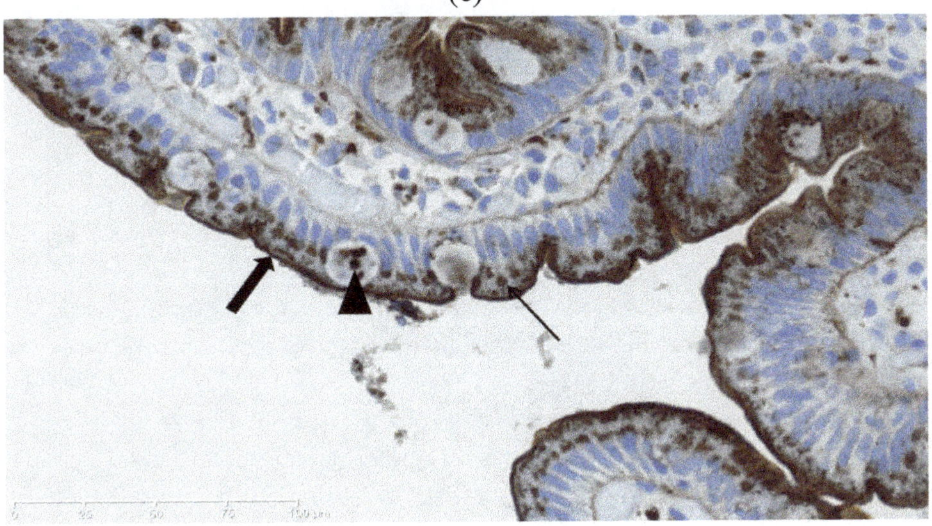

(d)

Table 2. Peanut agglutinin staining scores. Stained sections of biopsies from patients in Groups A (before and after remission), B, and C were scored as follows: 0 represents no staining of the epithelial cell layer, 1 represents staining in the cytoplasm of epithelial cells, 2 represents staining of cytoplasm and glycocalyx, and 3 represents staining of cytoplasm and glycocalyx, as well as goblet cells.

Group / Score	A CD + T1D Untreated	A CD + T1D GFD	B CD	C Non-CD
3	0	2	0	2
2	5	4	1	0
1	5	4	9	8
0	0	0	0	0
Median score	1.5	2	1	1

UEA staining patterns are illustrated in Figure 2 with samples from a non-CD patient, a CD + T1D patient before and after treatment with GFD, and a CD patient. UEA staining was observed in all patients except one: C4 (Figure 2a). A score of 1 (cytoplasmic staining alone) was not given to any samples (Table 3). In general, the UEA staining appeared more intense in comparison to PNA staining. This was especially evident in goblet cells (Figure 2b,d).

Figure 2. Ulex europaeus agglutinin (UEA) staining. (**a**) Patient C4 (non-CD), score 0; (**b**) Patient A1 (CD + T1D, untreated), score 3; (**c**) Patient A1 (CD + T1D, on GFD), score 2; (**d**) Patient B5 (CD), score 3. Thin arrows mark staining of cytoplasm of epithelial cells. Thick arrows mark staining of glycocalyx. Arrowheads mark staining in goblet cells.

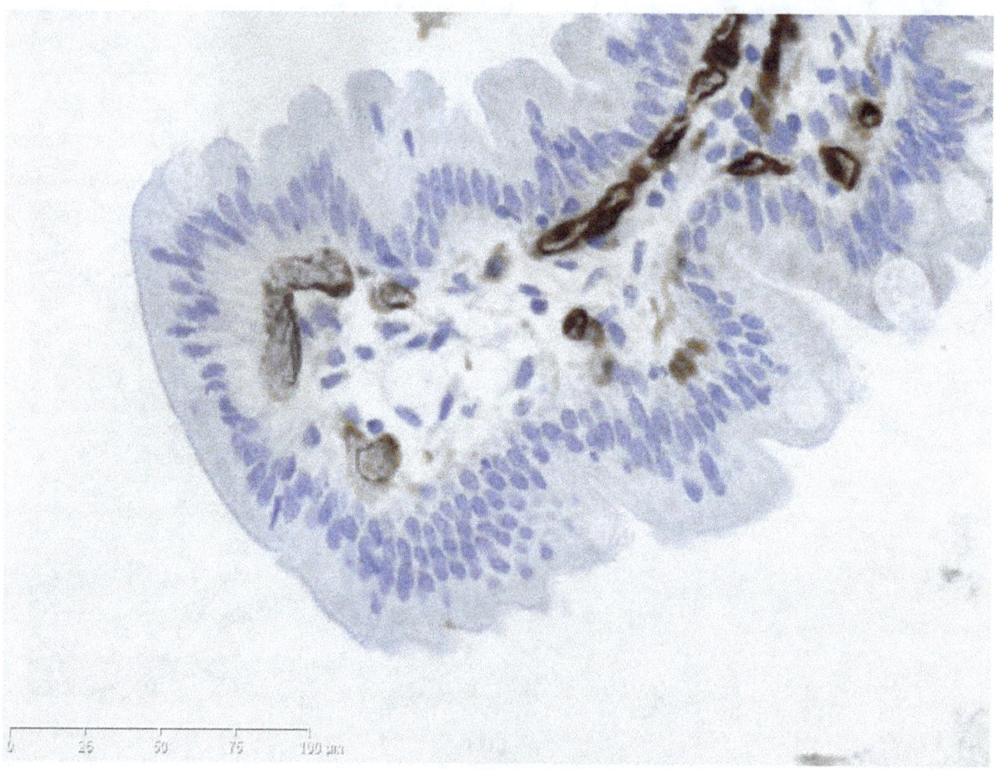

(**a**)

Figure 2. *Cont.*

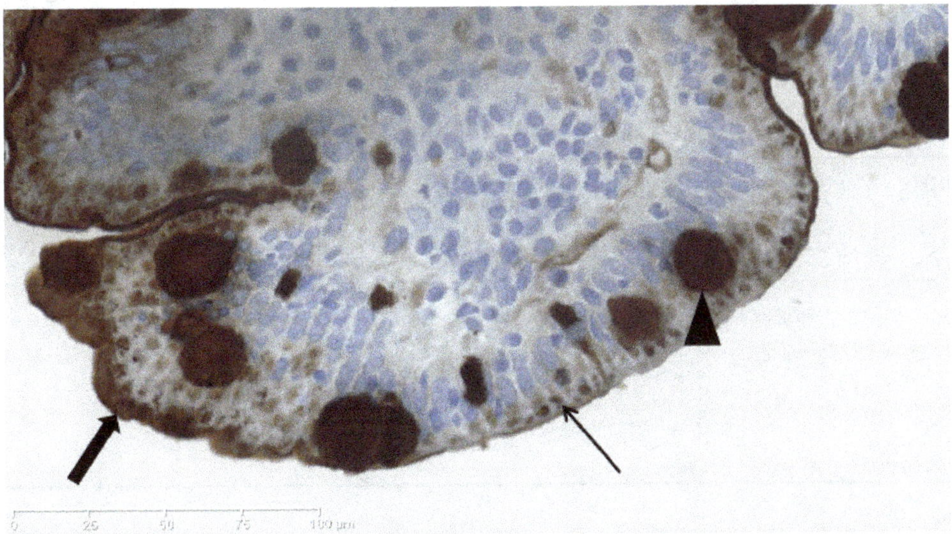

(**b**)

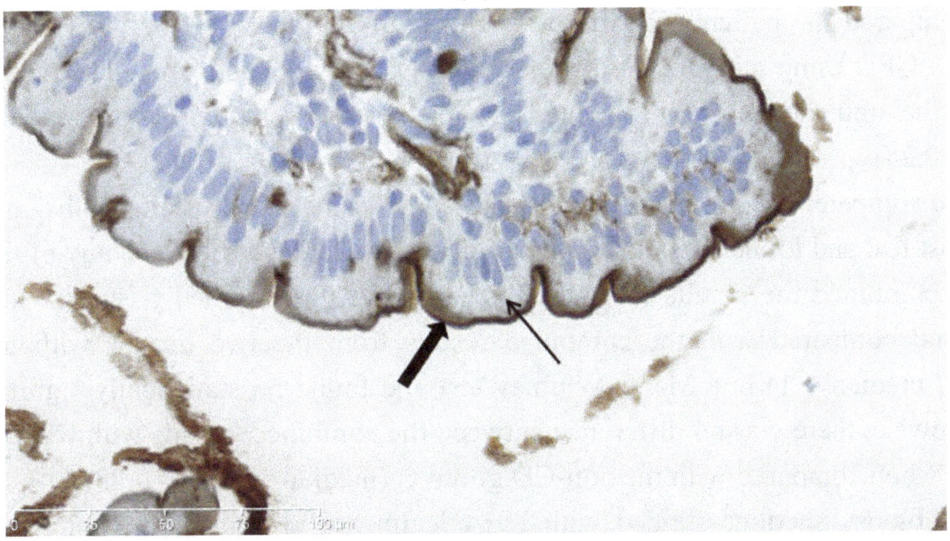

(**c**)

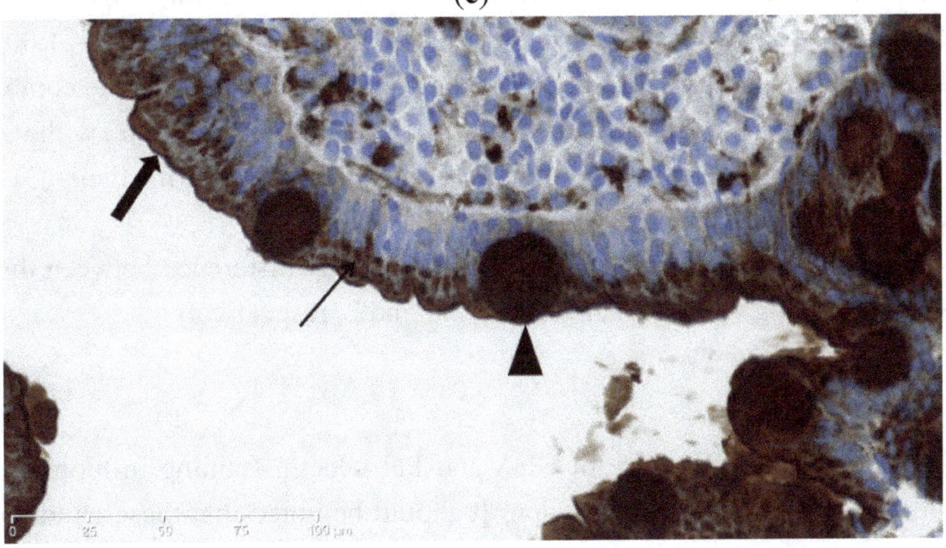

(**d**)

Table 3. Ulex europaeus agglutinin lectin staining scores. Stained sections of biopsies from patients in Groups A (before and after remission), B, and C were scored as follows: 0 represents no staining of the epithelial cell layer, 1 represents staining in the cytoplasm of epithelial cells; 2 represents staining of cytoplasm and glycocalyx; and 3 represents staining of cytoplasm and glycocalyx, as well as goblet cells.

Group / Score	A CD + T1D Untreated	A CD + T1D GFD	B CD	C Non-CD
3	5	4	10	5
2	5	6	0	4
1	0	0	0	0
0	0	0	0	1
Median score	2.5	2	3	2.5

Scores from biopsy sections stained with PNA lectin are presented in Table 2. We performed three sets of statistical analysis to test if the scores reflected differences between the groups.

First, we compared the patients in Group A with both CD and T1D before (untreated) and after treatment with a GFD using the Wilcoxon signed-rank test for matched pairs. The median scores were 1.5 and 2 for the untreated and GFD-treated groups, respectively, with no statistically significant difference ($p = 0.25$).

Secondly, we compared the groups A untreated, B and C using the Kruskal–Wallis one-way ANOVA with Dunn's post test and found no statistically significant differences between any of the groups.

Finally, we combined the results from the two groups with inflamed tissue (A untreated and B, median = 1) and compared with the combined results from the two groups without inflammation (A GFD and C, median = 1) in a Mann–Whitney test and found no statistically significant difference ($p = 0.38$). Likewise, there was no difference between the combined groups with CD (A untreated and B, median = 1) when compared with the non-CD group C (median = 1) ($p = 0.88$).

Scores from biopsy sections stained with UEA lectin are presented in Table 3. We performed statistical analyses analogous to the statistical tests described above for PNA lectin, and found no difference in the comparison between Group A untreated and GFD-treated ($p = 1.00$), no difference between any of the groups A untreated, B and C, and also no difference when the combined group with inflammation (median = 3) was compared with the combined group without inflammation (median = 2) ($p = 0.09$), or when the combined groups of CD patients (median = 3) were compared with the non-CD group C (median = 2.5) ($p = 0.23$).

Combining the results in Tables 2 and 3 did not indicate any difference between the four groups in combined PNA/UEA staining with medians of 2, 2, 2.5 and 2, respectively.

4. Discussion

In our study, we found no difference in UEA and PNA lectin staining in biopsies from the same pediatric CD patients before and after remission. It should be noted that these children also had T1D, another autoimmune disease whereby the composition of commensals in the gastrointestinal tract could be of pathogenic importance [14]. Likewise, we found no difference when biopsies showing CD-associated inflammation were compared to biopsies with normal histology.

Earlier work has shown somewhat conflicting results regarding the reactivity of PNA in CD biopsies. PNA has been reported to not show any reactivity at all in patients or controls [15], to be upregulated in goblet cells of CD patients compared to controls [16], or downregulated in the glycocalyx of CD patients in a study where no reactivity in goblet cells was noted [8]. There is more agreement with regards to UEA reactivity, which was shown to be upregulated in goblet cells of CD patients in two of these studies [8,15]. Some methodological differences between these studies and our own could in part explain the discrepancies: whether it is children or adults being studied, the origin of the biopsy (jejunum as opposed to duodenum), and the specific structures included in the analysis (e.g., crypt goblet cells *versus* villus goblet cells).

It has been well described that the bacterial microbiota is important for the function of the mucosal immune system, and proper development of gut-associated lymphoid tissue is dependent on bacterial presence and influenced by the composition of the microbiota [17–19]. Colonization of germ-free mice with *Bacteroides* modulated the expression of numerousl genes involved in diverse intestinal functions including maintenance of intestinal permeability [20]. In rats, it was shown that the composition of the commensal microbiota can modulate intestinal permeability with certain bacterial strains increasing permeability, and other (probiotic) strains reducing permeability [21]. Colonization with such probiotic strains of bacteria could potentially reduce intestinal inflammation [22], and be beneficial in the context of celiac disease, whereas colonization with other strains could be detrimental.

Characterization of the bacterial population in the human gastrointestinal tract is currently intensely investigated [23], and it remains an important issue to define how the composition of the commensal microbiota is determined. It is clear that the exposure to diverse bacterial strains in different environments plays an important role, but a genetic predisposition to colonization with particular bacterial strains is also likely to influence the composition of the microbiota [24,25]. Such a genetic component could be the result of inherited differences in the expression pattern of unique carbohydrate structures in the glycocalyx/mucous layer. This could influence bacterial composition if bacteria can utilize carbohydrates for colonization, as was proposed for *Bacteroides* using glycans [26]. Recently, it was found that the genetically determined AB0 blood group system can modulate the composition of the human intestinal microbiota [27]. Furthermore, the secretor status encoded by the FUT2 gene, which defines the expression of the AB0 blood group antigens in the mucus, is associated with the composition of intestinal bifidobacteria [28]. If the AB0 antigens are present in the mucosal layer, they could facilitate bacterial colonization by acting as attachment sites or carbon sources. In a Finnish study, it was found that 14.7% of a healthy control population was homozygous for a nonsense mutation in the FUT2 gene leading to non-secretor status [29]. The non-secretor status was positively associated with CD susceptibility, and the frequency of non-secretors was increased to 18% in the CD population.

It appears likely that the composition of the intestinal microbiota is associated with the development of CD [30], either through a genetic predisposition, environmental influence, or infection with pathogens [31]. Several studies point to differences in the microbiota between CD patients with active disease, CD patients in remission, and normal controls [32–34]. Moreover, animal models have demonstrated how gluten-induced enteropathy can be modulated by the bacterial microbiota [35,36]. The presence of rod-shaped bacteria in intestinal mucosa was shown to be frequently associated with pediatric CD patients regardless of disease status (patients with active disease, compared to another group of patients in remission), but not with controls [8]. This was linked with differences in lectin staining of biopsies from the three groups in the study with UEA staining being more intense and widespread in CD patients (active CD or treated) compared to controls, and PNA staining being less widespread and intense in both groups of CD patients compared to controls. These findings could be explained by either a genetic predisposition to express certain carbohydrates in people who develop CD, or by the effect that the components of the microbiota, such as the rod-shaped bacteria associated with CD patients, could have on glycosylation.

Although not evident in our study, there is indication that inflammatory processes can alter the expression of carbohydrates in the gut. A characterization of the human MUC2 mucin in colon revealed a complex glycosylation pattern in healthy individuals [37]. This pattern was altered with a shift towards smaller and less complex glycans in patients with active ulcerative colitis [38]. Interestingly, this effect was reversed after remission of disease, arguing against a genetic reason for the shift.

With respect to CD in future studies, it would be relevant to investigate other differences in mucus glycosylation that are not detected by UEA or PNA staining. Also, potential differences in other modifications, such as sulfation, could be relevant in CD [39]. Our limited study supports the notion that glycosylation is independent of disease activity as previously shown by Forsberg and colleagues [8]. In contrast to that study, however, we could not demonstrate a difference in lectin staining between CD patients, either with or without T1D or combined, when compared to non-CD controls.

5. Conclusions

In our study, we did not identify any differences in the staining pattern of the lectins PNA or UEA in duodenal biopsies between samples obtained before and after remission in the same children with both CD and T1D. Also, we did not observe any differences in lectin staining between children with both CD and T1D, children with CD alone, or non-CD controls. In conclusion, we found no indication that the presence of unique carbohydrate structures bound by PNA or UEA is involved in the susceptibility to CD, or that the inflammation caused by the disease affects the glycosylation process.

Acknowledgments

The authors would like to thank laboratory technician Mette Hviid and the staff of the Department of Pathology, Odense University Hospital for their valuable assistance. Financial support for this study was provided by The Danish Council for Strategic Research, Programme Commission on Health, Food and Welfare, and The Novo Nordisk Research Foundation.

References

1. Abadie, V.; Sollid, L.M.; Barreiro, L.B.; Jabri, B. Integration of genetic and immunological insights into a model of celiac disease pathogenesis. *Annu. Rev. Immunol.* **2011**, *29*, 493–525.

2. Dubois, P.C.; Trynka, G.; Franke, L.; Hunt, K.A.; Romanos, J.; Curtotti, A.; Zhernakova, A.; Heap, G.A.; Adany, R.; Aromaa, A.; *et al.* Multiple common variants for celiac disease influencing immune gene expression. *Nat. Genet.* **2010**, *42*, 295–302.
3. Kverka, M.; Tlaskalova-Hogenova, H. Two faces of microbiota in inflammatory and autoimmune diseases: Triggers and drugs. *Acta Pathol. Microbiol. Immunol. Scand.* **2013**, *121*, 403–421.
4. Le Chatelier, E.; Nielsen, T.; Qin, J.; Prifti, E.; Hildebrand, F.; Falony, G.; Almeida, M.; Arumugam, M.; Batto, J.M.; Kennedy, S.; *et al.* Richness of human gut microbiome correlates with metabolic markers. *Nature* **2013**, *500*, 541–546.
5. Robbe, C.; Capon, C.; Coddeville, B.; Michalski, J.C. Structural diversity and specific distribution of o-glycans in normal human mucins along the intestinal tract. *Biochem. J.* **2004**, *384*, 307–316.
6. Brinck, U.; Korabiowska, M.; Bosbach, R.; Gabius, H.J. Detection of inflammation- and neoplasia-associated alterations in human large intestine using plant/invertebrate lectins, galectin-1 and neoglycoproteins. *Acta Anat.* **1998**, *161*, 219–233.
7. Cheng, J.; Kalliomaki, M.; Heilig, H.G.; Palva, A.; Lahteenoja, H.; de Vos, W.M.; Salojarvi, J.; Satokari, R. Duodenal microbiota composition and mucosal homeostasis in pediatric celiac disease. *BMC Gastroenterol.* **2013**, *13*, 113.
8. Forsberg, G.; Fahlgren, A.; Horstedt, P.; Hammarstrom, S.; Hernell, O.; Hammarstrom, M.L. Presence of bacteria and innate immunity of intestinal epithelium in childhood celiac disease. *Am. J. Gastroenterol.* **2004**, *99*, 894–904.
9. Volta, U.; Tovoli, F.; Caio, G. Clinical and immunological features of celiac disease in patients with type 1 diabetes mellitus. *Expert Rev. Gastroenterol. Hepatol.* **2011**, *5*, 479–487.
10. Camarca, M.E.; Mozzillo, E.; Nugnes, R.; Zito, E.; Falco, M.; Fattorusso, V.; Mobilia, S.; Buono, P.; Valerio, G.; Troncone, R.; *et al.* Celiac disease in type 1 diabetes mellitus. *Ital. J. Pediatr.* **2012**, *38*, 10.
11. Antonioli, D.A. Celiac disease: A progress report. *Mod. Pathol.* **2003**, *16*, 342–346.
12. Roth, Z.; Yehezkel, G.; Khalaila, I. Identification and quantification of protein glycosylation. *Int. J. Carbohydr. Chem.* **2012**, *2012*, doi:10.1155/2012/640923.
13. *GraphPad Prism*, version 4.03 for Windows; GraphPad Software: San Diego, CA, USA, 2005.
14. Herold, K.C.; Vignali, D.A.; Cooke, A.; Bluestone, J.A. Type 1 diabetes: Translating mechanistic observations into effective clinical outcomes. *Nat. Rev. Immunol.* **2013**, *13*, 243–256.
15. Vecchi, M.; Torgano, G.; de Franchis, R.; Tronconi, S.; Agape, D.; Ronchi, G. Evidence of altered structural and secretory glycoconjugates in the jejunal mucosa of patients with gluten sensitive enteropathy and subtotal villous atrophy. *Gut* **1989**, *30*, 804–810.
16. Barresi, G.; Tuccari, G.; Tedeschi, A.; Magazzu, G. Lectin binding sites in duodeno-jejunal mucosae from coeliac children. *Histochemistry* **1988**, *88*, 105–112.
17. Gronlund, M.M.; Arvilommi, H.; Kero, P.; Lehtonen, O.P.; Isolauri, E. Importance of intestinal colonisation in the maturation of humoral immunity in early infancy: A prospective follow up study of healthy infants aged 0–6 months. *Arch. Dis. Childh. Fetal Neonatal Ed.* **2000**, *83*, F186–F192.
18. Lanning, D.; Sethupathi, P.; Rhee, K.J.; Zhai, S.K.; Knight, K.L. Intestinal microflora and diversification of the rabbit antibody repertoire. *J. Immunol.* **2000**, *165*, 2012–2019.

19. Rhee, K.J.; Sethupathi, P.; Driks, A.; Lanning, D.K.; Knight, K.L. Role of commensal bacteria in development of gut-associated lymphoid tissues and preimmune antibody repertoire. *J. Immunol.* **2004**, *172*, 1118–1124.
20. Hooper, L.V.; Wong, M.H.; Thelin, A.; Hansson, L.; Falk, P.G.; Gordon, J.I. Molecular analysis of commensal host-microbial relationships in the intestine. *Science* **2001**, *291*, 881–884.
21. Garcia-Lafuente, A.; Antolin, M.; Guarner, F.; Crespo, E.; Malagelada, J.R. Modulation of colonic barrier function by the composition of the commensal flora in the rat. *Gut* **2001**, *48*, 503–507.
22. Bai, A.P.; Ouyang, Q.; Zhang, W.; Wang, C.H.; Li, S.F. Probiotics inhibit TNF-α-induced interleukin-8 secretion of HT29 cells. *World J. Gastroenterol.* **2004**, *10*, 455–457.
23. Cox, M.J.; Cookson, W.O.; Moffatt, M.F. Sequencing the human microbiome in health and disease. *Hum. Mol. Genet.* **2013**, doi: 10.1093/hmg/ddt398.
24. Benson, A.K.; Kelly, S.A.; Legge, R.; Ma, F.; Low, S.J.; Kim, J.; Zhang, M.; Oh, P.L.; Nehrenberg, D.; Hua, K.; *et al.* Individuality in gut microbiota composition is a complex polygenic trait shaped by multiple environmental and host genetic factors. *Proc. Natl. Acad. Sci. USA* **2010**, *107*, 18933–18938.
25. McKnite, A.M.; Perez-Munoz, M.E.; Lu, L.; Williams, E.G.; Brewer, S.; Andreux, P.A.; Bastiaansen, J.W.; Wang, X.; Kachman, S.D.; Auwerx, J.; *et al.* Murine gut microbiota is defined by host genetics and modulates variation of metabolic traits. *PLoS One* **2012**, *7*, e39191.
26. Lee, S.M.; Donaldson, G.P.; Mikulski, Z.; Boyajian, S.; Ley, K.; Mazmanian, S.K. Bacterial colonization factors control specificity and stability of the gut microbiota. *Nature* **2013**, *501*, 426–429.
27. Makivuokko, H.; Lahtinen, S.J.; Wacklin, P.; Tuovinen, E.; Tenkanen, H.; Nikkila, J.; Bjorklund, M.; Aranko, K.; Ouwehand, A.C.; Matto, J. Association between the abo blood group and the human intestinal microbiota composition. *BMC Microbiol.* **2012**, *12*, 94.
28. Wacklin, P.; Makivuokko, H.; Alakulppi, N.; Nikkila, J.; Tenkanen, H.; Rabina, J.; Partanen, J.; Aranko, K.; Matto, J. Secretor genotype (FUT2 gene) is strongly associated with the composition of bifidobacteria in the human intestine. *PLoS One* **2011**, *6*, e20113.
29. Parmar, A.S.; Alakulppi, N.; Paavola-Sakki, P.; Kurppa, K.; Halme, L.; Farkkila, M.; Turunen, U.; Lappalainen, M.; Kontula, K.; Kaukinen, K.; *et al.* Association study of FUT2 (rs601338) with celiac disease and inflammatory bowel disease in the finnish population. *Tissue Antigens* **2012**, *80*, 488–493.
30. Sanz, Y.; de Pama, G.; Laparra, M. Unraveling the ties between celiac disease and intestinal microbiota. *Int. Rev. Immunol.* **2011**, *30*, 207–218.
31. Plot, L.; Amital, H. Infectious associations of celiac disease. *Autoimmun. Rev.* **2009**, *8*, 316–319.
32. Collado, M.C.; Donat, E.; Ribes-Koninckx, C.; Calabuig, M.; Sanz, Y. Specific duodenal and faecal bacterial groups associated with paediatric coeliac disease. *J. Clin. Pathol.* **2009**, *62*, 264–269.
33. Di Cagno, R.; de Angelis, M.; de Pasquale, I.; Ndagijimana, M.; Vernocchi, P.; Ricciuti, P.; Gagliardi, F.; Laghi, L.; Crecchio, C.; Guerzoni, M.E.; *et al.* Duodenal and faecal microbiota of celiac children: Molecular, phenotype and metabolome characterization. *BMC Microbiol.* **2011**, *11*, 219.

34. Nistal, E.; Caminero, A.; Herran, A.R.; Arias, L.; Vivas, S.; de Morales, J.M.; Calleja, S.; de Miera, L.E.; Arroyo, P.; Casqueiro, J. Differences of small intestinal bacteria populations in adults and children with/without celiac disease: Effect of age, gluten diet, and disease. *Inflamm. Bowel Dis.* **2012**, *18*, 649–656.
35. Cinova, J.; de Palma, G.; Stepankova, R.; Kofronova, O.; Kverka, M.; Sanz, Y.; Tuckova, L. Role of intestinal bacteria in gliadin-induced changes in intestinal mucosa: Study in germ-free rats. *PLoS One* **2011**, *6*, e16169.
36. D'Arienzo, R.; Stefanile, R.; Maurano, F.; Mazzarella, G.; Ricca, E.; Troncone, R.; Auricchio, S.; Rossi, M. Immunomodulatory effects of *Lactobacillus casei* administration in a mouse model of gliadin-sensitive enteropathy. *Scand. J. Immunol.* **2011**, *74*, 335–341.
37. Larsson, J.M.; Karlsson, H.; Sjovall, H.; Hansson, G.C. A complex, but uniform o-glycosylation of the human MUC2 mucin from colonic biopsies analyzed by nanoLC/MSn. *Glycobiology* **2009**, *19*, 756–766.
38. Larsson, J.M.; Karlsson, H.; Crespo, J.G.; Johansson, M.E.; Eklund, L.; Sjovall, H.; Hansson, G.C. Altered o-glycosylation profile of MUC2 mucin occurs in active ulcerative colitis and is associated with increased inflammation. *Inflamm. Bowel Dis.* **2011**, *17*, 2299–2307.
39. Brockhausen, I. Sulphotransferases acting on mucin-type oligosaccharides. *Biochem. Soc. Transact.* **2003**, *31*, 318–325.

12

Application of Dairy Proteins as Technological and Nutritional Improvers of Calcium-Supplemented Gluten-Free Bread

Urszula Krupa-Kozak [1,*], Natalia Bączek [1,2] and Cristina M. Rosell [2]

[1] Department of Chemistry and Biodynamics of Food, Institute of Animal Reproduction and Food Research of the Polish Academy of Sciences, Tuwima St., 10, Olsztyn 10-748, Poland; E-Mail: n.baczek@pan.olsztyn.pl

[2] Cereal Group, Institute of Agrochemistry and Food Technology (IATA-CSIC), Av Agustin Escardino 7, Paterna, Valencia 46980, Spain; E-Mail: crosell@iata.csic.es

* Author to whom correspondence should be addressed; E-Mail: u.krupa-kozak@pan.olsztyn.pl;

Abstract: Effect of dairy proteins on gluten-free dough behavior, and nutritional and technological properties of gluten-free bread was evaluated. Experimental doughs, containing dairy powders, showed low consistency. Obtained gluten-free breads were rich in proteins, and, regarding the energy value delivered by proteins, they could be considered as a source of proteins or high in proteins. Applied dairy proteins affected the technological properties of experimental breads causing a significant ($p < 0.05$) increase of the specific volume, crust darkening, and crumb lightness, depending on the dairy supplementation level, rather than the protein type. Dairy proteins incorporated at a 12% level, significantly ($p < 0.05$) decreased the hardness; nevertheless, the highest amount of proteins tested led to the opposite effect. These results indicate that milk proteins tested could be successfully added to gluten-free bread with beneficial effects on technological and nutritional properties.

Keywords: dairy proteins; gluten-free bread; dough consistency; technological properties; nutritional value; celiac disease

---

1. Introduction

Celiac disease (CD) is a chronic immune-mediated intestinal disorder that develops in individuals having genetic predispositions with multiple contributing genes. The most important are HLA-DQ2 and HLA-DQ8, however, non-HLA genes also contribute to the development of CD. Approximately 1% of the worldwide population is suffering from CD, and, thus, this disorder is classified as one of the most common food intolerances [1,2]. CD is related to permanent intolerance to gluten, a storage protein found in wheat (gliadin), rye (secalins), barley (hordeins), and, probably, in some oat (avenins) cultivars. A great deal is known on the sequential pathophysiological events driving the intestinal inflammatory cascade [3–5] The immune response in CD involves the adaptive, as well as the innate, and is characterized by the presence of anti-gluten and anti-transglutaminase 2 antibodies, lymphocytic infiltration in the epithelial membrane and the lamina propria, and expression of multiple cytokines and other signaling proteins. The disease leads to inflammation, villous atrophy, and crypt hyperplasia in the small intestine. Mentioned factors can contribute to malabsorption of several nutrients (iron, folic acid, calcium, and fat-soluble vitamins) [6], general malnutrition, and reduced body mass index (BMI) [7]. Currently, strict and life-long adherence to a gluten-free diet (GFD) remains the only effective treatment for CD.

Generally, gluten-free formulas and baked products are poor in proteins [8]. In traditional baking industry proteins derived from plants (proteins of soya) and animal origin (milk proteins and egg albumins) are frequently used [9,10]. Milk proteins are highly functional ingredients characterized by a significant nutritional value. They swell in a high level and are able to build up a network [11,12]. Next to the functional benefits, gluten-free products with milk proteins are affluent in calcium and proteins, and, thus, enriched in essential amino acids like lysine, methionine and tryptophan [13]. Milk proteins can be successfully added to gluten-free products with beneficial effects on the technological properties. Caseinates are good emulsifiers and stabilize the batter; isolated and concentrated whey proteins can form gels; high temperature skim milk powder exhibits high water-binding capacity [10]. Whey proteins increased the specific volume and decreased bread crumb hardness over time, while sodium caseinate demonstrated the opposite effect [14]. On the contrary, the addition of both - whey proteins concentrate and sodium caseinate to short biscuit formulation, raised hardness and intensified surface brownness [15]. To improve the nutritional value of gluten-free products by the addition of milk proteins particular attention should be paid to the lactose content [16]. Celiac patients are often susceptible to secondary lactose intolerance due to alterations of lactase secretion resulted from the villous atrophy [6]. The addition of high protein/low lactose dairy powders combined with optimal amount of water resulted in gluten-free breads rich in proteins, with dark crust and white crumb, good acceptability scores in sensory tests, an increase in loaf volume, and a decrease in crust and crumb hardness [17].

There is a justified need to improve the nutritional value of gluten-free products. The present study is a continuation of previous trials on the enhancement of the quality and nutritional value of gluten-free bread [18], this time focused on the fortification in proteins. The aim of the study was to enrich a gluten-free formulation, supplemented with calcium citrate in low-lactose dairy proteins, to evaluate its mixing and pasting behavior and to analyze the technological properties, overall quality, and sensory characteristics of obtained gluten-free bread.

2. Experimental Section

2.1. Materials

Corn starch (Huici Leidan SA, Huarte, Spain), potato starch (EPSA, Valencia, Spain), pectin (E 440(i), ZPOW Pectowin, Jasło, Poland), calcium citrate (Sigma-Aldrich, St. Louis, MO, USA), commercial sunflower oil, dried yeast (Lessaffre, Valladolid, Spain), sugar, salt, and tap water were used as the basic ingredients. Calcium citrate was added in an amount to provide 0.6% of elementary calcium. The diary components used were: calcium caseinate (CAS; PZH SM Lacpol, Murowana Goślina, Poland), sodium caseinate (NAS; POCh, Gliwice, Poland), spray dried whey protein isolate (ISO; Carbery Ballineen, Ireland), and hydrolyzed whey proteins (OPT; Carbery Ballineen, Ireland). The amount of protein components was determined on the basis of nutrition and health claims made on foods in such a way that the final gluten-free product was either a source of protein or high in protein [19].

2.2. Characteristic of Dairy Powders

2.2.1. Chemical Composition of Dairy Ingredients

The moisture, crude proteins (N × 6.25), and ash contents were evaluated using the standard methods [20–22]. The results presented are the mean values of at least two replicates.

2.2.2. Physical and Functional Properties of Dairy Ingredients

Particle size distribution was determined using a Mastersizer 2000 Particle Size Analyzer with a wet dispersion unit Hydro 2000 S (Malvern Instrument Ltd, Malvern, England). Samples (1–2 g) were suspended in isopropanol. In order to keep the sample suspended and homogenized, it was recirculated continuously through the measurement zone. Particle size distribution was assessed using the mean particle volume (D50) in six replicates for each sample.

The measurement of color was performed by using a Minolta colorimeter (Chroma Meter CR-400/410, Konica Minolta, Japan), equipped with a granular attachment after standardization with a white calibration plate. The color was expressed in accordance with CIE-$L^*a^*b^*$ uniform color space (CIE-Lab). The parameters determined were lightness L^* ($L^* = 0$ [black] and $L^* = 100$ [white]), a^* ($-a^*$ = greenness and $+a^*$ = redness), and b^* ($-b^*$ = blueness and $+b^*$ = yellowness). Values were the mean of nine replicates.

Water absorption index (WAI) and water solubility index (WSI) were determined according the method of Anderson *et al.* [23] at room temperature (RT) and after heating. Oil absorption capacity (OAC) was determined according to the method of Lin, Humbert, and Sosulski [24]. The values presented are the average of three measurements.

2.3. Mixolab® Measurements

Mixing and pasting behavior of the protein enriched gluten-free dough were evaluated using Mixolab® (Chopin, Tripette et Renaud, Paris, France) [25]. The Mixolab® curves were recorded to evaluate the effect of different dairy powders and variable amount of them. Potato starch (8.4 g), pectin (2.1 g), calcium citrate (3.0 g), sugar (2.6 g), and salt (0.8 g) were added to corn starch (31.4 g). The investigated protein powders (6.3 or 12.6 g) were added substituting the appropriate amount of corn starch and 41.7 mL of water. For the assays, 90 g sample was placed into the Mixolab® bowl and mixed (15 min/30 °C). Subsequently, the temperature was raised to 90 °C (increase of 4 °C/min) and at 90 °C was held for 8 min. In the cooling phase the temperature was reduced until 50 °C (decrease of 4 °C/min), and 50 °C was held for 2 min. The mixing speed during the entire assay was 80 rpm. The values obtained are the mean of two replicates. Parameters recorded included: initial pasting temperature where initial increase of consistency was detected, maximum torque during heating for potato (C3) and corn (C3′) starches, gelatinization rate for potato (β1) and corn (β2) starches, minimum dough torque during heating (C4), cooking stability rate (γ), final consistency after cooling until 50 °C (C5), and gelling rate (δ).

2.4. Breadmaking Process

Potato starch (16 g), pectin (4 g), and calcium citrate (5.8 g) were added to corn starch (60.3 g). The investigated protein powders (12 or 24 g) were added substituting the appropriate amount of corn starch. Subsequently, sugar (5 g), dried yeast (5 g), and salt (1.5 g) were dissolved separately in tap water (80 mL) and added to the dry ingredients together with oil (2.5 g). The batter was mixed for 12 min in a Brabender farinograph SEW (Brabender OHG, Duisburg, Germany). The resulting batter was proofed for 20 min in a proofing cabinet (35 °C/70% relative humidity). Then, the batter was divided into 200 g samples, placed in baking tins and proofed for another 20 min under the same conditions. The baking was carried out in convection oven at 200 °C for 25 min (Eurofours type 10AB20W2, Gommergnies, France). The obtained loaves were divided into two groups: the first was analyzed directly after cooling to room temperature (2 h); and the second was packed in polyethylene bags and stored 24 h at ambient temperature (22 ± 2 °C) for crumb structure analysis and sensory evaluation.

2.5. Characteristic of Gluten-Free Bread

2.5.1. Chemical Composition and Nutritional Value

Bread moisture [20], proteins [21], ash [22], and fat [26] contents were determined following the standard methods. Total carbohydrates were determined by difference subtracting 100 g minus the sum of protein, ash, and fat expressed in g/100 g. The energy value was calculated by multiplying the amount of each macronutrient by the corresponding conversion factor (4, 9, and 4 for protein, fat, and carbohydrates, respectively) [27]. The percentage of energy delivered by protein was calculated.

2.5.2. Technological Parameters

The bread loaf weight and volume (rapeseed displacement method) were determined. The specific volume and bake loss were calculated [18]. The height/width ratio of the central 10 mm slices was determined using Image J software (National Institutes of Health, Bethesda, MD, USA) [28]. The energy status of water in bread samples was measured as water activity (a_w) using an Aqua Lab Series 3 (Decagon Devices Pullman, USA) at 22 °C. The crust and crumb color was analyzed as previously described using a Minolta colorimeter. Values were the mean of nine replicates.

2.5.3. Crumb Texture Properties

Texture profile analysis (TPA test) of the 24-h stored bread crumbs was performed using Texture Analyzer TA-XT2i (Stable Micro Systems, Surrey, UK) equipped with a 30 kg load cell and 25 mm aluminum cylindrical probe. Three middle slices of each loaf were evaluated. A 10 mm thick bread slice underwent a double compression test up to 50% deformation of its original height at a crosshead speed of 1 mm/s and a 30 s gap between compressions. From the two-bite texture profile curve the following texture parameters were obtained: hardness, adhesiveness, springiness, cohesiveness, chewiness, and resilience.

2.6. Statistical Analysis

One-way analysis of variance (ANOVA) and Fisher's least significant difference test (LSD) using Statistica 7.1 (StatSoft, Kraków, Poland) were applied to define significant differences ($p < 0.05$) between samples.

3. Results and Discussion

3.1. Chemical, Physical and Functional Characteristic of Dairy Powders

Detailed characteristics of selected dairy powders (NAS, CAS, ISO, OPT), including chemical composition, and physical and functional properties, are provided in order to evaluate the effect of each individual powder on the gluten-free batter and bread (Table 1). High concentration of proteins was confirmed for all dairy ingredients tested (Table 1). Total proteins content exceeded 85%, with distinguishing concentration in sodium caseinate, containing over 94% of proteins. According to the suppliers, all dairy ingredients tested were poor in fat (1.0%–1.5%) and lactose (0.5%–2%). Caseinates (CAS and NAS) were richer in mineral compounds (ash; near 4%) than whey proteins tested.

The measurement of particle size showed that the mean size of whey proteins particles was significantly higher in comparison with particles of caseinates tested, and ISO showed the highest particle size (Table 1). The color parameters of dairy powders indicated that they were very light, white, or creamy powders, characterized by high L^* value, above 91, and in the case of NAS, near 94. The negative value of parameter a^* (below−2) indicated greenish color and the positive b^* values described the yellowish color, being significantly higher for the whey proteins.

The ability to bind and hold water without syneresis is critical in many foods, thus, hydration properties were determined in the dairy proteins. Results indicated that CAS followed by NAS showed the highest value of WAI at room temperature (Table 1), however, that trend was reversed when this parameter was determined after heating. Although caseins are relatively hydrophobic, they contain regions of high, medium, or low hydrophobicity [29] and they bind about 2 g water/g, which is typical of proteins [30]. Whey proteins in their native form exhibit little water-binding capacity [31]. Nevertheless, heat-denaturated whey proteins, although retaining most of their secondary structure, are linked together and can have a perceived hydration of over 10 g of water/g protein, compared with 0.2 g water/g protein for whey protein in their native globular state [29]. Processing has also a considerable impact on solubility of dairy proteins (Table 1). At room temperature, whey proteins tested were soluble in very high degree, however the heat treatment impaired the solubility of these proteins. WSI of ISO and OPT decreased by over 80% and 70%, respectively. Whey proteins are susceptible to denaturation at temperature higher that 70 °C. When heated, the tertiary structure of protein globules are destroyed, then unfolding of the protein molecules and new protein-protein interactions occur [32]. In case of both caseinates tested the opposite situation was observed. Here, after boiling the WSI values for CAS and NAS increased by more than 15%. Analyzing the OAC, significant differences were found between the dairy proteins tested (Table 1). The highest OAC was observed for CAS, followed by ISO, and OPT, whereas NAS has the lowest oil absorption capacity, probably due to its highest protein concentration. According to Kinsella [33], the mechanism of fat absorption has been attributed mostly to the physical entrapment of oil, but as well may be influenced by lipophilicity of the protein concentrate. In protein powder foods fat binding can be influenced by the size of powder particles [34], however in the dairy proteins tested such correlation was not observed.

3.2. *Effect of Dairy Powders on the Gluten-Free Dough Characteristics*

The effect of the dairy powders at two different levels (12% and 24%) on the rheology of gluten-free dough was studied by using the Mixolab, where dough behavior subjected to shear and temperature constraints is recorded [25]. The Mixolab plots obtained in the presence of the dairy powders are shown in Figure 1.

Gluten-free doughs showed very low consistency during mixing, which only increased after heating when starches present in the recipe started to gelatinize. Consistency enhanced during heating till the rupture of the starch granules where the maximum consistency was detected. Further heating led to a decrease in the consistency derived from the starches stability during cooking and when temperature decreased the amylose retrogradation associated to cooling was observed as a consistency increase. This pattern agrees with previous description of the compounds changes reported by Rosell *et al.* [25]. The trends observed on the plots indicated that gluten-free dough rheology was clearly governed by starch changes during heating and cooling. The consistency of the gluten-free dough is greatly dependent on the amount of water or hydration, showing very low consistency during mixing when water adsorption is higher than 90% [35]. It must be remarked that during heating two consistency peaks were detected that were associated to the different gelatinization temperature of corn and potato starches. Matos and Rosell [36] also detected different peaks depending on the type of starch and their diverse pasting temperatures, being 65.4 °C for potato starch, 69.9 °C for corn starch and 70.2 °C for rice flour. In addition, Krupa-Kozak *et al.* [18] observed two different slopes during heating, the first one detected around 28–31 min corresponded to potato starch gelatinization, whereas the second one observed from 31 to 36 min was ascribed to corn starch gelatinization, which agrees with results of the present study. The patterns obtained during mixing, overmixing, pasting, and gelling greatly varied with the protein source and the level of proteins (Figure 1). It was not possible to record the consistency of the 24% NAS containing dough with the Mixolab due to its high consistency. The inclusion of the dairy proteins decreased the dough consistency during the heating-cooling stages, with the exception of NAS added at 12% that showed higher consistency after cooling. Bonet *et al.* [37] found that the addition of protein sources (gelatin, egg, and lupine) to wheat flour significantly changed the Mixolab plot and the effect was attributable to the nature of the proteins. The presence of different proteins and starches modifies protein–protein interactions and also the starch gelatinization and the gelling processes [25,35,38]. Regarding the level of the proteins added, dough consistencies decreased with increasing level of proteins.

Figure 1. Effect of dairy proteins on the gluten-free dough consistency determined by Mixolab® device. Control: unfortified gluten-free dough; CAS 12: gluten-free dough with 12% of calcium caseinate; CAS 24: gluten-free dough with 24% of calcium caseinate; NAS 12: gluten-free dough with 12% of sodium caseinate; NAS 24: gluten-free dough with 24% of sodium caseinate: OPT 12: gluten-free dough with 12% of whey proteins hydrolysate; OPT 24: gluten-free dough with 24% of whey proteins hydrolysate; ISO 12: gluten-free dough with 12% of whey proteins isolate; ISO 24: gluten-free dough with 24% of whey proteins isolate. C3: maximum torque during heating of potato starch; C3′: maximum torque during heating of corn starch; C4: minimum dough torque during heating; C5: final viscosity after cooling till 50 °C; β1: gelatinization rate for potato starch; β2: gelatinization rate for corn starch; γ: cooking stability rate.

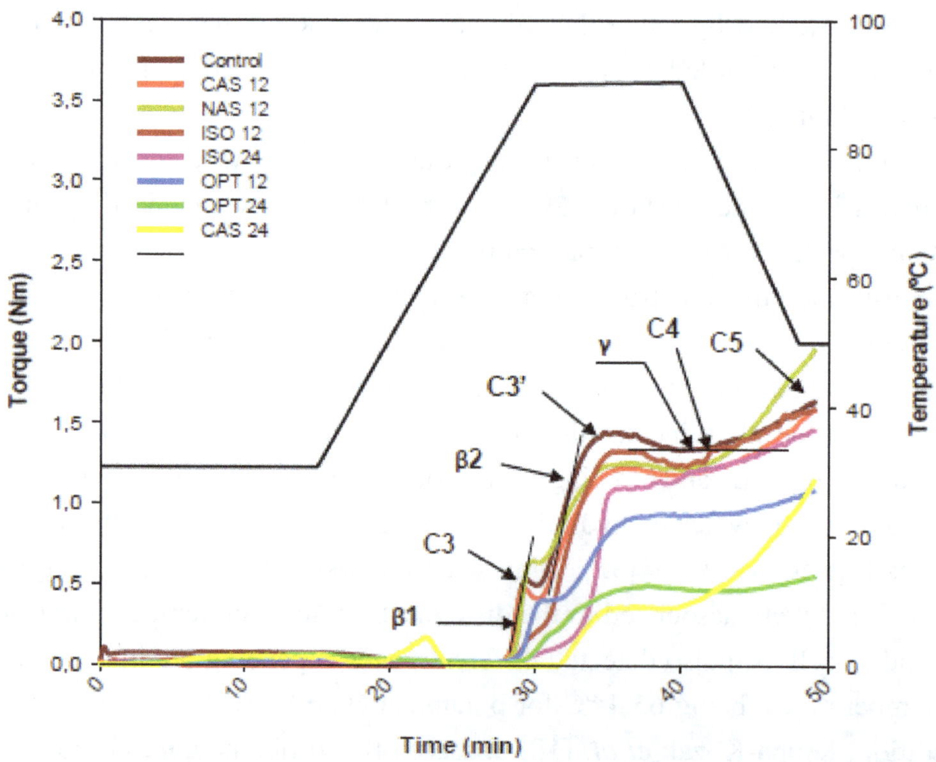

Primary and secondary parameters were extracted from the Mixolab curves to quantify the effect of the different dairy proteins on dough empirical rheology (Table 2). Proteins added to experimental doughs retarded the initial pasting temperature and the temperatures at which maximum dough consistency (C3 and C3′) was obtained; likely due to proteins compete with the starch for the available water, limiting the starch granule swelling and, therefore, promoting a delay in the pasting process as has been observed with hydrocolloids [39]. Consistency associated to potato starch gelatinization (C3) decreased in the presence of proteins, with the exception of NAS 12, and was barely noticeable when increasing protein level up to 24%. That effect was even more accentuated in the case of the consistency associated to corn starch gelatinization (C3′), since water will be even more limited after proteins hydration and potato starch gelatinization. Nevertheless, no relationship could be established between the consistency parameters during heating and the hydration properties of the dairy powders, likely the interaction between starches and proteins affected the ability of the proteins and starches to bind water. The final dough consistency after cooling (C5) was also significantly affected with the addition of the different protein powders, therefore, dairy powders modified amylose chains crystallization and in consequence, starch gelling, and the effect was dependent on the nature of the protein. NAS added at 12% increased the final consistency, whereas ISO at 12% did not modify that parameter and the other proteins decreased it. When increasing levels of proteins were added, the effect was a reduction of the final consistency. Considering the particle size of the proteins and also the hydration properties of the dairy proteins, there was no relationship between those properties and the dough behavior during heating and cooling. Regarding the secondary parameters, all doughs showed very low cooking stability range (C4–C3), whereas the cooling setback or gelling (C4–C5) was increased with the inclusion of dairy proteins, with the exception of the OPT that decreased that value.

Likely the hydrolyzed nature of this protein isolate hindered the amylose recrystallization, lowering the final dough consistency. The rate of the starches phenomena associated to heating ($\beta 1$, $\beta 2$, γ) and cooling (δ) were significantly affected in the presence of proteins. In general, starch gelatinization was slowed down in the presence of proteins, with the exception of NAS-12 in the case of $\beta 1$ or ISO-12 in the case of $\beta 2$. Again, no correlation could be established with the protein properties.

3.3. Chemical Composition and Nutritional Value of the Gluten-Free Breads Containing Different Dairy Powders

The addition of dairy proteins to gluten-free bread formulations is a common practice for increasing nutritional value, as in general, the commercial gluten-free formulas are poor in proteins [35,40]. Similarly to the results of our previous study [41], the control gluten-free bread, mainly composed of corn and potato starches, was poor in proteins (Table 3).

Table 1. Chemical, physical, and functional characteristic of dairy powders.

Sample	Moisture (%)	Protein [1] (% d.b.)	Fat [2] (% d.b.)	Lactose [2] (% d.b.)	Ash (% d.b.)	Particle size (μm)	Color parameters			WAI (g/g)		WSI (g/100 g)		OAC (g/g)
							L^*	a^*	b^*	RT	90 °C	RT	90 °C	
CAS	7.23^{a}	88.39^{b}	1.50^{a}	0.50^{c}	3.99^{a}	62.89^{a}	91.78^{b}	−2.09^{a}	9.42^{d}	2.81^{a}	1.21^{d}	56.84^{b}	72.78^{a}	
NAS	6.66^{b}	94.42^{a}	1.00^{b}	1.00^{b}	3.93^{a}	75.79^{b}	93.70^{a}	−2.46^{c}	6.77^{c}	1.84^{b}	1.54^{c}	50.61^{c}	67.95^{b}	
OPT	4.43^{c}	87.02^{b}	1.00^{b}	2.00^{a}	2.69^{b}	179.19^{c}	91.37^{c}	−2.48^{c}	11.05^{a}	0.96^{c}	5.30^{b}	81.88^{a}	22.34^{c}	
ISO	4.40^{c}	88.42^{b}	1.50^{a}	0.20^{d}	2.68^{b}	233.70^{d}	91.09^{d}	−2.32^{b}	10.86^{b}	0.82^{d}	6.12^{a}	81.85^{a}	14.17^{d}	

CAS: calcium caseinate; NAS: sodium caseinate; OPT: whey proteins hydrolysate; ISO: whey proteins isolate; [1] N × 6.25; [2] Provided by the supplier; RT: Room temperature; WAI: Water absorption index; WSI: Water solubility index; OAC: Oil absorption capacity; Mean values labeled with different letters in the same column are significantly different ($p < 0.05$).

Table 2. Effect of dairy powders on the gluten-free dough characteristics during mixing and heating determined by Mixolab® device.

Sample	Initial pasting temperature (°C)	Peak torque (potato) (C3) (Nm)	Temperature at C3 (°C)	Peak torque (corn) (C3′) (Nm)	Temperature at C3′ (°C)	β1 (potato) (Nm/min)	β2 (corn) (Nm/min)	C4 (Nm)	Γ (Nm/min)	C5 (Nm)	Cooking stability range (C4-C3) (Nm)	Gelling (C5-C4) (Nm)	δ (Nm/min)
Control	69.1^{d}	0.53^{b}	72.9^{e}	1.45^{a}	84.5^{b}	0.618^{a}	0.285^{b}	1.34^{a}	−0.026^{b}	1.68^{b}	−0.11^{b}	0.35^{c}	0.050
CAS 12	71.2^{c}	0.29^{d}	74.1^{d}	1.03^{c}	86.2^{a}	0.470^{b}	0.227^{c}	0.97^{b}	−0.025^{b}	1.45^{c}	−0.07^{ab}	0.49^{b}	0.065
NAS 12	72.4^{ab}	0.66^{a}	76.9^{b}	1.25^{b}	85.1^{b}	0.726^{a}	0.181^{d}	1.21^{a}	−0.012^{a}	2.05^{a}	−0.04^{a}	0.84^{a}	0.114
OPT 12	73.3^{a}	0.41^{c}	78.3^{a}	0.94^{c}	86.3^{a}	0.302^{c}	0.149^{e}	0.93^{b}	−0.007^{a}	1.12^{d}	−0.01^{a}	0.20^{d}	0.032
ISO 12	71.6^{bc}	0.17^{e}	75.3^{c}	1.34^{b}	86.6^{a}	0.134^{d}	0.360^{a}	1.24^{a}	−0.030^{b}	1.70^{b}	−0.11^{b}	0.47^{b}	0.039
Control	69.1^{C}	0.53^{A}	72.9^{C}	1.45^{A}	84.5^{D}	0.618^{A}	0.285^{B}	1.34^{A}	−0.026^{C}	1.68^{A}	−0.11^{B}	0.35^{B}	0.050
CAS 24	nd	nd	Nd	0.36^{D}	85.1^{C}	0.055^{C}	0.131^{C}	0.35^{D}	−0.005^{A}	1.28^{C}	−0.02^{A}	0.93^{A}	0.117
NAS 24						na							
OPT 24	77.4^{A}	0.21^{B}	79.9^{A}	0.50^{C}	86.5^{A}	0.096^{B}	0.095^{C}	0.47^{C}	−0.008^{B}	0.57^{D}	−0.03^{A}	0.11^{C}	0.020
ISO 24	71.9^{B}	0.09^{C}	77.8^{B}	1.11^{B}	85.4^{B}	0.047^{C}	0.770^{A}	1.09^{B}	−0.008^{B}	1.49^{B}	−0.03^{A}	0.40^{B}	0.039

Control: unfortified gluten-free dough; CAS 12: gluten-free dough with 12% of calcium caseinate; CAS 24: gluten-free dough with 24% of calcium caseinate; NAS 12: gluten-free dough with 12% of sodium caseinate; NAS 24: gluten-free dough with 24% of sodium caseinate: OPT 12: gluten-free dough with 12% of whey proteins hydrolysate; OPT 24: gluten-free dough with 24% of whey proteins hydrolysate; ISO 12: gluten-free dough with 12% of whey proteins isolate; ISO 24: gluten-free dough with 24% of whey proteins isolate; C3: maximum torque during heating for potato starch; C3′: maximum torque during heating for corn starch; C4: minimum dough torque during heating; C5: final consistency after cooling till 50 °C; β1: gelatinization rate for potato starch; β2: gelatinization rate for corn starch; γ: cooking stability rate; δ: gelling rate; nd: not detected; na: not available; Mean values labeled with different letters in the same column are signific different ($P < 0.05$). Lower case letters were used with the low-level protein addition and upper case letters are referred to the highest level of protein addition.

Table 3. Chemical composition and nutritional value of the gluten-free breads containing different dairy powders.

Sample	Moisture (%)	Proteins (% as is)	Fat (% as is)	Ash (% as is)	Energetic value (kcal as is)	Energy delivered by proteins (%)
Control	39.97 c	1.51 b	1.14 a	1.82 d	239 a	2.53 e
CAS 12	39.23 e	8.65 a	0.83 c	2.14 a	239 a	14.50 b
NAS 12	41.64 a	8.57 a	0.39 d	1.82 d	228 c	15.03 a
OPT 12	39.69 d	8.23 a	0.83 c	1.98 b	237 b	13.86 c
ISO 12	40.09 b	8.07 a	1.04 b	1.92 c	237 b	13.61 d
Control	39.97 C	1.51 C	1.14 D	1.82 D	239 C	2.53 D
CAS 24	40.59 A	14.49 B	1.29 C	2.20 A	235 D	24.63 B
NAS 24	39.37 D	15.75 A	1.21 CD	2.15 B	240 B	26.25 A
OPT 24	40.49 B	14.74 B	1.71 B	2.06 C	238 C	24.74 B
ISO 24	39.06 D	14.39 B	2.08 A	2.12 B	246 A	23.43 C

Control: unfortified gluten-free bread; CAS 12: gluten-free bread with 12% of calcium caseinate; CAS 24: gluten-free bread with 24% of calcium caseinate; NAS 12: gluten-free bread with 12% of sodium caseinate; NAS 24: gluten-free bread with 24% of sodium caseinate: OPT 12: gluten-free bread with 12% of whey proteins hydrolysate; OPT 24: gluten-free bread with 24% of whey proteins hydrolysate; ISO 12: gluten-free bread with 12% of whey proteins isolate; ISO 24: gluten-free bread with 24% of whey proteins isolate; Mean values labeled with different letters in the same column are significantly different ($p < 0.05$). Lower case letters were used with the low-level protein addition and upper case letters are referred to the highest level of protein addition.

As was expected, the proteins content in all experimental gluten-free breads with dairy powders increased significantly ($p < 0.05$). Breads supplemented with 12 g of milk powders were more than five-times richer in protein than the control. The increase of the level of supplementation with dairy proteins (up to 24 g) caused the further increase of protein content in the bread samples, especially in NAS 24 with sodium caseinate, which was ten-times richer in proteins than the control. Milk proteins have a high nutritional value [10,13] and the addition of milk proteins and essential amino acids, such as lysine, methionine and tryptophan also increases the nutritional value of the bakery products [14,15]. Within bread samples with dairy proteins addition, a fat content was low ranging from 0.39 to 2.08 (Table 3) as all dairy powders added were relatively poor in fat (Table 1). However, comparing with the control, experimental breads were more affluent in minerals, especially when 24 g of calcium caseinate was included to formulation (CAS 24). There are inconsistencies about CD patients being overweight at diagnosis and gaining weight while on GFD [42,43]. Taking this into account, the calorie content of gluten-free products is of importance [44]. Energetic value (in kcal) of experimental gluten-free bread with dairy proteins ranged from 228 to 246, and was comparable to unfortified control (239 kcal). Hager *et al.* [45] indicated that although the calorie content was higher in white and wholemeal wheat bread than in oat, buckwheat, maize, sorghum, teff, and rice, these breads were of inferior quality at the same time. In the present study the two levels of dairy proteins supplementation to experimental gluten-free bread were tested regarding the energy delivered by proteins (Table 3). In the case of experimental breads with lower amount (12 g) of caseinates and whey proteins powders, the proteins delivered around 15% or above 13% of energy, respectively. The higher threshold of proteins supplementation influenced further significant growth of energy delivered by proteins up to 26% in NAS 24. According to the European Parliament regulation on nutrition and health claims made on foods, a claim that a food is a source of protein may only be applied to food product where at least 12% of the energy value of the food is provided by protein, whereas a claim that a food is high in protein may only be made where at least 20% of the energy value of the food is provided by protein [19]. Based on that regulation, all experimental gluten-free breads with 12 g dairy proteins addition can be recognized as a source of proteins, whereas all experimental gluten-free breads with 24 g dairy proteins addition are high in protein.

3.4. Technological Parameters of Gluten-Free Breads with Dairy Powders

In general, milk products have been described as volume-depressing contributory factors of wheat bread [46,47]. In this study, the addition of 12 g dairy proteins to the experimental gluten-free formulations increased significantly the specific volume of all breads, comparing with the control bread, with distinguishing results obtained in bread NAS 12 (Table 4). Similarly, Gallagher *et al.* [17] indicated that addition of high protein/low lactose dairy powders resulted in gluten-free breads of improved overall shape and volume. Additionally, in the case of increase of sodium caseinate concentration in gluten-free formulation, the further increase of specific volume of bread NAS 24 was observed. In all remaining samples, the used of increased amount of dairy proteins (up to 24 g) affected specific volume in a different manner. Compared with the control, increased level of hydrolyzed whey proteins decreased significantly the volume of bread OPT 24, whereas a higher concentration of whey proteins isolate increased the specific value of bread ISO 24. Specific volume of bread CAS 24 was similar to the control. The volume of bread with dairy powders depends on the powder type and level of addition. Breads with addition of dairy supplements showed higher height/width ratio of central slices in comparison with the unfortified control (Table 4). However, only in the case of breads with the 12 g of proteins in formulation, the increase in the height/width ratio of slice was significant. Analyzing relationship between specific volume and H/W ratio a linear positively correlation (Pearson's $r = 0.49$) was found.

Applied dairy supplements, regardless of the amount, influenced the bake loss, defined as the amount of water and organic material lost during baking (Table 4). In comparison with the control, bake loss of all breads tested increased significantly. The opposite effect was observed only in bread OPT 24, where the value of bake loss was significantly reduced by higher concentration of hydrolyzed whey proteins. Crumb characteristic affects the rate of water transport [48]. Small size of crumb pore slowed down moisture migration [49], whereas a larger number of connections between gas cells would give a faster transport of water. Additionally, the number of connections of each gas cell increased with increased size of gas cell [50].

Table 4. Technological parameters of the gluten-free breads containing different dairy powders.

Sample	Specific volume (cm^3/g)	Height/width ratio	Bake loss (%)	aw (av. temp.)	Crust color parameters			Crumb color parameters		
					*L**	*a**	*b**	*L**	*a**	*b**
Control	3.11 ^{c}	0.80 ^{d}	17.28 ^{b}	0.981 (24.8) ^{a}	46.37 ^{a}	14.22 ^{a}	35.34 ^{a}	69.10 ^{ab}	−1.25 ^{b}	10.62 ^{c}
CAS 12	4.50 ^{a}	0.93 ^{a}	22.00 ^{a}	0.980 (24.8) ^{a}	32.97 ^{b}	11.75 ^{b}	20.20 ^{b}	66.02 ^{c}	−1.01 ^{a}	9.74 ^{d}
NAS 12	4.70 ^{a}	0.92 ^{a}	22.74 ^{a}	0.979 (24.9) ^{b}	30.25 ^{c}	8.31 ^{e}	13.02 ^{c}	69.92 ^{a}	−0.95 ^{a}	12.55 ^{a}
OPT 12	4.56 ^{a}	0.89 ^{b}	22.42 ^{a}	0.979 (25.0) ^{b}	27.56 ^{d}	9.76 ^{c}	11.54 ^{d}	68.79 ^{b}	−1.18 ^{b}	11.05 ^{b}
ISO 12	4.00 ^{b}	0.86 ^{c}	19.90 ^{ab}	0.979 (24.8) ^{b}	29.47 ^{c}	9.23 ^{d}	10.23 ^{e}	68.95 ^{ab}	−1.20 ^{b}	9.80 ^{d}
Control	3.11 ^{C}	0.80	17.28 ^{C}	0.981 (24.8) ^{A}	46.37 ^{A}	14.22 ^{A}	35.34 ^{A}	69.10 ^{C}	−1.25 ^{E}	10.62 ^{C}
CAS 24	3.10 ^{C}	0.92	19.29 ^{B}	0.979 (24.9) ^{B}	29.34 ^{B}	9.05 ^{B}	10.65 ^{B}	71.19 ^{B}	−0.27 ^{A}	14.55 ^{A}
NAS 24	5.07 ^{A}	0.86	22.13 ^{A}	0.977 (25.1) ^{D}	28.78 ^{B}	5.34 ^{E}	6.74 ^{C}	65.09 ^{D}	−0.53 ^{B}	14.37 ^{A}
OPT 24	2.43 ^{D}	1.00	15.50 ^{D}	0.976 (25.0) ^{E}	29.12 ^{B}	7.36 ^{C}	6.62 ^{C}	76.49 ^{A}	−0.88 ^{D}	14.81 ^{A}
ISO 24	3.58 ^{B}	0.85	19.11 ^{B}	0.978 (24.8) ^{C}	28.90 ^{B}	6.61 ^{D}	5.97 ^{D}	69.92 ^{C}	−0.80 ^{C}	11.10 ^{B}

Control: unfortified gluten-free bread; CAS 12: gluten-free bread with 12% of calcium caseinate; CAS 24: gluten-free bread with 24% of calcium caseinate; NAS 12: gluten-free bread with 12% of sodium caseinate; NAS 24: gluten-free bread with 24% of sodium caseinate: OPT 12: gluten-free bread with 12% of whey proteins hydrolysate; OPT 24: gluten-free bread with 24% of whey proteins hydrolysate; ISO 12: gluten-free bread with 12% of whey proteins isolate; ISO 24: gluten-free bread with 24% of whey proteins isolate; Mean values labeled with different letters in the same column are significantly different ($p < 0.05$). Lower case letters were used with the low-level protein addition and upper case letters are referred to the highest level of protein addition.

Incorporation of dairy powders affected the color of both, crust and crumb of experimental gluten-free breads (Table 4). Crust of the control bread was characterized by the highest lightness (L^* = 46.37), whereas the inclusion of dairy proteins resulted in crust darkening, influenced by the level of dairy proteins addition rather than the protein type. All gluten-free breads containing dairy supplements showed the significantly lower L^* value. Additionally, in the case of experimental gluten-free breads containing 12 g of dairy proteins, the further crust color diversification was observed. Crust of bread CAS 12 and NAS 12, containing calcium or sodium caseinate, respectively, was significantly lighter in comparison with dark crust of breads containing whey proteins, with distinguishing OPT12 where L^* value reached 27.56. The value of parameter a^* (red hue) was positive for crust of all experimental breads (Table 4). Comparing with the control, the incorporation of dairy powders to gluten-free formulation affected the significant decrease in redness, especially in breads containing sodium caseinate at both levels tested (NAS 12 and NAS 24). Crust of the control gluten-free bread obtained the highest b^* value (yellow hue). Whereas, the addition of dairy proteins to formulation produced a significant decrease of crust yellowness of breads obtained, however all the values were still positive. The crust yellowness was especially low in the case of breads with higher dairy proteins concentration. Observed darkening of crust color resulted probably from the Maillard browning, a chemical reaction between amino groups and reducing sugars. In the case of milk derivatives undergoing a high temperature treatment, lactose as a reducing sugar interacts mainly with lysine residues, resulting in the formation of brown melanoidins [51]. These non-enzymatic reactions are responsible for numerous changes on food properties. From the technological point of view, the brown crust formation on gluten-free bread is desirable and the resulting color, taste and flavor characteristics are generally experienced as pleasant. Crumb color was influenced by a level of dairy proteins addition. Lower concentration of proteins tested in the formulations resulted in bread of similar to control crumb lightness, with slightly distinguishing NAS 12 (Table 4). Only in CAS 12 the L^* was significantly reduced. Whereas, the lightness of bread crumb supplemented with 24 g of dairy proteins was higher in comparison with crumb of breads with 12 g dairy proteins addition, except for crumb of bread NAS 24. The a^* values for the crumbs were all negative, with the lowest redness detected in the control crumb.

Comparing with the control, increasing concentration of dairy powders increased significantly the value of a^* parameter of tested crumbs. This effect was especially visible in the case of breads containing calcium (CAS 24) and sodium (NAS 24) caseinate, where the a^* value reached −0.27 and −0.53, respectively. Yellowness (b^*) of all crumb samples was positive. Similarly to redness, also the value of b^* increased significantly with increased dairy proteins concentration. Gluten-free breads containing dairy powders had an appealing dark crust and white crumb appearance, and received good acceptability scores in sensory tests [14,17]. As a wide variety of dairy supplement are available, their application in baked product development need to be determined adequately. In addition to the type and the amount of dairy supplement, the choice must be based on their physicochemical and functional properties, which varies remarkably.

3.5. Textural Parameters of Gluten-Free Breads with Dairy Powders

The values obtained for the textural parameters of the bread crumbs are shown in Table 5. Wide variations in the crumb hardness (3.66 to 25.28 N) were observed among the gluten-free bread samples. These results reflect large differences depending on type of proteins used. Dairy proteins incorporated at 12% level significantly ($p < 0.05$) decreased the hardness, with the exception of NAS 12. Nevertheless, the addition of increasing amounts of proteins led to the opposite effect and only ISO 24 remained softer than the control crumb. NAS at any level of addition led to harder crumbs and the same effect was observed in chewiness. Nunes *et al.* [14] analyzed the influence of low lactose dairy powders on gluten-free bread quality indicated that sodium caseinate had a negative impact on crumb hardness, whereas whey proteins demonstrated the ability to increase significantly the specific volume of the breads and decrease its the hardness.

Table 5. Texture profile analysis of the gluten-free bread crumbs containing different dairy powders.

Sample	Hardness (N)	Springiness	Cohesiveness	Chewiness (g)	Resilience
Control	9.44 ^{b}	1.002 ^{a}	0.454 ^{ab}	431.70 ^{b}	0.195 ^{a}
CAS 12	3.66 ^{e}	1.007 ^{a}	0.460 ^{a}	169.80 ^{c}	0.186 ^{a}
NAS 12	11.43 ^{a}	0.981 ^{ab}	0.427 ^{b}	475.84 ^{a}	0.188 ^{a}
OPT 12	5.46 ^{c}	0.940 ^{c}	0.335 ^{c}	170.74 ^{c}	0.134 ^{b}
ISO 12	4.20 ^{d}	0.972 ^{b}	0.366 ^{c}	152.99 ^{c}	0.141 ^{b}
Control	9.44 ^{C}	1.002 ^{A}	0.454 ^{B}	431.70 ^{C}	0.195 ^{A}
CAS 24	11.60 ^{B}	0.979 ^{AB}	0.486 ^{A}	568.38 ^{B}	0.196 ^{A}
NAS 24	25.28 ^{A}	0.954 ^{B}	0.434 ^{B}	1071.26 ^{A}	0.184 ^{A}
OPT 24	11.06 ^{B}	0.872 ^{C}	0.376 ^{C}	368.83 ^{D}	0.133 ^{B}
ISO 24	6.35 ^{D}	0.959 ^{B}	0.446 ^{B}	282.34 ^{E}	0.181 ^{A}

Control: unfortified gluten-free bread; CAS 12: gluten-free bread with 12% of calcium caseinate; CAS 24: gluten-free bread with 24% of calcium caseinate; NAS 12: gluten-free bread with 12% of sodium caseinate; NAS 24: gluten-free bread with 24% of sodium caseinate: OPT 12: gluten-free bread with 12% of whey proteins hydrolysate; OPT 24: gluten-free bread with 24% of whey proteins hydrolysate; ISO 12: gluten-free bread with 12% of whey proteins isolate; ISO 24: gluten-free bread with 24% of whey proteins isolate; Mean values labeled with different letters in the same column are significantly different ($p < 0.05$). Lower case letters were used with the low-level protein addition and upper case letters are referred to the highest level of protein addition.

Springiness is associated with a fresh, aerated and elastic product, thus high springiness is desirable in this type of products. Low springiness value is indicative of brittleness and this reflects the tendency of the bread to crumble when is sliced. Although the proteins addition decreased the springiness, the effect was only significant in the presence of the protein isolates (ISO and OPT) at both levels tested. Marco and Rosell [35] found springiness values that ranged from 0.77 to 0.94 when study the protein enrichment of rice based gluten-free breads, and later on Matos and Rosell [8] reported springiness values from 0.76 to 1.00 in commercial gluten free breads. Therefore, springiness values obtained in the present study agree with reported ones.

Cohesiveness characterizes the extent to which a material can be deformed before it ruptures, reflecting the internal cohesion of the material. Bread with high cohesiveness is desirable because it forms a bolus rather than disintegrates during mastication, whereas low cohesiveness indicates increased susceptibility of the bread to fracture or crumble [8]. In case of breads containing caseinates (CAS and NAS) values obtained for cohesiveness were similar to control, while whey proteins (OPT and ISO) decreased, significantly, the value of this parameter ($p < 0.05$). Very low resilience values were obtained for experimental gluten-free breads, especially for breads with whey proteins, indicating a low elasticity. Values obtained agreed with results reported for commercial gluten-free bread where resilience ranged from 0.09 to 0.84 [8].

4. Conclusions

The present study has shown that the application of low-lactose dairy proteins in a gluten-free formulation influenced considerably the characteristic of experimental doughs and breads. Gluten-free doughs containing dairy proteins tested showed very low consistency during mixing stage and decreased consistency during the heating-cooling stages. Experimental breads were significantly richer in proteins and more affluent in minerals than the control one. Energetic value of experimental gluten-free bread with dairy proteins was comparable to unfortified control, however regarding the energy delivered by proteins they can be recognized as a source of proteins or as high in protein. Addition of dairy proteins to the experimental gluten-free formulations increased significantly ($p < 0.05$) the specific volume of all breads, with distinguishing results obtained in bread NAS 24. Inclusion of dairy proteins resulted in crust darkening and crumb lightness, influenced by the level of dairy proteins addition rather than the protein type. Dairy proteins incorporated at a 12% level significantly ($p < 0.05$) decreased the hardness, with the exception of NAS 12. Nevertheless, the addition of increasing amounts of proteins led to the opposite effect. Obtained results suggest that dairy proteins tested in this study could be used successfully in gluten-free recipes in order to obtain gluten-free bread of a pleasant color, taste, and flavor characteristics, and improved technological and nutritional properties.

Acknowledgments

Authors acknowledge the financial support of the Spanish Ministry of Economy and Competitiveness (Project AGL2011-23802), the European Regional Development Fund (FEDER) and Generalitat Valenciana (Project Prometeo 2012/064) and Project REFRESH - Unlocking the potential of the Institute of Animal Reproduction and Food Research for strengthening integration with the European Research Area and regional development of the 7th Framework Programme EU-Research Potential-Capacities-FP7-REGPOT-2010-1-264103. The authors would like to thank to Józef Warechowski from the Faculty of Food Sciences of the University of Warmia and Mazury in Olsztyn for the particle size distribution analysis.

References

1. Fasano, A.; Berti, I.; Gerarduzzi, T.; Not, T.; Colletti, R.B.; Drago, S.; Elitsur, Y.; Green, P.H.; Guandalini, S.; Hill, I.D.; *et al.* Prevalence of celiac disease in at-risk and not-at-risk groups in the United States: A large multicenter study. *Arch. Int. Med.* **2003**, *163*, 286–292.
2. Tommasini, A.; Not, T.; Kiren, V.; Baldas, V.; Santon, D.; Trevisiol, C.; Berti, I.; Neri, E.; Gerarduzzi, T.; Bruno, I.; *et al.* Mass screening for coeliac disease using anti-human transglutaminase antibody assay. *Arch. Dis. Child.* **2004**, *89*, 512–515.
3. Darewicz, M.; Dziuba, J.; Minkiewicz, P. Coeliac disease—Background, molecular, bioinformatics and analytical aspects. *Food Rev. Int.* **2008**, *24*, 311–329.
4. Lerner, A. New therapeutic strategies for celiac disease. *Autoimmun. Rev.* **2010**, *9*, 144–147.
5. Briani, C.; Samaroo, D.; Alaedini, A. Celiac disease: From gluten to autoimmunity. *Autoimmun. Rev.* **2008**, *7*, 644–650.
6. Murray, J.A. The widening spectrum of celiac disease. *Am. J. Clin. Nutr.* **1999**, *69*, 354–365.
7. Bianchi, M.L.; Bardella, M.T. Bone in celiac disease. *Osteoporos. Int.* **2008**, *19*, 1705–1716.
8. Matos, M.E.; Rosell, C.M. Relationship between instrumental parameters and sensory characteristics in gluten-free breads. *Eur. Food Res. Technol.* **2012**, *235*, 107–117.
9. Marco, C.; Rosell, C.M. Effect of different protein isolates and transglutaminase on rice flour properties. *J. Food Eng.* **2008**, *84*, 132–139.
10. Kenny, S.; Wehrle, K.; Stanton, C.; Arendt, E.K. Incorporation of dairy ingredients into wheat bread: Effects on dough rheology and bread quality. *Eur. Food Res. Technol.* **2000**, *210*, 391–396.
11. Stathopoulos, C.; O'Kennedy, B.T. A rheological evaluation of concentrated casein systems as replacement for gluten: Calcium effects. *Int. J. Dairy Technol.* **2008**, *61*, 397–402.
12. Stathopoulos, C.; O'Kennedy, B.T. The effect of salt on the rheology and texture of a casein based ingredient intended to replace gluten. *Milchwissenschaft* **2008**, *63*, 430–433.
13. Stathopoulos, C. Dairy-Based Ingredients. In *Gluten-Free Cereal Products and Beverages*; Arendt, E.K., Dal Bello, F., Eds.; Academic Press: San Diego, CA, USA, 2008; pp. 217–236.
14. Nunes, M.; Ryan, L.; Arendt, E.K. Effect of low lactose dairy powder addition on the properties of gluten-free batters and bread quality. *Eur. Food Res. Technol.* **2009**, *229*, 31–41.
15. Gallagher, E.; Kenny, S.; Arendt, E.K. Impact of dairy protein powders on biscuit quality. *Eur. Food Res. Technol.* **2005**, *221*, 237–243.
16. Ojetti, V.; Nucera, G.; Migneco, A.; Gabrielli, M.; Lauritano, C.; Danese, S.; Zocco, M.A.; Nista, E.C.; Cammarota, G.; de Lorenzo, A.; *et al.* High prevalence of celiac disease in patients with lactose intolerance. *Digestion* **2005**, *71*, 106–110.
17. Gallagher, E.; Kunkel, A.; Gormley, T.R.; Arendt, E.K. The effect of dairy and rice powder addition on loaf and crumb characteristics, and on shelf life (intermediate and long-term) of gluten-free breads stored in a modified atmosphere. *Eur. Food Res. Technol.* **2003**, *218*, 44–48.
18. Krupa-Kozak, U.; Altamirano-Fortoul, R.; Wronkowska, M.; Rosell, C.M. Breadmaking performance and technological characteristic of gluten-free bread with inulin supplemented with calcium salts. *Eur. Food Res. Technol.* **2012**, *235*, 545–554.
19. European Union. Regulation (EC) No 1924/2006 of the European Parliament and the Concil of 20 December 2006 on nutrition and health claims made on foods. *Off. J. Eur. Union* **2006**, *L404*, 9–25.

20. ICC Standard Method 110/1, Determination of the Moisture Content of Cereals and Cereal Products (Practical method), 1976. Available online: http://www.icc.or.at/standard_methods (accessed on 12 November 2013).
21. ICC Standard Method 105/2, Determination of Crude Protein in Cereals and Cereal Products for Food and for Feed, 1994. Available online: http://www.icc.or.at/standard_methods (accessed on 12 November 2013).
22. ICC Standard Method 104/1, Determination of Ash in Cereals and Cereal Products, 1990. Available online: http://www.icc.or.at/standard_methods (accessed on 12 November 2013).
23. Anderson, R.A.; Conway, H.F.; Pfeifer, V.F.; Griffin, E.L. Gelatinization of corn grits by roll and extrusion cooking. *Cereal Sci. Today* **1969**, *14*, 4–12.
24. Lin, M.J.Y.; Humbert, E.S.; Sosulski, F. Certain functional properties of sunflower meal products. *J. Food Sci.* **1974**, *39*, 368–370.
25. Rosell, M.C.; Collar, C.; Haros, M. Assessment of hydrocolloid effects on the thermo-mechanical properties of wheat using the Mixolab. *Food Hydrocoll.* **2007**, *21*, 452–462.
26. ICC Standard Methods, 136, Cereals and Cereal Products–Determination of Total Fat Content, 1984. Available online: http://www.icc.or.at/standard_methods (accessed on 12 November 2013).
27. Food and Agriculture Organization of the United Nations (FAO) recommendations. *Food Energy-Methods of Analysis and Conversion Factors*; Rome, Italy, 2003; pp. 57–60.
28. Gonzales-Barron, U.; Butler, F. A comparison of seven thresholding techniques with the k-means clustering algorithm for measurement of breadcrumb features by digital image analysis. *J. Food Eng.* **2006**, *74*, 268–278.
29. Carr, A.J.; Southward, C.R.; Creamer, L.K. Protein Hydratation and Viscosity of Dairy Proteins. In *Advanced Dairy Chemistry. Proteins. Part B*; Fox, P.F., McSweeney, P.L.H., Eds.; Kluver Academic/Plenum Publishers: New York, NY, USA, 2003; pp. 1289–1318.
30. Fox, P.F.; McSweeney, P.L.H. *Dairy Chemistry and Biochemistry*; Blackie Academic: London, UK, 1998.
31. Cayot, P.; Lorient, D. *Food Proteins and their Applications*; Damodaran, S., Paraf, A., Eds.; Marcel Decker: New York, NY, USA, 1997.
32. Mulvihill, D.M.; Ennis, M.P. Functional Milk Proteins: Production and Utilization. In *Advanced Dairy Chemistry. Proteins. Part B*; Fox, P.F., McSweeney, P.L.H., Eds.; Kluver Academic/Plenum Publishers: New York, NY, USA, 2003; pp. 1175–1219.
33. Kinsella, J.E. Functional properties of soybean proteins. *J. Am. Oil Chem. Soc.* **1979**, *56*, 242–258.
34. Zayas, J.F. *Functionality of Proteins in Food*; Zayas, J.F., Ed.; Springer: Berlin/Heidelberg, Germany, 1997.
35. Marco, C.; Rosell, C.M. Breadmaking performance of protein enriched gluten free breads. *Eur. Food Res. Technol.* **2008**, *227*, 1205–1213.
36. Matos, M.E.; Rosell, C.M. Quality indicators of rice based gluten-free bread-like products: Relationships between dough rheology and quality characteristics. *Food Bioprocess Technol.* **2013**, *6*, 2331–2341.

37. Bonet, A.; Blaszczak, W.; Rosell, C.M. Formation of homopolymers and heteropolymers between wheat flour and several protein sources by transglutaminase catalyzed crosslinking. *Cereal Chem.* **2006**, *83*, 655–662.
38. Rosell, C.M.; Santos, E.; Collar, C. Physical characterization of fiber-enriched bread doughs by dual mixing and temperature constraint using the Mixolab®. *Eur. Food Res. Technol.* **2010**, *231*, 535–544.
39. Rosell, C.M.; Yokoyama, W.; Shoemaker, C. Rheology of different hydrocolloids-rice starch blends. Effect of successive heating-cooling cycles. *Carbohyd. Polym.* **2011**, *84*, 373–382.
40. Wronkowska, M.; Soral-Śmietana, M. Buckwheat flour-a valuable component of gluten-free formulations. *Pol. J. Food Nutr. Sci.* **2008**, *58*, 59–63.
41. Krupa-Kozak, U.; Troszyńska, A.; Bączek, N.; Soral-Śmietana, M. Effect of organic calcium supplements on the technological characteristic and sensory properties of gluten-free bread. *Eur. Food Res. Technol.* **2011**, *232*, 497–508.
42. Valletta, E.; Fornaro, M.; Cipolli, M.; Conte, S.; Bissolo, F.; Danchielli, C. Celiac disease and obesity: Need for nutritional follow-up after diagnosis. *Eur. J. Clin. Nutr.* **2010**, *64*, 1371–1372.
43. Brambilla, P.; Picca, M.; Dilillo, D.; Meneghin, F.; Cravidi, C.; Tischer, M.C.; Vivaldo, T.; Bedoni, G.; Zuccotti, G.V. Changes of body mass index in celiac children on a gluten-free diet. *Nutr. Metab. Cardiovasc.* **2013**, *23*, 177–182.
44. Matos, M.E.; Rosell, C.M. Chemical composition and starch digestibility of different gluten-free breads. *Plant Food Hum. Nutr.* **2011**, *66*, 224–230.
45. Hager, A-S.; Wolter, A.; Czerny, M.; Bez, J.; Zannini, E.; Arendt, E.K.; Czerny, M. Investigation of product quality, sensory profile and ultrastructure of breads made from a range of commercial gluten-free flours compared to their wheat counterparts. *Eur. J. Food Res. Technol.* **2012**, *235*, 333–344.
46. Singh, N.; Kaur, B.I.; Singh, G.H. Effect of different additives on mixograph and bread making properties of Indian wheat flour. *J. Food Eng.* **2003**, *56*, 89–95.
47. Esteller, M.S.; Zancanaro, O.; Palmeira, C.N.S.; da Silva Lannes, S.C. The effect of kefir addition on microstructure parameters and physical properties of porous white bread. *Eur. Food Res. Technol.* **2006**, *222*, 26–31.
48. Roca, E.; Guillard, V.; Guilbert, S.; Gontard, N. Moisture migration in a cereal composite food at high water activity: Effects of initial porosity and fat content. *J Cereal Sci.* **2006**, *43*, 144–151.
49. Labbuza, T.P.; Hyman, C.R. Moisture migration and control in multi-domain foods *Trends Food Sci. Technol.* **1998**, *9*, 47–55.
50. Van Dalen, G.; Notenboom, P.; van Vliet, L.J.; Voortman, L.; Esveld, E. 3-D imaging analysis and modeling of porous cereal products using X-ray microtomography. *Image Anal. Stereol.* **2007**, *26*, 169–177.
51. Calligaris, S.; Manzocco, L.; Anese, M.; Nicoli, M.C. Effect of heat-treatment on the antioxidant and pro-oxidant activity of milk. *Int. Dairy J.* **2004**, *14*, 421–427.

13

Gluten-Free Diet in Children: An Approach to a Nutritionally Adequate and Balanced Diet

Francesca Penagini *, Dario Dilillo, Fabio Meneghin, Chiara Mameli, Valentina Fabiano and Gian Vincenzo Zuccotti

Department of Pediatrics, University of Milan, Luigi Sacco Hospital, Milan 20157, Italy;
E-Mails: dilillo.dario@hsacco.it (D.D.); meneghin.fabio@hsacco.it (F.M.);
mameli.chiara@hsacco.it (C.M.); fabiano.valentina@hsacco.it (V.F.);
gianvincenzo.zuccotti@unimi.it (G.V.Z.)

* Author to whom correspondence should be addressed; E-Mail: frapenagini@tiscali.it;

Abstract: Gluten-free diet (GFD) is the cornerstone treatment for celiac disease (CD). GFD implies a strict and lifelong elimination from the diet of gluten, the storage protein found in wheat, barley, rye and hybrids of these grains, such as kamut and triticale. The absence of gluten in natural and processed foods, despite being the key aspect of GFD, may lead to nutritional consequences, such as deficits and imbalances. The nutritional adequacy of GFD is particularly important in children, this the age being of maximal energy and nutrient requirements for growth, development and activity. In recent years, attention has focused on the nutritional quality of gluten-free products (GFPs) available in the market. It is well recognized that GFPs are considered of lower quality and poorer nutritional value compared to the gluten-containing counterparts. The present review focuses on the nutritional adequacy of GFD at the pediatric age, with the aim being to increase awareness of the potential complications associated with this diet, to identify strategies in order to avoid them and to promote a healthier diet and lifestyle in children with CD.

Keywords: celiac disease; gluten-free diet; children; nutritional complications; balanced diet

1. Introduction

Celiac disease (CD) is a chronic systemic autoimmune disorder caused by a permanent intolerance to gluten proteins in genetically susceptible individuals. Gluten is a general term used to describe a mixture of storage proteins, including prolamins, hordeins and secalins found in wheat, barley and rye, respectively. These proteins may exert a toxic effect on intestinal mucosa in genetically susceptible individuals by triggering an immune-mediated response, responsible for the typical villous atrophy and lymphocyte infiltrate in small intestine mucosa seen in CD. In fact, these proteins contain epitopes that undergo deamidation, an important process for the binding of the CD associated human leukocyte antigen (HLA) DQ2/DQ8 haplotypes with T-lymphocytes, activating an autoimmune response [1–3].

A lifelong strict gluten-free diet (GFD) is the only available treatment for CD. Adherence to GFD leads to regression of symptoms, normalization of histological and laboratory findings and reduces the risk of CD associated complications [4]. Within the range of gluten-free foods, a distinction must be made between those that are naturally gluten-free and those that are made gluten-free through a process of purification. There are several foods that are naturally gluten-free, such as rice, corn, potatoes and a number of different grains, seeds and legumes. Historically, rice, corn and potatoes have been the first natural substitutes for gluten-containing grains. Today, a number of different grains, including pseudo-cereals, offer increased variety, improved palatability to GFD and are a good source of carbohydrates, protein, dietary fiber, vitamins and polyunsaturated fatty acids [5,6]. The commercially available gluten-free (GF) products are processed foods purified of gluten. The elimination of this storage protein inevitably alters the macro- and micro-nutrient composition, thus the nutritional value. First, wheat is not only a major source of protein, but also of iron, folates and B vitamins (thiamin, riboflavin and niacin); in fact, GF products are often low in these nutrients, as opposed to their gluten containing equivalents [7–9]. The various gluten-free and gluten containing foods are listed in Table 1.

Table 1. Gluten-free and gluten containing cereals and other foods.

Gluten-Free Cereals	Gluten Containing Cereals
Cereals and minor cereals	
Corn	
Rice	Wheat
Sorghum	Barley
Oats *	Rye
Teff	Kamut
Millet	Malt
Pseudo-cereals	Triticale
Amaranth	
Quinoa	
Buckwheat	
Vegetable foods	Bread
Vegetables	Pasta
Fruits	Snacks
Nuts	Biscuits

Table 1. *Cont.*

Other plant foods Potatoes Tapioca Soybean Vegetable oils **Animal foods** Dairy products Egg Meat Fish	All foods produced with any of the gluten containing cereals mentioned above. Numerous foods available in supermarkets and grocery stores, including meat products, sweets and beer, contain gluten.

* Controversial; see paragraph on oats.

1.1. Macronutrients

Studies show that gluten-free products (GFPs) often have a greater carbohydrate and lipid content than their gluten containing equivalents [10–13]. Segura *et al.* analyzed the nutritional composition of a range of GF breads and found that these are starchy-based foods with a high glycemic index (estimated between 83.3 and 96.1 *vs.* 71 for white wheat flour bread), with low protein and high fat content [9]. With regards to lipid content and composition, Caponio *et al.* showed that commercially available GF biscuits are richer in saturated fatty acids compared to the gluten containing equivalents [13]. All these characteristics have a negative effect on health, and this should be seriously taken into account, because the limited choice of food products in the diet of children with CD induces a high consumption of packaged GFPs, such as snacks and biscuits.

1.2. Micronutrients and Minerals

It has been shown that some commercially available GFPs have a lower content of folates, iron and B vitamins or are not consistently enriched/fortified compared to their gluten containing counterparts [7–9]. Thompson [7,8] conducted two studies on US commercially available GFPs. The author analyzed the folate, iron and B vitamins (thiamin, riboflavin and niacin) composition of these products and compared them with the composition of their gluten containing counterparts, finding that GFPs were significantly lower in folates, iron and B vitamins.

1.3. Dietary Fiber

Some studies have reported that GFD is associated with a lower intake of dietary fiber than a standard gluten containing diet [14,15]. A study conducted in the USA on adults showed that the diet of CD patients on GFD was low in fiber intake [15]. This phenomenon is likely to be related to the composition of many GF foods made with starches and/or refined flours with low content in fiber. In fact, during the refining process, the outer layer of grain containing most of the fiber is removed, leaving only the starchy inner layer.

2. Nutritional Imbalances in Children with Celiac Disease Following a GFD

Studies conducted in adults and children show that approximately 20%–38% of patients with CD have nutritional complications, such as calorie/protein imbalance, dietary fiber, mineral and vitamin deficiencies [16–19]. These complications may be encountered both at diagnosis and during follow-up, whilst on GFD [9,18]. At diagnosis, the deficiencies are often secondary to nutrient malabsorption due to mucosal damage. Studies show that the more pronounced the villous atrophy, the greater the nutritional deficiencies, with lower levels of iron, copper, folate, vitamin B-12 and zinc [19]. For CD patients on GFD, the nutritional complications are likely to be caused by the poor nutritional quality of the GFPs mentioned above and by the incorrect alimentary choices of CD patients. The most common nutritional deficiencies encountered in adults with CD, at diagnosis and during GFD, are described in Table 2.

Table 2. Common nutrient deficiencies in adults with celiac disease (CD) at diagnosis and after Gluten-free diet (GFD). Modified from Cynthia Kupper [20].

Common Nutrient Deficiencies in Subjects with Celiac Disease			
At Diagnosis	**GFD**	**GFD Products**	**Long-Term GFD**
Calorie/protein			
Fiber	Fiber	Fiber	Fiber
Iron	Iron	Iron	
Calcium	Calcium		
Vitamin D	Vitamin D		
Magnesium	Magnesium		
Zinc			
Folate, niacin, vitamin B12	Folate, niacin, vitamin B12	Folate, niacin, vitamin B12	Folate, niacin, vitamin B12
Riboflavin	Riboflavin	Riboflavin	Riboflavin

Numerous studies focus their attention specifically on the nutrient intakes of CD children and adolescents on GFD. Mariani *et al.* [21] studied the nutritional habits of 47 adolescents (aged 10–20 years) affected by CD, by means of a three-day alimentary diary. A comparison with the Italian and American recommended daily allowance (RDAs) was done for the intakes of macronutrients, fiber, iron and calcium. The results showed that CD subjects followed a high-protein and high-lipid diet with low intakes of carbohydrates, iron, calcium and fiber compared to the recommended daily intakes. Furthermore, Hopman *et al.* [22] studied the nutrient intake of 37 adolescents with CD (aged 13–16 years) following a strict GFD and compared the intakes with a control group in the same age category. In the CD group, the intake of saturated fat was significantly higher than recommended by both the American and Dutch RDAs; the intake of fiber and iron was significantly lower than recommended. Furthermore, the comparison between the two groups showed that the intake of fiber and iron was lower in the CD group compared to controls ($p < 0.05$). Öhlund *et al.* [23] conducted a study in 2010 on 30 children aged 4–17 years with CD and on GFD, using a five-day food record. High intakes of saturated fat and sucrose and low intakes of dietary fiber, vitamin D and magnesium compared to recommendations (New Nordic Nutrition Recommendations, 2004) was observed.

An elegantly conducted study by Zuccotti *et al.* compared the dietary intake of CD children on GFD to a group of healthy children (healthy controls, HC) and evaluated the contribution of commercially available GFPs on the observed nutritional intake [24]. The study showed that the daily intake of vitamin D was significantly lower in the CD compared to the HC group (vitamin D median value 3.1 μg + 0.6 *vs.* 3.1 μg + 2.8, $p < 0.01$). With regards to macronutrients, the intake of simple sugars, fats and protein exceeded the national recommendations for health in both the CD and HC groups. The total daily energy intake was significantly higher in the CD group compared to HCs (8961.8 KJ day^{-1} *vs.* 5761.0 KJ day^{-1}; $p < 0.001$). In the CD group, the carbohydrate-derived energy was higher, while the lipid-derived energy was lower, compared to the HC group. Protein-derived energy did not differ between the two groups. In the CD group, the contribution of commercially available GFPs on daily energy intake was studied. The main finding was that these products provided 36.3% of the total daily energy intake (3253.1 KJ day^{-1} out of 8961.8 KJ day^{-1}) in these patients. Analyzing the contribution of the macronutrients derived from GFPs on the total daily energy intake, it was observed that protein derived from GFPs accounted for 7.3% of the total energy derived from protein, representing 18% of total daily energy intake. With regards to lipids, GFPs contributed a median of 12.9 g day^{-1} of the median total daily fat intake of 73.0 g, which is equivalent to 17.7% of energy from fat. Furthermore, Mariani *et al.* [21] conducted a nutritional analysis of children with CD. The author found that children complying with a strict GFD had significantly greater nutritional imbalance in their diet than did children cheating on their GFD. More troubling, the incidence of children who were overweight or obese was more frequent (72%) in the strict GFD group compared with the children not following a strict GFD (51%) and healthy age-matched controls (47%). A study conducted by Ferrara *et al.* [25] compared the caloric intake and fat consumption of 50 children with CD following a GFD with 50 healthy children. A significant increase in fat consumption was observed in children with CD compared to healthy children (72.5 + 37.2 g *vs.* 52.9 + 35.4 g per 100 g of food, $p < 0.008$). Furthermore, a significant difference in fat intake was observed between the two groups (10.21 + 3.15 g per 100 g of food in CD group *vs.* 7.46 + 2.91 g/100 g in control group, $p = 0.004$).

3. Effects of Gluten-Free Diet on Anthropometric Parameters

The scientific literature on anthropometric parameters in children with CD on GFD provide contrasting data. On the one hand, there is evidence that good compliance with GFD is associated with a positive effect on anthropometric parameters, including: the reduction of fat and the recovery of lean body mass [26], normalization of body mass index (BMI) in both previously underweight and overweight subjects [27] and acceleration of linear growth [28]. A study conducted in children with CD and obesity at diagnosis showed a significant reduction in BMI after 12 months of GFD [29]. Another study conducted by Brambilla *et al.* found a lower frequency of being overweight and of obesity in children with CD, both at diagnosis and during GFD, compared to healthy controls [30]. Even though the frequency of being overweight and of obesity in the CD group increased on GFD, it remained lower than observed in the general population.

On the other hand, there are also studies that suggest that GFD may have a negative effect on body composition and anthropometric parameters in subjects with CD [31]. Mariani *et al.* [21] first reported the high prevalence of being overweight and of obesity in CD adolescents on GFD; the authors found that more than 50% of CD adolescents were overweight during GFD. However, in the latter paper, the authors used a relative body weight >110%, rather than BMI, to define being overweight, probably leading to an overestimation of being overweight. Furthermore, a study conducted by Valletta *et al.* showed that the frequency of being overweight in children with CD was nearly doubled after one year of GFD [32]. Potential explanations for the undesirable weight gain and obesity observed in these studies are possible overfeeding as the intestinal mucosa heals, consumption of less complex carbohydrates and fiber and more sugars, proteins and saturated fats in GFD. The conflicting data may in part be caused by differences in the timing of anthropometric assessment. Many children with CD, after introduction of GFD, may initially gain excessive weight and only thereafter start to show catch-up growth and normalization of weight. Even though the effect of GFD on body weight and BMI remains a controversial issue, it remains fundamental for pediatricians to be aware of the possible nutritional consequences of GFD for which early recognition can be crucial in the prevention of obesity-related complications.

4. Dietary Advices for a Nutritionally Adequate and Balanced Diet in Children with Celiac Disease

4.1. Education and Compliance

The first step towards a balanced diet starts from early education on CD and GFD, possibly provided by a skilled dietitian and/or by a physician with expert knowledge in CD. The diet is complicated and can be overwhelming if not presented using a thorough and proactive approach. Early education is fundamental to promote adherence to GFD. In fact, studies focusing on compliance to GFD indicate that adherence is compromised by a number of factors, including a lack of education and continued support by a physician and dietitian [33,34]. In a study conducted by Charalampopoulos *et al.* on determinants of the adherence of GFD in children with CD, baseline education was one of the main determinant factors influencing compliance, suggesting the importance for frequent reinforcement and an accurate explanation of dietary recommendations [34].

4.2. Dietary Intake

In CD children on GFD, the recommended distribution of daily calorie intake for a healthy and balanced diet does not differ from that recommended to the general population. According to the dietary reference intake values (DRI), the total daily dietary calories should be ideally obtained as 55% from complex and simple carbohydrates, 15% from dietary protein and 25%–30% or less from lipids. The intake of unsaturated fat (monounsaturated and polyunsaturated) should be preferred. Monounsaturated and polyunsaturated fatty acids should provide more than 15% and 10% of total calories, respectively. They are found in foods, such as vegetable oils, nuts, seeds and fish high in lipid content, such as salmon, trout and herring. Thus, it is important to inform and recommend children with CD on the ideal distribution of the daily calorie intake.

4.3. Gluten-Free Foods

It is advisable to prefer consumption of naturally GF foods, since it has been shown that they are more balanced and complete under both the macro- and micro-nutrient point of view. In fact, these foods are considered to have a higher nutritional value in terms of energy provision, lipid composition and vitamin content as opposed to the commercially purified GF products. Within the range of naturally GF foods, it is preferable to consume those rich in iron and folic acid, such as leafy vegetables, legumes, fish and meat. During explanation of naturally GF foods to patients, it is a good approach for healthcare professionals to bear in mind the local food habits and recipes of each country. This may provide tailored dietary advice, improving acceptance and compliance to GFD. Furthermore, increasing awareness on the availability of the local naturally GF foods may help promote their consumption, resulting in a more balanced and economically advantageous diet. Indeed, these aspects should always be addressed during dietary counseling. With regards to the commercially purified GFPs, it is recommended to pay special attention to the labeling and chemical composition. In European countries, the currently accepted definition of GF is the one designed by Codex Alimentarius (the gluten-free certification organization, 2007) [35]. The term "gluten-free" refers only to foods containing less than 20 ppm of gluten. In addition, the claim "very low gluten" is used for foods, such as bread, produced using cereals that have been specially processed to remove most of the gluten and containing less than 30 mg daily. Furthermore, some GFPs are enriched/fortified with vitamins and/or minerals, thus the choice of these products is preferred, to prevent the deficiencies associated with GFD, mentioned above. Clear labeling of GFPs and education of CD patients on how to interpret them is fundamental to helping CD subjects make safer and more informed food choices.

4.4. Pseudo-Cereals and Minor-Cereals

Pseudo-cereals, such as amaranth, quinoa and buckwheat, and other minor cereals represent a healthy alternative to frequently used ingredients in gluten-free products. They are a good source of carbohydrates, protein, dietary fiber, vitamins and polyunsaturated fatty acids [36]. In fact, the fiber content in these grains ranges from seven to 10 g/100 g [37], which is higher compared to those of other plant foods and cereals and approximately the same as the content in wheat (fiber 9.5 g/100 g). Furthermore, they are a valid source of protein, as their content is superior to that of wheat in terms of the quantity and quality of proteins: in particular, lysine, arginine, histidine, methionine and cysteine can be found in high amounts [38,39]. Although the lipid content of pseudo-cereals is higher compared to other plant foods, they are characterized by a higher content of unsaturated fatty acids, in particular, α-linolenic acid [40,41], beneficial for the prevention of cardiovascular diseases. In addition, higher concentrations of folic acid have been found in quinoa (78.1 μg/100 g) and amaranth (102 μg/100 g) with respect to wheat (40 μg/100 g). Furthermore, both amaranth and quinoa are also good sources of riboflavin, vitamin C and vitamin E [42]. In addition, pseudo-cereals permit a wider variety of foods, broadening the choice for CD children when selecting foods. Under the economic point of view, these grains offer a less expensive alternative with respect to standard gluten-free choices; also, this aspect could help increase dietary compliance by reducing the economic burden of the diet [43]. The nutritional advantages of pseudo-cereals are listed in Table 3.

Table 3. Nutritional advantages of pseudo-cereals (amaranth, buckwheat and quinoa).

Nutritional Characteristics of Amaranth, Buckwheat and Quinoa
High fiber content, 7–10 g/100 g, approximately the same as wheat fiber 9.5 g/100 g.
High protein content, 10.9%–15.2% of dry mass *vs.* 11.7% of dry mass in wheat.
High quality amino acids: lysine, arginine, histidine, methionine and cysteine.
Source of unsaturated fatty acids, in particular, α-linolenic acid.
High content of folic acid: quinoa and amaranth, 78.1 μg/100 g and 102 μg/100 g, respectively, *vs.* 40 μg/100 g in wheat.
Source of vitamins: B2, B6, riboflavin, vitamin C and E.
Source of minerals: the content is twice as high as in other cereals.

4.5. Oats

The inclusion of oats in the GFD has been, for many years, and still is a matter of debate, because it was thought that avenin (the storage protein found in oats) was also toxic to CD patients. Moreover, attention has been focused on the issue of the frequent cross-contamination of oats with gluten-containing grains. Studies have demonstrated that when consumed in moderation, oats free from cross-contamination are well tolerated by most children [44,45]. Under the nutritional point of view, oats represent a good source of iron, dietary fiber, thiamin and zinc and, in addition, have a good palatability [46]. A study conducted by Størsund *et al.* in CD children suggests that oats may improve the nutritional value of GFD and, in view of the good palatability, may also help increase compliance [47]. Recently, Lee *et al.* demonstrated that adding three servings of gluten-free alternative grains, including oats, positively impacts the nutrient profile (fiber, thiamin, riboflavin, niacin, folate and iron) of the grain portion of the gluten-free diet [48].

4.6. Vitamins and Minerals

Meat, fish, fruit and vegetables are an important natural source of vitamins, minerals and trace elements. In view of the possible micronutrient deficiencies associated with GFPs, an appropriate consumption of these foods should be advised in children with CD. In particular, fruit and vegetables are low in energy and rich in vitamins and minerals; moreover, they contain phytochemicals and antioxidant compounds that exert a protective effect against diseases associated with oxidative damage [49]. The intake of at least five portions of fruit and vegetables a day should be recommended in children with CD. Minerals (calcium, phosphorus, sodium, potassium, chloride and magnesium) and trace elements (iron, zinc and selenium) are also contained in a significant amount in pseudo-cereals, in which the content can be twice as high as in other cereals. For example, in teff, iron and calcium contents (11–33 mg/100 g and 100–150 mg/100 g, respectively) are higher than those of wheat, barley, sorghum and rice.

4.7. Nutritional Follow-Up

Continuous long-term follow-up is crucial to promote adherence to GFD and for early identification of nutritional deficiencies and/or metabolic imbalances. Ideally, a skilled dietitian with knowledge in CD and GFD should be an integral part of the healthcare team. A child's nutritional status should be accurately assessed at diagnosis and at each follow-up, which ideally should be performed at six months post commencement of GFD and then annually, post-diagnosis. The evaluation of nutritional status should start from a thorough and accurate dietary history and include the assessment of anthropometric parameters (weight, height and body mass index). Adherence to GFD should be assessed, and information on how to safely broaden food choices and interpret food labeling should be given. Early identification and correction of nutritional deficiencies should be regularly addressed. Table 4 summarizes the key points of nutritional follow-up in children with CD.

Table 4. Recommended timing for nutritional follow-up. BMI: body mass index.

Nutritional Follow-Up	
When?	**How?**
Diagnosis 6 months post commencement of GFD Annually post diagnosis	Accurate dietary history Evaluation of nutritional status Anthropometric parameters, (weight, height, BMI) Physical examination (attention to signs of malnutrition)

Figure 1. Schematic representation of proposed approach to a nutritionally adequate and balanced gluten-free diet.

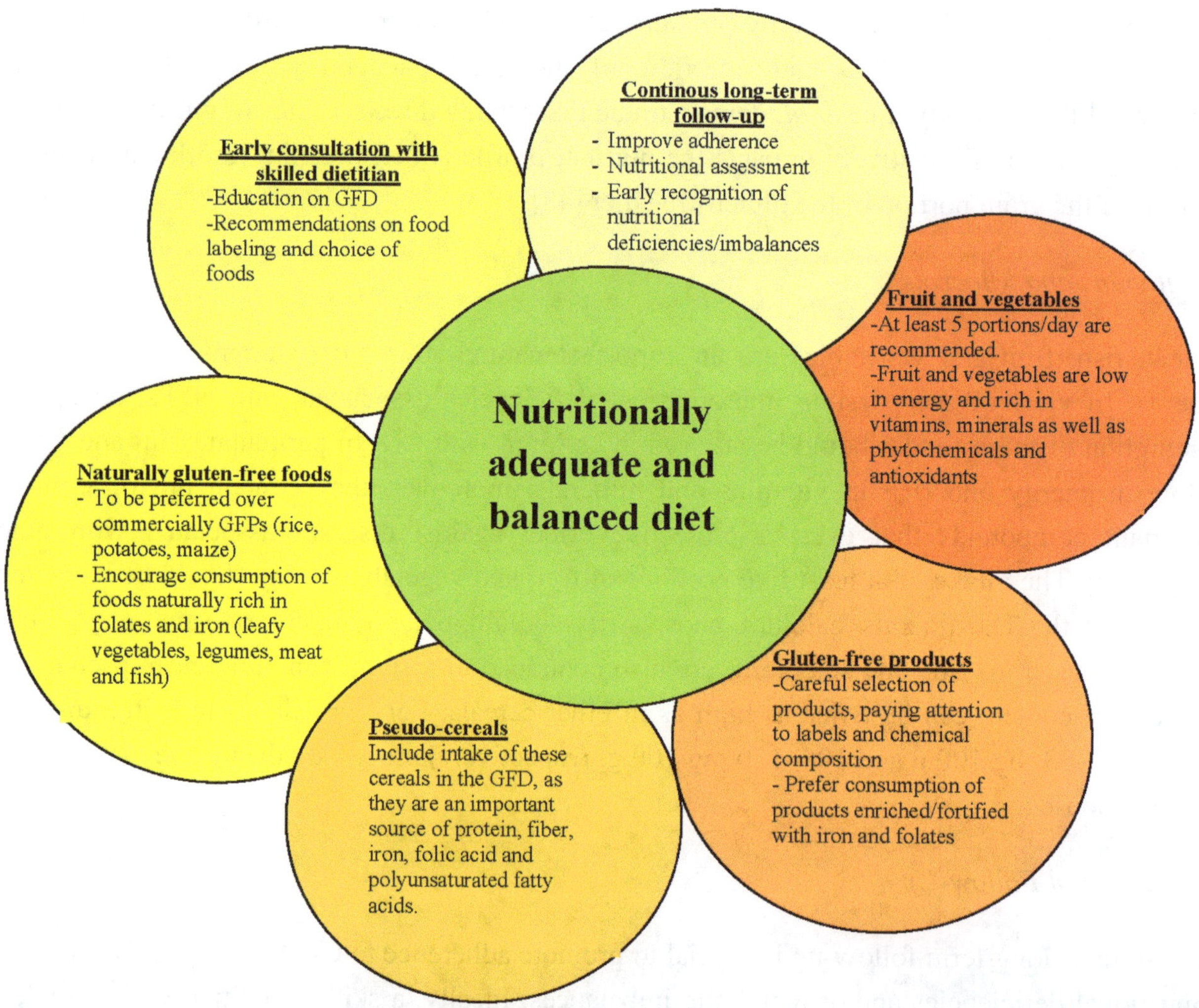

5. Conclusions

Gluten-free diet, the only available treatment for CD, if not carried out with attention, may paradoxically lead to nutritional imbalances, which should be avoided, particularly at the pediatric age, the phase of maximal growth and development. Increasing awareness on the possible nutritional deficiencies associated with GFD may help healthcare professionals and families tackle the issue by starting from early education on GFD and clear dietary advice on how to choose the most appropriate gluten-free foods. Figure 1 summarizes, by means of a schematic representation, a proposed approach towards a nutritionally adequate and balanced gluten-free diet. Further studies on the technological and nutritional properties of the alternative cereals as wheat replacements are needed to confirm their role in improving the intake of protein, iron, calcium and fiber and reducing nutritional deficiencies in children with CD. Their role in the economic burden of the diet and their effect on compliance should also be further investigated. Furthermore, a promising field for gluten-free diet is food biotechnologies. By means of this science, it would be worth considering genetically modifying the amino acid sequence of gluten storage proteins, in order to make them free of those domains high in prolines and glutamines, which are responsible for the toxicity.

References

1. Sjöström, H.; Lundin, K.E.; Molberg, O.; Körner, R.; McAdam, S.N.; Anthonsen, D.; Quarsten, H.; Norén, O.; Roepstorff, P.; Thorsby, E.; *et al.* Identification of a gliadin T-cell epitope in celiac disease: General importance of gliadin deaminidation for intestinal T cell recognition. *Scand. J. Immunol.* **1998**, *48*, 111–115.
2. Maiuri, L.; Ciacci, C.; Ricciardelli, I.; Vacca, L.; Raia, V.; Auricchio, S.; Picard, J.; Osman, M.; Quarantino, S.; Londei, M. Association between innate response to gliadin and activation of pathogenic T cells in coeliac disease. *Lancet* **2003**, *362*, 30–37.
3. Mowat, A.M. Coeliac disease—A meeting point for genetics, immunology and protein chemistry. *Lancet* **2003**, *361*, 1290–1292.
4. Ciacci, C.; Cirillo, M.; Cavallaro, R.; Mazzacca, G. Long-term follow-up of celiac adults on gluten-free diet: Prevalence and correlates of intestinal damage. *Digestion* **2002**, *66*, 178–185.
5. Alvarez-Jubete, L.; Arendt, E.K.; Gallagher, E. Nutritive value and chemical composition of pseudocereals as gluten-free ingredients. *Int. J. Food Sci. Nutr.* **2009**, *60*, 240–257.
6. Vega-Gàlvez, A.; Miranda, M.; Vergara, J.; Uribe, E.; Puente, L.; Martìnez, E.A. Nutrition facts and functional potential of quinoa (*Chenopodium quinoa* willd.), an ancient Andean grain: A review. *J. Sci. Food Agric.* **2010**, *90*, 2541–2547.
7. Thompson, T. Thiamin, riboflavin, and niacin contents of the gluten-free diet: Is there cause for concern? *J. Am. Diet. Assoc.* **1999**, *99*, 858–862.
8. Thompson, T. Folate, iron, and dietary fiber contents of the gluten-free diet. *J. Am. Diet. Assoc.* **2000**, *100*, 1389–1396.

9. Hallert, C.; Grant, C.; Grehn, S.; Grännö, C.; Hultén, S.; Midhagen, G.; Strön, M.; Svensson, H.; Valdimarsson, T. Evidence of poor vitamin status in celiac patients on a gluten-free diet for 10 years. *Aliment. Pharmacol. Ther.* **2002**, *16*, 1333–1339.
10. Segura, M.E.; Rosell, C.M. Chemical composition and starch digestibility of different gluten-free breads. *Plant Foods Hum. Nutr.* **2011**, *66*, *3*, 224–230.
11. Jenkins, D.J.; Thorne, M.J.; Wolever, T.M.; Jenkins, A.L.; Rao, A.V.; Thompson, L.U. The effect of starch-protein interaction in wheat on the glycaemic response and rate of *in vitro* digestion. *Am. J. Clin. Nutr.* **1987**, *45*, 946–951.
12. Berti, C.; Riso, P.; Monti, L.D.; Porrini, M. *In vitro* starch digestibility and *in vivo* glucose response of gluten-free foods and their gluten counterparts. *Eur. J. Nutr.* **2004**, *43*, 198–204.
13. Caponio, F.; Summo, C.; Clodoveo, M.L.; Pasqualone, A. Evaluation of the nutritional quality of the lipid fraction of gluten-free biscuits. *Eur. Food Res. Technol.* **2008**, *223*, 135–139.
14. Thompson, T.; Dennis, M.; Higgins, L.A.; Lee, A.R.; Sharrett, M.K. Gluten-free diet survey: Are Americans with celiac disease consuming recommended amounts of fibre, iron, calcium and grain food? *J. Hum. Nutr. Diet.* **2005**, *18*, 163–169.
15. Wild, D.; Robins, G.G.; Burley, V.J.; Howdle, P.D. Evidence of high sugar intake and low fiber and mineral intake in the gluten–free diet. *Aliment. Pharmacol. Ther.* **2010**, *32*, 573–581.
16. Kemppainen, T.; Uusitupa, M.; Janatuinen, E.; Järvinen, R.; Julkunen, R.; Pikkarainen, P. Intakes of nutrients and nutritional status in celiac patients. *Scand. J. Gastroenterol.* **1995**, *30*, 575–579.
17. Kinsey, L.; Burden, S.T.; Bannerman, E. A dietary survey to determine if patients with celiac disease are meeting current healthy eating guidelines and how their diet compares to that of British general population. *Eur. J. Clin. Nutr.* **2008**, *62*, 1333–1342.
18. Bardella, M.T.; Fredella, C.; Prampolini, L.; Molteni, N.; Giunta, A.M.; Bianchi, P.A. Body composition and dietary intakes in adult celiac disease patients consuming a strict gluten-free diet. *Am. J. Clin. Nutr.* **2000**, *72*, 937–939.
19. Jameson, S. Coeliac, insulin-like growth factor, bone mineral density, and zinc. *Scand. J. Gastroenterol.* **2000**, *35*, 894–896.
20. Kupper, C. Dietary guidelines and implementation for celiac disease. *Gastroenterology* **2005**, *128*, S121–S127.
21. Mariani, P.; Viti, M.G.; Montuori, M.; La Vecchia, A.; Cipolletta, E.; Calvani, L.; Bonamico, M. The gluten-free diet: A nutritional risk factor for adolescents with celiac disease? *J. Pediatr. Gastroenterol. Nutr.* **1998**, *27*, 519–523.
22. Hopman, E.G.; Le Cessie, S.; von Blomberg, B.M.; Mearin, M.L. Nutritional management of the gluten-free diet in young people with coeliac disease in The Netherlands. *J. Paediatr. Gastroenterol. Nutr.* **2006**, *43*, 102–108.
23. Öhlund, K.; Olsson, C.; Hernell, O.; Öhlund, L. Dietary shortcomings in children on a gluten-free diet. *J. Hum. Nutr. Diet.* **2010**, *23*, 294–300.
24. Zuccotti, G.; Fabiano, V.; Dilillo, D.; Picca, M.; Cravidi, C.; Brambilla, P. Intakes of nutrients in Italian children with celiac disease and the role of commercially available gluten-free products. *J. Hum. Nutr. Diet.* **2013**, *26*, 436–444.

25. Ferrara, P.; Cicala, M.; Tiberi, E.; Spadaccio, C.; Marcella, L.; Gatto, A.; Calzolari, P.; Castelluccio, G. High fat consumption in children with celiac disease. *Acta Gastroenterol. Belg.* **2009**, *72*, 296–300.
26. Barera, G.; Mora, S.; Brambilla, P.; Ricotti, A.; Menni, L.; Beccio, S.; Bianchi, C. Body composition in children with celiac disease and the efffects of a gluten-free diet: A prospective case-control study. *Am. J. Clin. Nutr.* **2000**, *72*, 71–75.
27. Cheng, J.; Brar, P.S.; Lee, A.R.; Green, P.H.; Body mass index in celiac disease: Beneficial effect of a gluten-free diet. *J. Clin. Gastroenterol.* **2010**, *44*, 267–271.
28. Radlović, N.; Mladenović, M.; Leković, Z.; Zivanović, D.; Brdar, R.; Radlović, V.; Ristić, D.; Pavlović, M.; Stojsić, Z.; Vuletić, B.; *et al.* Effect of gluten-free diet on the growth and nutritional status of children with coeliac disease. *Srp. Arh. Celok. Lek.* **2009**, *137*, 632–637.
29. Venkatasubramani, N.; Telega, G.; Werlin, S.L. Obesity in pediatric celiac disease. *J. Pediatr. Gastroenterol. Nutr.* **2010**, *51*, 295–297.
30. Brambilla, P.; Picca, M.; Dilillo, D.; Meneghin, F.; Cravidi, C.; Tischer, M.C.; Vivaldo, T.; Bedogni, G.; Zuccotti, G.V. Changes of body mass index in celiac children on a gluten-free diet. *Nutr. Metab. Cardiovasc. Dis.* **2013**, *23*, 177–182.
31. Kabbani, T.A.; Goldberg, A.; Kelly, C.P.; Pallav, K.; Tariq, S.; Peer, A.; Hasen, J.; Dennis, M.; Leffler, D.A. Body mass index and the risk of obesity in coeliac disease treated with gluten-free diet. *Aliment. Pharmacol. Ther.* **2012**, *35*, 723–729.
32. Valletta, E.; Fornaro, M.; Cipolli, M.; Conte, S.; Bissolo, F.; Danchielli, C. Celiac disease and obesity: Need for nutritional follow-up after diagnosis. *Eur. J. Clin. Nutr.* **2010**, *64*, 1371–1372.
33. Roma, E.; Roubani, A.; Kolia, E.; Panayiotou, J.; Zellos, A.; Syriopoulou, V.P. Dietary compliance and life style of children with celiac disease. *J. Hum. Nutr. Diet.* **2010**, *23*, 176–182.
34. Charalampopoulos, D.; Panayiotou, J.; Chouliaras, G.; Zellos, A.; Kyritsi, E.; Roma, E. Determinants of adherence to gluten-free diet in Greek children with celiac disease: A cross-sectional study. *Eur. J. Clin. Nutr.* **2013**, *67*, 615–619.
35. Codex Alimentarius Commission. *Draft Revised Codex Standard for Foods for Special Dietary Use for Persons Intolerant to Gluten Joint FAO/WHO Food Standards Programme*; WHO: Geneva, Switzerland, 2007.
36. Dyner, L.; Drago, S.R.; PiÑeiro, A.; Sànchez, H.; Gonzàlez, R.; Villaamil, E.; Valencia, M.E. Composition and potential contribution of iron, calcium and zinc of bread and pasta made with wheat and amaranth flours. *Arch. Latinoam. Nutr.* **2007**, *57*, 69–77.
37. Ötles, S.; Cagindi, Ö. Cereal based functional foods and nutraceuticals. *Acta Sci. Pol. Technol. Aliment.* **2006**, *5*, 107–112.
38. Gorinstein, S.; Pawelzik, E.; Delgado-Licon, E.; Haruenkit, R.; Weisz, M.; Trakhtenberg, S. Characterization of pseudocereal and cereal proteins by protein and amino acid analyses. *J. Sci. Food Agric.* **2002**, *82*, 886–891.
39. Abdel-Aal, E.S.M.; Hucl, P. Amino acid composition and *in vitro* protein digestibility of selected ancient wheats and their products. *J. Food Comp. Anal.* **2002**, *15*, 737–747.
40. Yànez, E.; Zacarìas, I.; Granger, D.; Vàsquez, M.; Estèvez, A.M. Chemical and nutritional characterization of amaranthus (*Amaranthus cruentus*). *Arch. Latinoam. Nutr.* **1994**, *44*, 57–62.

41. Adeyeye, A.; Ajewole, K. Chemical composition and fatty acid profiles of cereals in Nigeria. *Food Chem.* **1992**, *44*, 41–44.
42. Coulter, L.; Lorenz, K. Quinoa-composition, nutritional value, food applications. *Lebensm. WissTechnol.* **1990**, *23*, 203–207.
43. Stevens, L.; Rashid, M. Gluten-free and regular foods: A cost comparison. *Can. J. Diet. Pract. Res*. **2008**, *69*, 147–150.
44. Hoffenberg, E.J.; Haas, J.; Drescher, A.; Barnhurst, R.; Osberg, I.; Bao, F.; Eisenbarth, G. A trial of oats in children with newly diagnosed celiac disease. *J. Pediatr.* **2000**, *137*, 361–366.
45. Höberg, L.; Laurin, P.; Faith-Magnusson, K.; Grant, C.; Grodzinsky, E.; Jansson, G.; Ascher, H.; Browaldh, L.; Hammersjö, J.A.; Lindberg, E.; *et al.* Oats to children with newly diagnosed celiac disease: A randomized double-blind study. *Gut* **2004**, *53*, 649–654.
46. Sadiq Butt, M.; Tahir-Nadeem, M.; Khan, M.K.; Shabir, R.; Butt, M.S. Oat: Unique among the cereals. *Eur. J. Nutr*. **2008**, *47*, 68–79.
47. Størsund, S.; Hulthèn, L.R.; Lenner, R.A. Beneficial effects of oats in the gluten-free diet of adults with special reference to nutrient status, symptoms and subjective experiences. *Br. J. Nutr*. **2003**, *90*, 101–107.
48. Lee, A.R.; Ng, D.L.; Dave, E.; Ciaccio, E.J.; Green, P.H. The effect of substituting alternative grains in the diet on the nutritional profile of the gluten-free diet. *J. Hum. Nutr. Diet*. **2009**, *22*, 359–363.
49. Stevenson, D.E.; Hurst, R.D. Polyphenolic phytochemicals—Just antioxidants or much more? *Cell Mol. Life Sci*. **2007**, *64*, 2900–2916.

14

Is Dietitian Use Associated with Celiac Disease Outcomes?

SriHari Mahadev, Suzanne Simpson, Benjamin Lebwohl, Suzanne K. Lewis, Christina A. Tennyson and Peter H. R. Green *

Celiac Disease Center, Columbia University College of Physicians and Surgeons, 180 Fort Washington Avenue, Suite 934, New York, NY 10032, USA; E-Mails: sm3455@columbia.edu (S.M.); sms2246@columbia.edu (S.S.); bl114@columbia.edu (B.L.); skl3@columbia.edu (S.K.L.); ct2398@columbia.edu (C.A.T.)

* Author to whom correspondence should be addressed; E-Mail: pg11@columbia.edu;

Abstract: A gluten-free diet (GFD) is the treatment for celiac disease (CD), but due to its complexity, dietitian referral is uniformly recommended. We surveyed patients with CD to determine if dietitian use is associated with quality of life, symptom severity, or GFD adherence. The survey utilized three validated CD-specific instruments: the CD quality of life (CD-QOL), CD symptom index (CSI) and CD adherence test (CDAT). Four hundred and thirteen patients with biopsy-proven CD were eligible for inclusion. The majority (77%) were female and mean BMI was 24.1. Over three-quarters of patients (326, 79%) had seen a dietitian, however, 161 (39%) had seen a dietitian only once. Age, sex, and education level were not associated with dietitian use; nor was BMI (24.6 *vs*. 24.0, $p = 0.45$). On multivariate analysis, adjusting for age gender, education, duration of disease, and body mass index, dietitian use was not associated with CD-QOL, CSI, or CDAT scores. Our survey did not show an association between dietitian use and symptom severity, adherence, or quality of life. Delay in diagnosis was associated with poorer outcomes. This is a preliminary study with several limitations, and further prospective analysis is needed to evaluate the benefits and cost-effectiveness of dietitian-referral in the care of celiac disease patients.

Keywords: celiac disease; dietary services; quality of life; quality improvement

---

1. Introduction

Celiac disease (CD) is a common multi-system autoimmune disease, affecting approximately 1% of people worldwide [1]. Predisposed individuals develop an immune response to gluten, a protein found in the cereal grains: wheat, barley and rye. Autoimmune intestinal damage is the cardinal feature of CD, and typically involves villous atrophy, crypt hyperplasia, and increased intraepithelial lymphocytes [2]. Symptoms may be subclinical, varying from gastrointestinal upset to severe malabsorption [3,4]. Skin, nervous system, and multisystem involvement is also recognized. Strict avoidance of gluten-containing foods can reverse both enteric and extra-intestinal manifestations of the disease.

CD is unique in that its treatment consists of a dietary intervention: lifelong exclusion of gluten. A gluten-free diet (GFD) is highly effective at improving symptoms of CD in the majority of patients [5]. Nevertheless, a significant proportion remains symptomatic, and lack of strict adherence to GFD is the primary cause [6]. Those patients with celiac disease who follow a GFD frequently have persistent villous atrophy which may result from persistent gluten contamination and, in rare cases, can predispose patients to serious sequelae including T-cell lymphoma [7].

Although straightforward in principle, strict avoidance of gluten is challenging in practice. Gluten-containing products are ubiquitous and contamination may occur both consciously and unintentionally [8]. Poor labeling can make it difficult to determine which foods are gluten free, and options may be limited when eating out and traveling [9]. Moreover, a GFD is significantly more expensive, and may be deficient in certain nutrients, when compared to a regular diet [10,11]. Given the complexity of maintaining a strict GFD, multiple guidelines recommend dietetic referral for patients diagnosed with CD [12–15]. Dietitian involvement was recommended in the National Institutes of Health (NIH) Consensus Development Conference on celiac disease (2004) [16]. There is evidence that when asked to choose among several referral options, patients themselves express a preference for dietetic follow-up [17]. Nevertheless, availability of expert dietetic counselors is limited and may impact upon patient outcomes [18]. Membership in celiac advocacy groups, and regular dietetic follow-up has previously been reported to be correlate with higher rates of GFD adherence [19,20]. However there have been no studies that have directly examined the impact of dietitian use on celiac disease outcomes in the United States. As such, we sought to determine if dietitian use was associated with quality of life, symptom severity, or GFD adherence in patients with celiac disease.

2. Methods

Approval was obtained from the Institutional Review Board of Columbia University Medical Center prior to initiation of the study.

Adults (≥18 years of age) with celiac disease were recruited to participate in a survey either via email or in-person. A link to an online questionnaire, hosted by SurveyMonkey, was distributed by the Celiac Disease Center of Columbia University to an email list of patients affiliated with the Center. In addition, the questionnaire was administered to attendees at celiac support group conferences in Iowa, California, and New York, and patients additionally completed the questionnaire on-paper during an office visit. Data was collected between November 2010 and July 2011. Prior to distribution, the questionnaire was administered to a group of ten patients and subsequently modified for clarity.

The survey consisted of questions on demographics, celiac disease onset, symptoms, and dietitian use. It also included three validated celiac disease-specific instruments to assess quality of life, disease activity, and GFD adherence respectively [21–23]. Patients were asked how many times they had seen a dietitian: never, once, or more than once. Patients were excluded from the analysis if they did not have biopsy-proven celiac disease, or omitted the items on gender, age, or dietitian use.

The celiac disease-specific quality of life instrument (CD-QOL) was used to assess quality of life [21]. This validated instrument consists of 20 questions across four clinically relevant subscales (celiac disease-related limitations, dysphoria, health concerns, and inadequate treatment), and asks the respondent to indicate the frequency of celiac disease-related symptoms over the previous 30 days. The questions are graded on a 5-point Likert scale labeled 1 through 5, where 1 = not at all, 2 = slightly, 3 = moderately, 4 = quite a bit, and 5 = a great deal. The responses were reverse-coded and summed, with a higher score (up to a maximum of 100) suggestive of higher quality of life. No clear cut-off point has been established to dichotomize CD-QOL scores; hence membership in the lowest quartile of CD-QOL was taken to indicate poorer quality of life.

The Celiac Symptom Index (CSI) was employed to assess celiac disease-specific symptom severity [23]. The CSI consists of 16 questions on a 5-point Likert scale; with scores ≤30 and ≥45 suggestive of clinical remission and ongoing active disease respectively. For the purpose of our analysis; a single cutoff of ≥35 (suggestive of ongoing disease) was used to dichotomize patients.

The Celiac Disease Dietary Adherence Test (CDAT) was used to assess adherence to a GFD [22]. This validated 7-question instrument employs a 5-point Likert scale, with additive scores ranging from 7 to 35, where higher scores indicate worse adherence. For the purposes of dichotomization, scores ≥13 were taken to be indicative of poor adherence.

Univariate analysis was used to identify associations between demographics, dietitian use, and CD-QOL, CSI, and CDAT. The Chi-square and Fisher exact tests were used to compare proportions of categorical variables. The Mann-Whitney U test was used to compare continuous variables. Logistic regression was performed to develop a multivariate model identifying variables predictive of three outcomes as determined by these validated scores: poor quality of life, high symptom activity, and poor adherence. Two-sided *p*-values <0.05 were considered significant. All statistical calculations were performed with SAS 9.2 (Cary, NC, USA).

3. Results

3.1. Patient Characteristics

Of 600 respondents, 413 with biopsy-proven celiac disease were eligible for inclusion (Table 1). Roughly equal numbers of patients completed the survey online (47%) *versus* on paper (49%). The majority (77%) of subjects were female, with almost one-quarter over the age of 60 (24%). The cohort was highly educated, with 88% having attained a college degree, and 40% having a graduate or higher degree.

Table 1. Patient characteristics.

	***n* (%)**
Total number	413
Age	
18–30	80 (19)
31–40	67 (16)
41–50	75 (18)
51–60	93 (23)
61–70	67 (16)
>70	31 (8)
Gender	
Male	94 (23)
Female	319 (77)
Educational level	
High school or less	43 (10)
College	197 (48)
Graduate school	167 (40)
Presentation	
Classical	166 (40)
Atypical	204 (49)
None	32 (8)
Years since diagnosis	
<1	55 (13)
1–4	149 (36)
5–10	115 (28)
>10	93 (23)
Delay to diagnosis in years	
<1	51 (12)
1–4	149 (36)
5–10	115 (28)
>10	93 (23)
Mean Body Mass Index	24.1
Symptoms improved on GFD	
Yes	288 (70)
Somewhat	73 (18)
No	28 (7)
Filled in survey	
Online	195 (47)
Paper	204 (49)

3.2. Disease Characteristics

Regarding CD presentation, almost half of patients (49%) reported atypical symptoms of fatigue, anemia or osteoporosis; 40% reported classical diarrhea-predominant symptoms, and 8% reported no symptoms. Most patients' symptoms were either improved (70%) or somewhat improved (13%) with GFD. Mean body mass index (BMI) was in the normal-weight range (24.1). The median time since diagnosis was 5–10 years, and the median delay from onset of symptoms to diagnosis was also 5–10 years.

3.3. Dietitian Use

Of the 413 patients in the analysis, 326 (79%) reported having seen a dietitian, but 161 (39%) had only seen a dietitian once. One hundred and sixty-four patients (40%) agreed with the statement "it is hard to find a dietitian knowledgeable about GFD". One hundred and ninety-one patients (46%) reported gaining weight since starting a GFD. Demographic factors, including age, sex, and education level, were not associated with dietitian use (Table 2). There was no significant difference in BMI between patients who had and had not seen a dietitian (24.0 *vs.* 25.6, $p = 0.45$). Patients who had not seen a dietitian were more likely to agree with the statement "health insurance limits my ability to see a dietitian" (55% *vs.* 43%; $p = 0.04$).

Table 2. Patient characteristics by dietitian use.

	Not seen *n* (%)	**Seen *n* (%)**	*p*
Total number	87 (100)	326 (100)	
Age ≥60	20 (23)	78 (24)	0.96
Female gender	72 (83)	247 (76)	0.21
College educated	75 (86)	289 (89)	0.53
Symptoms improved on GFD	63 (72)	225 (69)	0.54
Mean BMI	25.6	24.0	0.45

3.4. Quality of Life, Disease Activity, and Dietary Adherence

Dietitian use was not associated with CD-QOL, CDAT, or CSI on univariate analysis (Table 3). Multivariate analysis (Table 4) identified two covariates associated with low CD-QOL, indicative of poor quality of life: a long delay (>10 years *vs.* <1 year) from symptom onset to CD diagnosis (OR 3.92, 95% CI 1.45–0.63), and underweight *vs.* normal weight (OR 3.46, 1.12–10.68). Older age (>60) and time since diagnosis (>10 years *vs.* <1 year) were protective for disease activity as measured by CSI (OR 0.35, 95% CI 0.17–0.71 and OR 0.34, 95% CI 0.13–0.87 respectively). Dietitian use was not associated with CD-QOL, CSI, or CDAT scores on multivariate analysis (see Table 4).

Table 3. Mean validated scores and use of a dietitian.

	Not seen	**Seen**	*p*
CD-QOL	75.4	72.6	0.08
CSI	33.5	33.3	0.62
CDAT	12.9	12.1	0.11

Table 4. Multivariate analysis of factors associated with low celiac disease quality of life (CD-QOL), high CD symptom index (CSI), and high CD adherence test (CDAT).

Covariate	Low CD-QOL		High CSI		High CDAT	
	OR	95% CI	OR	95% CI	OR	95% CI
Seen a dietitian	1.49	0.68–3.24	0.86	0.45–1.63	0.85	0.47–1.55
Older age (>60)	0.60	0.26–1.37	0.35	0.17–0.71	0.53	0.28–1.01
Male gender	1.29	0.61–2.72	1.24	0.58–2.64	0.92	0.48–1.77
College educated	3.65	0.97–13.7	1.33	0.53–3.38	0.74	0.32–1.71
Time since diagnosis [1]	0.38	0.13–1.10	0.34	0.13–0.87	0.48	0.20–1.13
Delayed diagnosis [1]	3.92	1.45–10.63	2.08	0.98–4.41	1.05	0.53–2.07
Underweight *vs.* normal	3.46	1.12–10.68	2.52	0.79–8.04	1.90	0.66–5.51
Overweight *vs.* normal	1.31	0.62–2.75	0.60	0.31–1.16	0.66	0.36–1.21
Obese *vs.* normal	0.86	0.33–2.23	0.75	0.32–1.76	0.65	0.29–1.46

[1] >10 years *vs.* <1 year.

4. Discussion

To our knowledge, this is the first study to examine dietitian use and outcomes as measured by validated CD-specific instruments. We were surprised at the lack of association between dietitian use, dietary adherence and quality of life. The study has several limitations, including selection bias, self-reported outcomes, and poor generalizability, however prior literature addressing these issues is similarly limited. While our findings are preliminary, they should provide impetus to further study the role of dietary counseling in CD management.

Several studies have examined dietitian use in CD, with frequently divergent results. Ukkola *et al.* [24] surveyed 698 newly diagnosed CD patients on their perceptions of living with CD, and found no correlation between dietitian follow-up and patients' knowledge of GFD or experience of their disease. A similar proportion of patients in this cohort (76%) had received dietitian counseling as in our sample (79%). The authors note that despite a lack of correlation, patients often requested more detailed dietary counseling when asked to indicate in their own words their wishes/needs, suggesting insufficient dietitian contact.

One outcome measure that has been demonstrated to be associated with dietitian use is improved GFD adherence, but this was not seen in our cohort. Wylie *et al.* [25] concluded in a prospective cohort of 99 patients that annual review within the context of a dietitian-led celiac clinic can significantly improve adherence as well as other nutritional markers. In a systemic review of 38 studies examining factors associated with adherence to GFD, Hall *et al.* [19] also concluded that regular dietetic follow-up and annual review in a dietitian-led clinic can improve adherence. Membership of a patient support group has been associated with adherence, and studies with cohorts recruited from patient support groups trend towards higher adherence rates (66%–90% strict adherence) than clinical samples (42%–91%) [26]. There are several possible reasons why these results might diverge from that of our study. First, dietitian use was common in our study (approaching 80%), leading to a small sample size for patients who had not seen a dietitian, and hence decreased ability to detect a difference. Our cohort was very highly educated, with almost 90% of patients having a college degree or higher qualification, as compared to a US-wide average of

28% [27]. It may be that university-educated patients may have less to gain from dietitian referral: they are more health-literate at baseline, and are better equipped to seek out and utilize information from other sources in addition to their health professional. As such, the high prevalence of highly educated patients in our cohort may have reduced the effect size of dietitian exposure. Hall *et al.* [19] included studies that assessed GFD adherence via a trained nutritionist assessment, which may be more sensitive for differences than use of the self-reported CDAT questionnaire. Last, cultural factors can influence response to dietary interventions. In a cross-sectional survey from 2004, Butterworth *et al.* [20] noted that South Asian patients with CD were much less likely than Caucasians to be members of a support group (53% *vs.* 80%, $p = 0.02$), were more frequently dissatisfied with dietetic advice (30% *vs.* 6%, $p = 0.01$), and exhibited a trend towards poorer dietetic follow-up (31% *vs.* 60%, p = NS). Dietetic follow-up correlated with GFD compliance for Caucasians but not for South Asians in that study. It is unclear to what extent these cultural issues apply to our cohort.

Although dietitian use was common in this study, almost half of these patients had only seen a dietitian once, possibly at diagnosis, falling short of CD treatment guidelines. Guidelines published by several authorities generally recommend annual dietitian review. The American Gastroenterological Association position statement on diagnosis and management of CD advises consultation with an experienced dietitian at initiation of a treatment plan and ongoing evaluation at regular intervals by a health care team including a dietitian [12]. Several other organizations also publish guidelines recommending ongoing dietitian involvement, including the NIH, the United States Department of Health and Human Services Agency for Healthcare Research and Quality, the National Institute for Health and Clinical Excellence in the United Kingdom, and the World Gastroenterology Association [14,16,28,29]. Given a median time since diagnosis of 5–10 years in this cohort, dietitian involvement fell well short of recommendations in a significant proportion of patients and insufficient dietitian follow-up may have contributed to the lack of effect on outcomes.

A long delay of >10 years from symptom onset to diagnosis of CD was associated with poor quality of life in this cohort. Prior studies have addressed the influence of delayed diagnosis on CD outcomes. In a survey of over 1000 patients with CD from Sweden, the mean delay to diagnosis from first symptoms was 9.7 years, and 5.8 years from the first doctor visit [30]. A long delay was associated with lower quality-adjusted life year scores prior to treatment; however delay in diagnosis had no effect on scores following initiation of GFD. The study concluded that untreated CD resulted in poor quality of life, which returned to baseline with treatment. Our findings of persistent quality of life impairment even following initiation of GFD are novel and warrant further study.

The limitations of this study include recruitment from a tertiary referral center (the Celiac Disease Center of Columbia University) and support groups, leading to a cohort that is likely to have greater health literacy than average. The sample size for patients who had not seen a dietitian was low, limiting our power to detect a difference in CD outcomes. The actual response rate of the survey is unable to be determined as the survey link may have been electronically forwarded by subjects to other members of support groups or known contacts with celiac disease. In addition we did not have information on the quality, nor expertise and practice setting of the dietitians used by the respondents.

5. Conclusions

In this survey of patients with celiac disease, more than 20% of respondents had never seen a dietitian, and 39% only saw a dietitian once. Dietitian follow-up fell short of published guidelines, which may relate to insurance access issues. Dietitian exposure was not associated with symptom severity, adherence, or quality of life, while delay in diagnosis was associated with poorer quality of life. Further prospective analysis is needed to evaluate the benefits and cost-effectiveness of dietitian referral in the care of patients with celiac disease.

Acknowledgements

The Celiac Disease Center thanks its supporters for their ongoing contribution.

References

1. Green, P.H.R.; Cellier, C. Celiac disease. *N. Engl. J. Med.* **2007**, *357*, 1731–1743.
2. Oberhuber, G.; Granditsch, G.; Vogelsang, H. The histopathology of coeliac disease: Time for a standardized report scheme for pathologists. *Eur. J. Gastroenterol. Hepatol.* **1999**, *11*, 1185–1194.
3. Corazza, G.R.; Frisoni, M.; Treggiari, E.A.; Valentini, R.A.; Filipponi, C.; Volta, U.; Gasbarrini, G. Subclinical celiac sprue. Increasing occurrence and clues to its diagnosis. *J. Clin. Gastroenterol.* **1993**, *16*, 16–21.
4. Ciacci, C.; Cirillo, M.; Sollazzo, R.; Savino, G.; Sabbatini, F.; Mazzacca, G. Gender and clinical presentation in adult celiac disease. *Scand. J. Gastroenterol.* **1995**, *30*, 1077–1081.
5. Murray, J.A.; Watson, T.; Clearman, B.; Mitros, F. Effect of a gluten-free diet on gastrointestinal symptoms in celiac disease. *Am. J. Clin. Nutr.* **2004**, *79*, 669–673.
6. Abdulkarim, A.S.; Burgart, L.J.; See, J.; Murray, J.A. Etiology of nonresponsive celiac disease: Results of a systematic approach. *Am. J. Gastroenterol.* **2002**, *97*, 2016–2021.
7. Cellier, C.; Delabesse, E.; Helmer, C.; Patey, N.; Matuchansky, C.; Jabri, B.; Macintyre, E.; Cerf-Bensussan, N.; Brousse, N. Refractory sprue, coeliac disease, and enteropathy-associated T-cell lymphoma. French Coeliac Disease Study Group. *Lancet* **2000**, *356*, 203–208.
8. Ciacci, C.; Mazzacca, G. Unintentional gluten ingestion in celiac patients. *Gastroenterology* **1998**, *115*, 243.
9. Zarkadas, M.; Cranney, A.; Case, S.; Molloy, M.; Switzer, C.; Graham, I.D.; Butzner, J.D.; Rashid, M.; Warren, R.E.; Burrows, V. The impact of a gluten-free diet on adults with coeliac disease: Results of a national survey. *J. Hum. Nutr. Diet.* **2006**, *19*, 41–49.
10. Stevens, L.; Rashid, M. Gluten-free and regular foods: A cost comparison. *Can. J. Diet. Pract. Res.* **2008**, *69*, 147–150.

11. Thompson, T.; Dennis, M.; Higgins, L.A.; Lee, A.R.; Sharrett, M.K. Gluten-free diet survey: Are Americans with coeliac disease consuming recommended amounts of fibre, iron, calcium and grain foods? *J. Hum. Nutr. Diet.* **2005**, *18*, 163–169.
12. AGA Institute. AGA Institute Medical Position Statement on the Diagnosis and Management of Celiac Disease. *Gastroenterology* **2006**, *131*, 1977–1980.
13. Centre for Clinical Practice at NICE (UK). *Coeliac Disease: Recognition and Assessment of Coeliac Disease*; National Institute for Health and Clinical Excellence: London, UK, 2009.
14. Bai, J.; Zeballos, E.; Fried, M.; Corazza, G.R.; Schuppan, D.; Farthing, M.; Catassi, C.; Greco, L.; Cohen, H.; Krabshuis, J.H. WGO-OMGE practice guideline celiac disease. *World Gastroenterol. News* **2005**, *10*, 1–8.
15. Hill, I.D.; Dirks, M.H.; Liptak, G.S.; Colletti, R.B.; Fasano, A.; Guandalini, S.; Hoffenberg, E.J.; Horvath, K.; Murray, J.A.; Pivor, M.; Seidman, E.G. North American Society for Pediatric Gastroenterology, Hepatology and Nutrition Guideline for the diagnosis and treatment of celiac disease in children: Recommendations of the North American Society for Pediatric Gastroenterology, Hepatology and Nutrition. *J. Pediatr. Gastroenterol. Nutr.* **2005**, *40*, 1–19.
16. *NIH Consensus Development Conference on Celiac Disease*; U.S. Department of Health and Human Services: Bethesda, MD, USA, 2004.
17. Bebb, J.R.; Lawson, A.; Knight, T.; Long, R.G. Long-term follow-up of coeliac disease—What do coeliac patients want? *Aliment. Pharmacol. Ther.* **2006**, *23*, 827–831.
18. Nelson, M.; Mendoza, N.; McGough, N. A survey of provision of dietetic services for coeliac disease in the UK. *J. Hum. Nutr. Diet.* **2007**, *20*, 403–411.
19. Hall, N.J.; Rubin, G.; Charnock, A. Systematic review: Adherence to a gluten-free diet in adult patients with coeliac disease. *Aliment. Pharmacol. Ther.* **2009**, *30*, 315–330.
20. Butterworth, J.R.; Banfield, L.M.; Iqbal, T.H.; Cooper, B.T. Factors relating to compliance with a gluten-free diet in patients with coeliac disease: Comparison of white Caucasian and South Asian patients. *Clin. Nutr.* **2004**, *23*, 1127–1134.
21. Dorn, S.D.; Hernandez, L.; Minaya, M.T.; Morris, C.B.; Hu, Y.; Leserman, J.; Lewis, S.; Lee, A.; Bangdiwala, S.I.; Green, P.H.R.; Drossman, D.A. The development and validation of a new coeliac disease quality of life survey (CD-QOL). *Aliment. Pharmacol. Ther.* **2010**, *31*, 666–675.
22. Leffler, D.A.; Dennis, M.; Edwards George, J.B.; Jamma, S.; Magge, S.; Cook, E.F.; Schuppan, D.; Kelly, C.P. A simple validated gluten-free diet adherence survey for adults with celiac disease. *Clin. Gastroenterol. Hepatol.* **2009**, *7*, 530–536.
23. Leffler, D.A.; Dennis, M.; Edwards George, J.; Jamma, S.; Cook, E.F.; Schuppan, D.; Kelly, C.P. A validated disease-specific symptom index for adults with celiac disease. *Clin. Gastroenterol. Hepatol.* **2009**, *7*, 1328–1334.
24. Ukkola, A.; Mäki, M.; Kurppa, K.; Collin, P.; Huhtala, H.; Kekkonen, L.; Kaukinen, K. Patients' experiences and perceptions of living with coeliac disease—Implications for optimizing care. *J. Gastrointestin. Liver Dis.* **2012**, *21*, 17–22.
25. Wylie, C.; Geldart, S.; Winwood, P. Dietitian-led coeliac clinic: A successful change in working practice in modern healthcare. *Gastroenterol. Today* **2005**, *15*, 11–12.

26. Leffler, D.A.; Edwards George, J.; Dennis, M.; Schuppan, D.; Cook, F.; Franko, D.L.; Blom-Hoffman, J.; Kelly, C.P. Factors that influence adherence to a gluten-free diet in adults with celiac disease. *Dig. Dis. Sci.* **2008**, *53*, 1573–1581.
27. *Educational Attainment in the United States: 2009*; U.S. Department of Commerce, Economics and Statistics Administration, U.S. Census Bureau: Washington, DC, USA, 2012; pp. 1–17.
28. Rostom, A.; Dube, C.; Cranney, A.; Saloojee, N.; Sy, R.; Garritty, C.; Sampson, M.; Zhang, L.; Yazdi, F.; Mamaladze, V.; *et al.* Celiac disease. *Evid. Rep. Technol. Assess. (Summ.)* **2004**, *104*, 1–6.
29. Richey, R.; Howdle, P.; Shaw, E.; Stokes, T.; Guideline Development Group. Recognition and assessment of coeliac disease in children and adults: Summary of NICE guidance. *BMJ* **2009**, *338*, b1684.
30. Norström, F.; Lindholm, L.; Sandström, O.; Nordyke, K.; Ivarsson, A. Delay to celiac disease diagnosis and its implications for health-related quality of life. *BMC Gastroenterol.* **2011**, *11*, 118.

15

2013 Update on Celiac Disease and Eosinophilic Esophagitis

Rinaldo Pellicano [1,*], Claudio De Angelis [1], Davide Giuseppe Ribaldone [1], Sharmila Fagoonee [2] and Marco Astegiano [1]

[1] Department of Gastro-Hepatology, Molinette Hospital, C.so Bramante 88, 10126 Turin, Italy; E-Mails: eusdeang@hotmail.com (C.D.); davrib_1998@yahoo.com (D.G.R.); mastegiano@cittadellasalute.to.it (M.A)

[2] Molecular Biotechnology Center, University of Turin, 10126 Turin, Italy; E-Mail: sharmila.fagoonee@unito.it

* Author to whom correspondence should be addressed; E-Mail: rinaldo_pellican@hotmail.com;

Abstract: Celiac disease is a chronic, immune-mediated disorder, characterized by small intestinal inflammation and villous atrophy after the ingestion of gluten by genetically susceptible individuals. Several extraintestinal manifestations have been associated to celiac disease. Eosinophilic esophagitis is a primary disorder of the esophagus characterized by upper gastrointestinal symptoms, absence of gastroesophageal reflux disease and more than 15 eosinophils per high-power field in biopsy specimens. Both celiac disease and eosinophilic esophagitis are caused by aberrant, but distinct, immune responses to ingested antigens and can be responsive to restricted food intake. The aim of this review is to assess whether there is an association between these two pathologies. In the majority of the studies examined, including the studies in pediatric population, the prevalence of eosinophilic esophagitis in subjects with celiac disease was about 10-times that of the general population. We suggest searching for eosinophilic esophagitis in all children undergoing endoscopy for suspicious celiac disease.

Keywords: celiac disease; eosinophilic esophagitis; food allergy; autoimmune disorders

---

1. Introduction

Celiac disease is a chronic, immune-mediated disorder, characterized by malabsorption of nutrients after the ingestion of wheat gluten or related proteins from rye and barley by genetically susceptible individuals expressing the human leukocyte antigen (HLA) class II molecules DQ2 or DQ8 [1] resulting in villus atrophy of the small intestinal mucosa. Prompt clinical and histologic improvement is observed following strict adherence to a gluten-free diet, and clinical and histologic relapse occurs when gluten is reintroduced [2]. Several extraintestinal manifestations, including anemia, osteopenia, neurologic symptoms, menstrual abnormalities, infertility, recurrent spontaneous abortions, growth retardation, dermatitis herpetiformis, aphthous stomatitis, dental defects, have been associated with celiac disease [3].

Eosinophilic esophagitis was first described in 1978 [4]; however, it became recognized as a distinct clinical entity in 1995 [5]. It is a chronic inflammatory primary disorder of the esophagus, presenting with dysphagia and symptoms mimicking those of gastroesophageal reflux disease, including vomiting, regurgitation, nausea and epigastric pain. This disorder is characterized by esophageal mucosal biopsy containing more than 15 eosinophils per high-power field (Figure 1) and absence of gastroesophageal reflux disease, as shown by normal pH monitoring or lack of response to high-dose proton pump inhibitory therapy [6].

Figure 1. Classic histological findings of eosinophilic esophagitis: hypereosinophilia, usually with >15–20 eosinophils per high-powered field. Eosinophils in the squamous mucosa are visible (arrows). (Courtesy of Dr. Ezio David, MD, Molinette Hospital, Turin, Italy.)

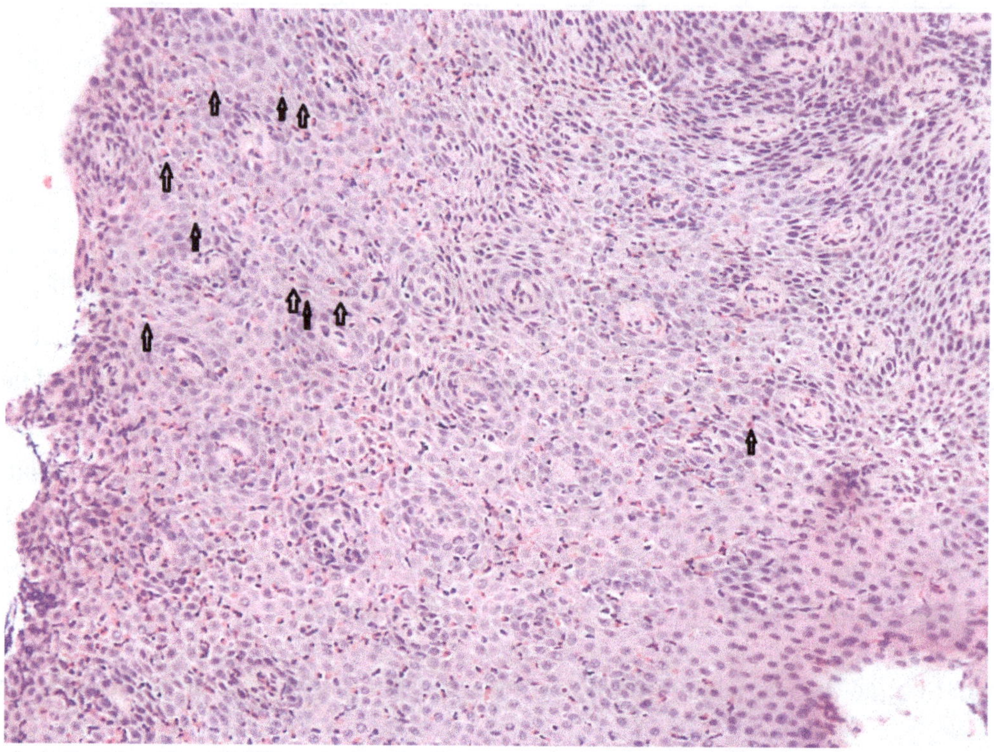

There are some classic endoscopic features including adherent whitish plaques, esophageal concentric rings, linear furrowing, but the esophagus can appear only slightly altered in some patients [7]. The squamous epithelium of the esophagus is normally devoid of eosinophils, but various disorders cause eosinophils to infiltrate the esophageal epithelium: parasitic infections, autoimmune disease, vasculitis, medications, gastroesophageal reflux disease [8]. When first described, eosinophilic esophagitis was believed to be a predominantly pediatric condition; however, it is now commonly diagnosed in adults as well as in children [9]. The clinical presentation of eosinophilic esophagitis may vary depending on age: younger children, generally present with non-specific symptoms of gastroesophageal reflux disease, abdominal pain or failure to thrive [10]; older children often present with dysphagia and esophageal food impaction [11]; however, asymptomatic low-grade counts of epithelial eosinophils (less than 15 eosinophils per high-power field) may be more common than has been estimated, but are of uncertain clinical significance [12]. A subset of patients with eosinophilic esophagitis responds to acid suppressive therapy, indicating some overlap between eosinophilic esophagitis and gastroesophageal reflux disease [6]; this is now considered as a separate entity labelled "proton pump inhibitors (PPI) responsive oesophageal eosinophilia" [13] In children, eosinophilic esophagitis has been shown to be associated with IgE- and non-IgE-mediated food allergy, and the majority of cases respond to elemental diets or specific food protein elimination [6]. By contrast, in adults the response to dietary interventions is less predictable, and the treatment more commonly relies on swallowed corticosteroid aerosols [6]. The poor response rate to dietary interventions in adults may be due to a lower prevalence of food allergy, and sensitization to inhalant allergens may play a more significant etiological role [6]. The data about the incidence of eosinophilic esophagitis range from 0.5 cases per 10,000 [14] to 1 in 10,000 in Ohio, USA [15] and the prevalence range from 0.89/10,000 in Western Australia [16] to four cases per 10,000 in Ohio, USA [15] and 5.5 cases per 10,000 in Olmsted County, Minnesota, USA [17]. The incidence seems to be increasing in both adults and children, though it is as yet unclear whether this is solely attributable to increasing awareness and detection of the disease or whether it represents a genuine phenomenon [18]. There is a male predominance, with 76% of adult and 66% of pediatric cases being diagnosed in males [6]. Since both celiac disease and eosinophilic esophagitis are caused by aberrant, but distinct, immune responses to ingested antigens and can be responsive to food elimination diets, the objective of our study was to verify if there is an association between these two conditions.

2. Experimental Section

Articles regarding the association of these two diseases were identified through MEDLINE search using the terms "celiac disease or celiac sprue or gluten AND eosinophilic esophagitis". The search was also performed using reference lists from published articles. The titles of these publications and their abstracts were scanned in order to eliminate duplicates and irrelevant articles. The final date of the MEDLINE search was June 19, 2013.

3. Results

The search identified 30 publications (from November 2001 to May 2013) on this subject. We read the abstracts of all articles and selected the 13 original articles in which associations between the two diseases were addressed; three were excluded because there were no data about the prevalence of the diseases. Celiac disease and eosinophilic esophagitis have been described in the same patient for the first time in a case report of 2007 [19] in a 7-year old black male with reactive airway disease, eczema and type 1 diabetes mellitus referred to the gastroenterology clinic for positive celiac serologic findings in recurrent abdominal pain. The eosinophilic esophagitis responded to an elimination diet with normalization of esophageal histology and subsequently recurred with reintroduction of cow's milk protein (while celiac disease's histology remained in remission with gluten-free diet). A second report of three associated cases was described in the same year [20] with a reported prevalence of eosinophilic esophagitis in patients with celiac disease of 9%, nine times higher than that expected in the general population (1:100) [21]. In one patient eosinophilic esophagitis disappeared after gluten-free diet; in the other two cases, the gluten-free diet did not have any effect on the eosinophilic infiltrate, but both subjects were not compliant to the gluten-free diet. Another study [22] reported a 35% of prevalence of celiac disease in 17 patients affected by eosinophilic esophagitis investigated for upper gastrointestinal symptoms, with a significant clinical and histological remission on gluten-free diet compared to the group of patients with eosinophilic esophagitis without celiac disease. In an Australian study regarding seven children with eosinophilic esophagitis and celiac disease [23], no patients with food allergy were reported; the prevalence of eosinophilic esophagitis in the cohort of patients with celiac disease was 3.1%; two of seven patients who underwent repeated endoscopic examinations showed improved duodenal histology but persistent eosinophilic esophagitis on gluten-free diet. In another Australian study published in 2010 [24], the prevalence of esophageal eosinophilia in children with celiac disease who had concurrent esophageal biopsies was 8.2% (10 of 121), 60% males, 30% had normal-appearing esophageal mucosa at endoscopy; children who had undergone repeated endoscopic examinations showed recovery of duodenal mucosa but no resolution of esophageal eosinophilia on a gluten-free diet alone. The association of celiac and eosinophilic esophagitis may not be a true association but a matter of biased enrollment in the above studies: regarding HLA DQ2 and/or DQ8, a study [25] showed that these alleles were not present in eosinophilic esophagitis at a greater rate than in healthy controls. But a recent study [26] demonstrated, a clear association between celiac disease and eosinophilic esophagitis in both pediatric and adult populations: the standardized incidence ratio of eosinophilic esophagitis in patients with celiac disease was 16.0 (95% CI, 8.7–25.5). A general population-based study on adults [27] did not find any association between eosinophilic esophagitis and celiac disease, whereas the latest one [28] showed a prevalence of 1.2% of eosinophilic esophagitis in children with celiac disease (Table 1).

Table 1. Published study about prevalence of eosinophilic esophagitis (EoE) in patients affected by celiac disease (CD).

Study	Country	Prevalence of EoE in CD population	% of Pediatric patients	% of Male in EoE patients	Population
A [22]	Australia	3.1% (7 of 221)	100	43	Tertiary center
B [23]	Australia	8.2% (10 of 121)	100	60	Tertiary center
C [25]	USA	0.97% (14 of 1439)	20.6	57	Tertiary center
D [27]	Canada	1.2% (3 of 245)	100	100	General population

4. Discussion

Both celiac disease and eosinophilic esophagitis are distinct clinical entities except for a few minor similarities. Celiac disease is a Th1 mediated disorder which aligns with autoimmunity, triggered by the ingestion of food containing gluten and affects females:males at a ratio of 2:1 [29]. By contrast, eosinophilic esophagitis has been shown to be a Th2-mediated disorder, which is triggered by exposure to dietary allergens causing infiltration of the esophageal mucosa by T lymphocytes, mast cells and eosinophils and predominates in males, with a 3:1 ratio to females. There is also an overexpression of eotaxin-3 and interleukin-5 [6] in the latter. Affliction of 8% of first-degree relatives of patients with celiac disease is similar to that reported in 10% of first-degree relatives of patients with eosinophilic esophagitis [30]. The genetic basis for celiac disease (*i.e.*, HLA DQ2) is well established and differs from that of eosinophilic esophagitis [25] whose etiology is far from clear, but in nearly 50% of the cases, it is associated with an allergy to food or to aeroallergens [15]. In children, IgE-dependent mechanism for eosinophilic esophagitis is supported; for instance, it was shown that affected patients have IgE sensitization to a wide variety of foods, although not all patients had evidence of food-specific IgE [31]. In one study, a higher level of IgE sensitization to food allergens was observed in patients with eosinophilic esophagitis alone compared to patients with both pathologies, and this led the authors to hypothesize that patients with both pathologies have elevated esophageal eosinophils for reasons different from allergy, with a significant clinical and histological remission on gluten-free diet [22]. Increased intestinal mucosal permeability secondary to celiac disease has been suggested as a contributing factor in the development of atopy [32,33]. Damaged intestinal barrier may expose the local intestinal immune system to macromolecules and lead to transport of these undigested proteins to other body sites, hence facilitating development of hypersensitivity reactions in a predisposed individual in and away from the gastrointestinal tract [23]. By contrast, in adults, the response to dietary interventions is less predictable, and treatment more commonly relies on swallowed corticosteroid aerosols [6]. The clinical significance of eosinophilic esophagitis as an incidental finding is uncertain; if the main treatment goal is suppression of clinical symptoms, asymptomatic eosinophilic esophagitis may not require any therapy, but as the natural history of eosinophilic esophagitis in largely unknown, it is unclear what proportion is at risk of developing esophageal strictures and dysphagia in the long term [34].

5. Conclusions

In summary, although there are fundamental differences in the pathophysiological mechanisms involved in eosinophilic esophagitis and celiac disease, these conditions may coexist and the prevalence is higher than anticipated. Our review highlights the importance of obtaining routine esophageal biopsies in children undergoing endoscopy for diagnosis of celiac disease irrespective of whether the esophagus appears normal or abnormal at endoscopy; however, asymptomatic low-grade counts of epithelial eosinophils are of uncertain clinical significance.

References

1. Fasano, A. Clinical presentation of celiac disease in the pediatric population. *Gastroenterology* **2005**, *128*, 68–73.
2. Farrell, R.J.; Kelly, C.P. Celiac sprue. *N. Engl. J. Med.* **2002**, *346*, 180–188.
3. Ribaldone, D.G.; Astegiano, M.; Fagoonee, S.; Rizzetto, M.; Pellicano, R. Epilepsy and celiac disease. *Panminerva Med.* **2011**, *53*, 213–216.
4. Landres, R.T.; Kuster, G.G.; Strum, W.B. Eosinophilic esophagitis in a patient with vigorous achalasia. *Gastroenterology* **1978**, *74*, 1298–1301.
5. Kelly, K.J.; Lazenby, A.J.; Rowe, P.C.; Yardley, J.H.; Perman, J.A.; Sampson, H.A. Eosinophilic esophagitis attributed to gastroesophageal reflux: Improvement with amino acid-based formula. *Gastroenterology* **1995**, *109*, 1503–1512.
6. Furuta, G.T.; Liacouras, C.A.; Collins, M.H.; Gupta, S.K.; Justinich, C.; Putnam, P.E.; Bonis, P.; Hassall, E.; Straumann, A.; Rothenberg, M.E.; *et al.* Eosinophilic esophagitis in children and adults: A systematic review and consensus recommendations for diagnosis and treatment. *Gastroenterology* **2007**, *133*, 1342–1363.
7. Nurko, S.; Teitelbaum, J.E.; Husain, K.; Buonomo, C.; Fox, V.L.; Antonioli, D.; Fortunato, C.; Badizadegan, K.; Furuta, G.T. Association of Schatzki ring with eosinophilic esophagitis in children. *J. Pediatr. Gastroenterol. Nutr.* **2004**, *38*, 436–441.
8. Feldman, M.; Friedman, L.S.; Brandt, L.J. *Gastrointestinal and Liver Disease*, 9th ed.; Saunders Elsevier: Philadelphia, PA, USA, 2010; p. 427.
9. Potter, J.W.; Saeian, K.; Staff, D.; Massey, B.T.; Komorowski, R.A.; Shaker, R.; Hogan, W.J. Eosinophilic esophagitis in adults: An emerging problem with unique esophageal features. *Gastrointest. Endosc.* **2004**, *59*, 355–361.
10. Orenstein, S.R.; Shalaby, T.M.; Di Lorenzo, C.; Putnam, P.E.; Sigurdsson, L.; Mousa, H.; Kocoshis, S.A. The spectrum of pediatric eosinophilic esophagitis beyond infancy: A clinical series of 30 children. *Am. J. Gastroenterol.* **2000**, *95*, 1422–1430.
11. Desai, T.K.; Stecevic, V.; Chang, C.H.; Goldstein, N.S.; Badizadegan, K.; Furuta, G.T. Association of eosinophilic inflammation with esophageal food impaction in adults. *Gastrointest. Endosc.* **2005**, *61*, 795–801.
12. Ronkainen, J.; Talley, N.J.; Aro, P.; Storskrubb, T.; Johansson, S.E.; Lind, T.; Bolling-Sternevald, E.; Vieth, M.; Stolte, M.; Walker, M.M.; *et al.* Prevalence of oesophageal eosinophils and eosinophilic oesophagitis in adults: The population-based Kalixanda study. *Gut* **2007**, *56*, 615–620.
13. Liacouras, C.A.; Furuta, G.T.; Hirano, I.; Atkins, D.; Attwood, S.E.; Bonis, P.A.; Burks, A.W.; Chehade, M.; Collins, M.H.; Dellon, E.S.; *et al.* Eosinophilic esophagitis: Updated consensus recommendations for children and adults. *J. Allergy Clin. Immunol.* **2011**, *128*, 3–20.
14. Hruz, P.; Straumann, A.; Bussmann, C.; Heer, P.; Simon, H.U.; Zwahlen, M.; Beglinger, C.; Schoepfer, A.M. Escalating incidence of eosinophilic esophagitis: A 20-year prospective, population-based study in Olten County, Switzerland. *J. Allergy Clin. Immunol.* **2011**, *128*, 1349–1350.
15. Noel, R.J.; Putnam, P.E.; Rothenberg, M.E. Eosinophilic esophagitis. *N. Engl. J. Med.* **2004**, *351*, 940–941.

16. Cherian, S.; Smith, N.M.; Forbes, D.A. Rapidly increasing prevalence of eosinophilic oesophagitis in Western Australia. *Arch. Dis. Child.* **2006**, *91*, 1000–1004.
17. Prasad, G.A.; Alexander, J.A.; Schleck, C.D.; Zinsmeister, A.R.; Smyrk, T.C.; Elias, R.M.; Locke, G.R.; Talley, N.J. Epidemiology of eosinophilic esophagitis over three decades in Olmsted County, Minnesota. *Clin. Gastroenterol. Hepatol.* **2009**, *7*, 1055–1061.
18. Straumann, A.; Simon, H.U. Eosinophilic esophagitis: Escalating epidemiology? *J. Allergy Clin. Immunol.* **2005**, *115*, 418–419.
19. Kagalwalla, A.F.; Shah, A.; Ritz, S.; Melin-Aldana, H.; Li, B.U. Cow's milk protein-induced eosinophilic esophagitis in a child with gluten-sensitive enteropathy. *J. Pediatr. Gastroenterol. Nutr.* **2007**, *44*, 386–388.
20. De Angelis, P.; Dall'Oglio, L.; Di Leo, G.; Ventura, A. Eosinophilic oesophagitis and coeliac disease: Is it just a casual association? *Gut* **2007**, *56*, 1029–1030.
21. Verzegnassi, F.; Bua, J.; Tommasini, A.; Not, T.; Kiren, V.; Baldas, V.; Santon, D.; Trevisiol, C.; Berti, I; Neri, E.; *et al.* Mass screening for coeliac disease using antihuman transglutaminase antibody assay. *Arch. Dis. Child.* **2004**, *89*, 512–515.
22. Quaglietta, L.; Coccorullo, P.; Miele, E.; Pascarella, F.; Troncone, R.; Staiano, A. Eosinophilic oesophagitis and coeliac disease: Is there an association? *Aliment. Pharmacol. Ther.* **2007**, *26*, 487–493.
23. Ooi, C.Y.; Day, A.S.; Jackson, R.; Bohane, T.D.; Tobias, V.; Lemberg, D.A. Eosinophilic esophagitis in children with celiac disease. *J. Gastroenterol. Hepatol.* **2008**, *23*, 1144–1148.
24. Leslie, C.; Mews, C.; Charles, A.; Ravikumara, M. Celiac disease and eosinophilic esophagitis: A true association. *J. Pediatr. Gastroenterol. Nutr.* **2010**, 50, 397–399.
25. Lucendo, A.J.; Arias, Á.; Pérez-Martínez, I.; López-Vázquez, A.; Ontañón-Rodríguez, J.; González-Castillo, S.; De Rezende, L.C.; Rodrigo, L. Adult patients with eosinophilic esophagitis do not show an increased frequency of the HLA-DQ2/DQ8 genotypes predisposing to celiac disease. *Dig. Dis. Sci.* **2011**, *56*, 1107–1111.
26. Thompson, J.S.; Lebwohl, B.; Reilly, N.R.; Talley, N.J.; Bhagat, G.; Green, P.H. Increased incidence of eosinophilic esophagitis in children and adults with celiac disease. *J. Clin. Gastroenterol.* **2012**, *46*, 6–11.
27. Ludvigsson, J.F.; Aro, P.; Walker, M.M.; Vieth, M.; Agréus, L.; Talley, N.J.; Murray, J.A.; Ronkainen, J. Celiac disease, eosinophilic esophagitis and gastroesophageal reflux disease, an adult population-based study. *Scand. J. Gastroenterol.* **2013**, *48*, 804–814.
28. Stewart, M.J.; Shaffer, E.; Urbanski, S.J.; Beck, P.L.; Storr, M.A. The association between celiac disease and eosinophilic esophagitis in children and adults. *BMC Gastroenterol.* **2013**, *13*, 96.
29. Green, P.H.; Cellier, C. Celiac disease. *N. Engl. J. Med.* **2007**, *357*, 1731–1743.
30. Rothenberg, M.E. Eosinophilic gastrointestinal disorders (EGID). *J. Allergy Clin. Immunol.* **2004**, *113*, 11–28.
31. Spergel, J.M.; Beausoleil, J.L.; Mascarenhas, M.; Liacouras, C.A. The use of skin prick tests and patch tests to identify the causative foods in eosinophilic esophagitis. *J. Allergy Clin. Immunol.* **2002**, *109*, 363–368.
32. Van Elburg, R.M.; Uil, J.J.; Mulder, C.J.; Heymans, H.S. Intestinal permeability in patients with coeliac disease and relatives of patients with coeliac disease. *Gut* **1993**, *34*, 354–357.

33. Bischoff, S.C.; Mayer, J.; Nguyen, Q.T.; Stolte, M.; Manns, M.P. Immunohistological assessment of intestinal eosinophil activation in patients with eosinophilic gastroenteritis and inflammatory bowel disease. *Am. J. Gastroenterol.* **1999**, *94*, 3521–3529.
34. Heine, R.G. Eosinophilic esophagitis in children with celiac disease: New diagnostic and therapeutic dilemmas. *J. Gastroenterol. Hepatol.* **2008**, *23*, 993–994.

Permissions

All chapters in this book were first published by MDPI; hereby published with permission under the Creative Commons Attribution License or equivalent. Every chapter published in this book has been scrutinized by our experts. Their significance has been extensively debated. The topics covered herein carry significant findings which will fuel the growth of the discipline. They may even be implemented as practical applications or may be referred to as a beginning point for another development.

The contributors of this book come from diverse backgrounds, making this book a truly international effort. This book will bring forth new frontiers with its revolutionizing research information and detailed analysis of the nascent developments around the world.

We would like to thank all the contributing authors for lending their expertise to make the book truly unique. They have played a crucial role in the development of this book. Without their invaluable contributions this book wouldn't have been possible. They have made vital efforts to compile up to date information on the varied aspects of this subject to make this book a valuable addition to the collection of many professionals and students.

This book was conceptualized with the vision of imparting up-to-date information and advanced data in this field. To ensure the same, a matchless editorial board was set up. Every individual on the board went through rigorous rounds of assessment to prove their worth. After which they invested a large part of their time researching and compiling the most relevant data for our readers.

The editorial board has been involved in producing this book since its inception. They have spent rigorous hours researching and exploring the diverse topics which have resulted in the successful publishing of this book. They have passed on their knowledge of decades through this book. To expedite this challenging task, the publisher supported the team at every step. A small team of assistant editors was also appointed to further simplify the editing procedure and attain best results for the readers.

Apart from the editorial board, the designing team has also invested a significant amount of their time in understanding the subject and creating the most relevant covers. They scrutinized every image to scout for the most suitable representation of the subject and create an appropriate cover for the book.

The publishing team has been an ardent support to the editorial, designing and production team. Their endless efforts to recruit the best for this project, has resulted in the accomplishment of this book. They are a veteran in the field of academics and their pool of knowledge is as vast as their experience in printing. Their expertise and guidance has proved useful at every step. Their uncompromising quality standards have made this book an exceptional effort. Their encouragement from time to time has been an inspiration for everyone.

The publisher and the editorial board hope that this book will prove to be a valuable piece of knowledge for researchers, students, practitioners and scholars across the globe.

List of Contributors

Carmela Lamacchia and Aldo Di Luccia
Department of Food Science, University of Foggia, Via Napoli 25, 71100 - Foggia, Italy

Alessandra Camarca and Stefania Picascia
Institute of Food Sciences-CNR, Carmen Gianfrani, ISA-CNR, Via Roma 64, 83100 - Avellino, Italy

Carmen Gianfrani
Institute of Food Sciences-CNR, Carmen Gianfrani, ISA-CNR, Via Roma 64, 83100 - Avellino, Italy
Institute of Protein Biochemistry-CNR, Via P. Castellino, 111, 80131 – Naples, Italy

Antonella Diamanti, Maria Sole Basso, Fabio Panetta and Francesca Bellucci
Gastroenterology-Hepatology and Nutrition Unit, "Bambino Gesù" Children's Hospital, Piazza Sant'Onofrio 4, Rome 00165, Italy

Teresa Capriati
Gastroenterology-Hepatology and Nutrition Unit, "Bambino Gesù" Children's Hospital, Piazza Sant'Onofrio 4, Rome 00165, Italy
Gastroenterology Unit, Pediatric Clinic of University, Piazza Giulio Cesare 11, Bari 70124, Italy

Fernanda Cristofori and Ruggiero Francavilla
Gastroenterology Unit, Pediatric Clinic of University, Piazza Giulio Cesare 11, Bari 70124, Italy
Interdisciplinary Department of Medicine, University of Bari, Bari 70124, Italy

Vincenzo Maria Di Ciommo Laurora
Epidemiology and Biostatistics Unit, "Bambino Gesù" Children's Hospital, Piazza Sant'Onofrio 4, Rome 00165, Italy

Preeti Rajpoot and Govind K. Makharia
Departments of Gastroenterology and Human Nutrition, All India Institute of Medical Sciences, New Delhi 110029, India

Michele Di Stefano, Caterina Mengoli, Manuela Bergonzi and Gino Roberto Corazza
1st Department of Internal Medicine, University of Pavia, IRCCS "S.Matteo" Hospital Foundation, Pavia 27100, Italy

Simona Gatti, Nicole Caporelli, Tiziana Galeazzi and Carlo Catassi
Department of Pediatrics, Università Politecnica delle Marche, 60121 Ancona, Italy

Maria Barbato
Department of Pediatrics, "Sapienza" University of Rome, 00161 Roma, Italy

Paola Roggero
Neonatal Intensive Care Unit, Department of Clinical Sciences and Community Health, Fondazione IRCCS Ca' Granda Ospedale Maggiore Policlinico, University of Milan, 20122 Milano, Italy

Basilio Malamisura
Department of Pediatrics, S. Maria dell'Olmo Hospital Cava de' Tirreni, 84013 Salerno, Italy

Giuseppe Iacono
Pediatric Gastroenterology Unit, "G. Di Cristina" Children Hospital, 90134 Palermo, Italy

Andrea Budelli
R&D Heinz Italia S.p.A, 04100 Latina, Italy

Rosaria Gesuita
Department of Epidemiology, Biostatistics and Medical Information Technology, Università Politecnica delle Marche, 60121 Ancona, Italy

Elena Lionetti
Department of Pediatrics, Università di Catania, 95123, Catania, Italy

Maaike J. Bruins
DSM Biotechnology Center, Alexander Fleminglaan 1, Delft 2613AX, The Netherlands

Julio C. Bai
Departamento de Medicina, Hospital de Gastroenterología "Dr. Carlos Bonorino Udaondo", Buenos Aires 1264, Argentina

Bruno Bonaz
Department of Gastroenterology and Liver Diseases, CHU Grenoble 38043, France

Gerd Bouma
Department of Gastroenterology and Hepatology, Vrije Universiteit Medical Center, Amsterdam 1081 HV, The Netherlands

Antonio Calabrò
Gastroenterology Unit, Department of Experimental and Clinical Biomedical Sciences, University of Florence, Florence 50134, Italy

Antonio Carroccio
Department of Internal Medicine, "Giovanni Paolo II" Hospital, Sciacca (AG) and University of Palermo, Sciacca 92019, Italy

Gemma Castillejo
Pediatric Gastroenterology Unit, Hospital Universitari de Sant Joan de Reus, Universitat Rovira i Virgili, Tarragona 43204, Spain

Carolina Ciacci
Department of Medicine and Surgery, University of Salerno, Baronissi Campus, Salerno 84081, Italy

Jernej Dolinsek
Gastroenterology Unit, Department of Pediatrics, University Medical Centre Maribor, Maribor 2000, Slovenia

Luca Elli
Centro Prevenzione e Diagnosi Malattia Celiaca Fondazione IRCCS Ca Granda, Milan 20122, Italy

Peter Green
Department of Medicine, Celiac Disease Center, Columbia University Medical Center, New York, NY 10032, USA

Wolfgang Holtmeier
Division of Gastroenterology and Internal Medicine, Hospital Porz am Rhein, Köln 51149, Germany

Peter Koehler
German Research Center for Food Chemistry, Leibniz Institute, Freising 85354, Germany

Sibylle Koletzko
Division of Pediatric Gastroenterology and Hepatology, Dr. von Hauner Children's Hospital, University of Munich Medical Center, Munich 80337, Germany

Christof Meinhold
Practice of Nutrition Therapy Meinhold & Team, Köln 50674, Germany

David Sanders
Department of Gastroenterology and Hepatology, Royal Hallamshire Hospital and University of Sheffield Medical School, Sheffield S10 2JF, UK

Michael Schumann and Reiner Ullrich
Department of Gastroenterology, Rheumatology and Infectiology, Charité University Medicine, Berlin 10203, Germany

Victor Zevallos
Department of Medicine I, University Medical Center, Johannes Gutenberg University Mainz, Mainz 55131, Germany

Detlef Schuppan
Department of Medicine I, University Medical Center, Johannes Gutenberg University Mainz, Mainz 55131, Germany
Division of Gastroenterology and Celiac Center, Beth Israel Deaconess Medical Center and Harvard Medical School, Boston, MA 02215, USA

Andreas Vécsei
St. Anna Children's Hospital, Vienna 1090, Austria

Umberto Volta
Department of Medical and Surgical Sciences, University of Bologna, Bologna 40138, Italy

Anna Sapone
Department of Gastroenterology, Second University of Naples, Naples 80136, Italy

Alessio Fasano
Pediatric Gastroenterology and Nutrition, Mass General Hospital for Children, Boston, MA 02129, USA

Nicolette J. Wierdsma, Marian A. E. van Bokhorst-de van der Schueren and Marijke Berkenpas
Department of Nutrition and Dietetics, VU University Medical Centre, Amsterdam 1007 MB, The Netherlands

Chris J. J. Mulder and Ad A. van Bodegraven
Department of Gastroenterology, Celiac Centre Amsterdam, VU University Medical Centre, Amsterdam 1007 MB, The Netherlands

Isabel Comino, María de Lourdes Moreno, Ana Real and Carolina Sousa
Departamento de Microbiología y Parasitología, Facultad de Farmacia, Universidad de Sevilla, c/ Profesor García González 2, 41012 Sevilla, Spain

Alfonso Rodríguez-Herrera
Instituto Hispalense de Pediatría, c/Guadalbullón 2, 41013 Sevilla, Spain

Francisco Barro
Instituto de Agricultura Sostenible (C.S.I.C.), Alameda del Obispo s/n, 14004 Córdoba, Spain

Letizia Saturni
Centro Interdipartimentale di Educazione Sanitaria e Promozione alla Salute, Ancona, 60035 Italy

Gianna Ferretti and Tiziana Bacchetti
Centro Interdipartimentale di Educazione Sanitaria e Promozione alla Salute, Ancona, 60035 Italy
Dipartimento di Biochimica, Biologia e Genetica - Università Politecnica delle Marche - Ancona, 60035, Italy

Steffen Husby
Hans Christian Andersen Children's Hospital, Odense University Hospital, Sdr. Boulevard 29, Odense 5000, Denmark

Henrik Toft-Hansen
Hans Christian Andersen Children's Hospital, Odense University Hospital, Sdr. Boulevard 29, Odense 5000, Denmark
Department of Clinical Immunology, Odense University Hospital, Sdr. Boulevard 29, Odense 5000, Denmark

Christian Nielsen and Søren T. Lillevang
Department of Clinical Immunology, Odense University Hospital, Sdr. Boulevard 29, Odense 5000, Denmark

Matteo Biagini
Department of Pathology, Odense University Hospital, J.B. Winsløws Vej 15, 2., Odense 5000, Denmark

Urszula Krupa-Kozak
Department of Chemistry and Biodynamics of Food, Institute of Animal Reproduction and Food Research of the Polish Academy of Sciences, Tuwima St., 10, Olsztyn 10-748, Poland

Natalia Bączek
Department of Chemistry and Biodynamics of Food, Institute of Animal Reproduction and Food Research of the Polish Academy of Sciences, Tuwima St., 10, Olsztyn 10-748, Poland
Cereal Group, Institute of Agrochemistry and Food Technology (IATA-CSIC), Av Agustin Escardino 7, Paterna, Valencia 46980, Spain

Cristina M. Rosell
Cereal Group, Institute of Agrochemistry and Food Technology (IATA-CSIC), Av Agustin Escardino 7, Paterna, Valencia 46980, Spain

Francesca Penagini, Dario Dilillo, Fabio Meneghin, Chiara Mameli, Valentina Fabiano and Gian Vincenzo Zuccotti
Department of Pediatrics, University of Milan, Luigi Sacco Hospital, Milan 20157, Italy

SriHari Mahadev, Suzanne Simpson, Benjamin Lebwohl, Suzanne K. Lewis, Christina A. Tennyson and Peter H. R. Green
Celiac Disease Center, Columbia University College of Physicians and Surgeons, 180 Fort Washington Avenue, Suite 934, New York, NY 10032, USA

Rinaldo Pellicano, Claudio De Angelis, Davide Giuseppe Ribaldone and Marco Astegiano
Department of Gastro-Hepatology, Molinette Hospital, C.so Bramante 88, 10126 Turin, Italy

Index

www.ingramcontent.com/pod-product-compliance
Lightning Source LLC
LaVergne TN
LVHW060535210926
848485LV00005B/1200